CONTEMPORARY TOPICS IN MOLECULAR IMMUNOLOGY

VOLUME 5

Contemporary Topics in Molecular Immunology

A Continuation Order Plan is available for this series. A continuation order will bring delivery of each new volume immediately upon publication. Volumes are billed only upon actual shipment. For further information please contact the publisher.

Contemporary Topics in Molecular Immunology

Volume 5

EDITED BY

H. N. Eisen

Massachusetts Institute of Technology
and
Harvard–MIT Program for Health Sciences and Technology
Cambridge, Massachusetts

and

R. A. Reisfeld

Scripps Clinic and Research Foundation
La Jolla, California

PLENUM PRESS • NEW YORK AND LONDON

The Library of Congress cataloged the first volume of this title as follows:

Contemporary topics in molecular immunology. v. 2–
New York, Plenum Press, 1973–

  v. illus. 24 cm.

  Continues Contemporary topics in immunochemistry.

  1. Immunochemistry—Collected works. 2. Immunology—Collected works.

QR180.C635   574.2′9′05   73–648513
ISSN 0090–8800   MARC-S

Volume 1 of this series was published under the title
Contemporary Topics in Immunochemistry

Library of Congress Catalog Card Number 73-648513

ISBN 0-306-36105-1

Contributors

Ettore Appella *Laboratory of Cell Biology*
National Cancer Institute
Bethesda, Maryland

Paul D. Gottlieb *Department of Biology and Center for Cancer Research*
Massachusetts Institute of Technology
Cambridge, Massachusetts

L. Hood *Division of Biology*
California Institute of Technology
Pasadena, California

Lloyd W. Law *Laboratory of Cell Biology*
National Cancer Institute
Bethesda, Maryland

Fred Karush *Department of Microbiology*
School of Medicine
University of Pennsylvania
Philadelphia, Pennsylvania

John J. Marchalonis *Molecular Immunology Laboratory*
The Walter and Eliza Hall Institute of Medical Research
Royal Melbourne Hospital, Victoria, Australia

Roald Nezlin *Institute of Molecular Biology*
USSR Academy of Sciences
Moscow, USSR

Jack H. Pincus *Life Sciences Division*
Stanford Research Institute
Menlo Park, California

Oscar Rokhlin *Institute of Molecular Biology*
USSR Academy of Sciences
Moscow, USSR

David H. Sachs *Transplantation Biology Section*
Immunology Branch
National Cancer Institute
National Institutes of Health
Bethesda, Maryland

J. Silver *Division of Biology*
California Institute of Technology
Pasadena, California

Preface

Immunochemistry, recently rechristened molecular immunology, has been preoccupied throughout its long history with the structure and function of antibodies and the specificity of antibody–antigen reactions. With the recent X-ray diffraction analyses of several crystallized immunoglobulin (Ig) fragments and a whole Ig molecule, the three-dimensional structure of antibodies and their ligand-combining sites has been realized, marking the concluding stages of a phase of immunological research that can be traced back at least 75 years.

At the same time chemically minded immunologists have been moving in new directions. A substantial beginning in one direction has been made with the purification of messenger RNAs (mRNAs) for Ig chains. Hybridization of these RNAs (or their DNA copies made with the enzyme reverse transcriptase) to cell DNA is beginning to provide convincing estimates of the number of germ-line Ig genes. And some hybridization studies have already yielded suggestive evidence for translocation of V and C genes from separate to contiguous positions in DNA isolated from cells at different stages of differentiation. Moreover, *in vitro* translation of Ig mRNAs has revealed a remarkably hydrophobic stretch of about 20 amino acids at the *N*-terminus of the nascent Ig chain. This extra piece is absent in the Ig extracted from or secreted by plasma cells, presumably because it is rapidly cleaved from the "preimmunoglobulin" chain within the cell, but the extra piece probably plays a key role in directing the synthesis of preIg to the cell's secretory pathway.

This volume emphasizes another new direction: the structure and function of cell surface antigen-binding receptors and cell surface antigens, particularly those specified by genes of the major histocompatibility locus. At first glance these surface elements appear to be much the same as the soluble antibodies and antigens with which immunologists are familiar. But there are likely to be profound differences, for conventional antibodies and antigens exist and react in solution, an aqueous three-dimensional space, whereas cell surface elements exist and react in or on the hydrophobic, nearly two-dimensional space of cell membranes. The differences could have far-reaching consequences, and the technology developed for studies of immune reactions in solution may have to be substantially altered for analyses of the corresponding reactions in or on cell surfaces.

In the present volume the chapter by Sachs provides a clear overview of the genetic and serologic basis for identification of Ia antigens. These polymorphic antigens are coded for by the I region of the major histocompatibility complex (MHC) of the mouse. Their role in cell–cell interactions, especially in T cell regulation of B cell differentiation, is of considerable interest. Silver and Hood focus on the glycoprotein specified by K and D loci of the MHC. They describe isolation procedures and new microsequencing techniques; and on the basis of preliminary N-terminal amino acid sequences they consider several genetic models to account for the homology between K and D gene products and their homology with products of the corresponding human complex (HLA).

Law and Appella emphasize other aspects of the K and D alloantigens of the mouse MHC. They show that their isolated K and D molecules retain biological activity, inducing specific cellular and humoral unresponsiveness and eliciting specific immunological enhancement. In addition, they describe some structural properties of these molecules and their subunits. Pincus discusses theoretical problems connected with the solubilization of biologically active cell surface antigens. His treatment of cell source materials, solubilization schemes, and isolation of plasma membrane glycoproteins is particularly thorough. The critical evaluation of the mode and efficacy of hypertonic salt extraction for the solubilization of histocompatibility antigens is particularly valuable in view of the widespread use of such approaches to the extraction of many cell surface components.

The antigen-binding receptors on lymphocytes were originally conceived of as simply surface representatives of the antibody molecules that are eventually secreted by antigen-stimulated cells. The receptors have, however, turned out to be rather special molecules. Marchalonis' contribution examines closely the evidence for 7 S IgMs and IgD-like molecules on mouse B cells, and marshals the still controversial evidence that the T cell receptor is also a special immunoglobulin.

The binding of antigen by antibody or antibody-like receptors on lymphocytes is usually discussed in terms of the reactants' mutual affinity, but the quantitative subtleties of affinity are not widely appreciated. The quantitative aspects are even less clear in the case of the multivalent binding associated with particles (cells, microbes) that have repeating copies of antigen on their surface. In his chapter on multivalent binding, Karush deals in his characteristically lucid way with *intrinsic affinity*, associated with monovalent binding, and what he designates as *functional affinity*, the corresponding property of multivalent binding.

Gottlieb's chapter considers in detail a genetic marker in the V region of mouse immunoglobulin light chains. The detail is justified by Gottlieb's discovery that this Ig marker is linked genetically with a distinctive surface antigen on T cells. this antigen (Ly 3.1) is especially notable because is associated with a small set of peripheral T cells with killer and suppressor activities. Finally, in the only chapter that has no direct bearing on lymphocyte surfaces, Nezlin and Rokhlin describe the use of allotypic immunoglobulin markers to study antibody synthesis. The mode of inheritance, molecular localization, and chemical differences of allelic variants, combined with data detailing their interaction in Ig biosynthesis, illustrate how allotypic markers contribute to the understanding of the antibody molecules.

H. N. Eisen
September, 1976   R. A. Reisfeld

Contents

The Ia Antigens

David H. Sachs

Preliminary Amino Acid Sequences of Transplantation Antigens: Genetic and Evolutionary Implications

J. Silver and L. Hood

Biological and Biochemical Properties of Solubilized
Histocompatibility-2 (H-2) Alloantigens
Lloyd W. Law and Ettore Appella

Allotypes of Light Chains of Rat Immunoglobulins and Their Application to the Study of Antibody Biosynthesis

Roald Nezlin and Oscar Rokhlin

Genetic and Structural Studies of a V-Region Marker in Mouse Immunoglobulin Light Chains

Paul D. Gottlieb

Multivalent Binding and Functional Affinity

Fred Karush

The Ia Antigens

David H. Sachs

Transplantation Biology Section
Immunology Branch
National Cancer Institute
National Institutes of Health
Bethesda, Maryland

I. INTRODUCTION

Histocompatibility loci determine polymorphic cell surface antigens capable of causing rejection of tissue grafts between animals which are genetically dissimilar at such loci. While the number of histocompatibility loci within any species is probably quite large (Bailey and Mobraaten, 1969), every mammalian species that has so far been examined possesses one such locus which has overwhelming importance in determining the fate of an allograft. This locus has been termed the "major histocompatibility complex" (MHC) (Bach, 1973), and within each species a particular system of nomenclature has been adopted. As an experimental model, the MHC of the mouse, known as the *H-2* complex, is the best defined in terms of genetic fine structure. Four major regions of the *H-2* complex have been defined and have been mapped linearly in the murine IXth linkage group (chromosome No. 17) in the order

$$K - - - I - - - S - - - D$$

with respect to the centromere (Klein, 1970) of that chromosome.

The *K* and the *D* regions determine serologically defined antigens which are present on virtually all murine tissues and which are the analogue of the serologically defined antigens in man known as the HL-A antigens. The *S* region was defined on the basis of an immunologically detectable substance in mouse serum, the levels of which were found to be genetically determined by genes mapping between various *H-2* serological specificities (Shreffler and David,

1

1972). The *I* region was defined by the immune response of inbred mouse strains to certain chemically well-defined antigens, the control of which was found to be determined by genes mapping between the *K*-region specificities and the *S* region (McDevitt *et al.*, 1972). In addition, the *I* region has quite recently been shown to code for a large number of cell surface antigens with more restricted tissue distribution than the antigens determined by the *K* and the *D* regions. These have been termed the "Ia" antigens, standing for "Ir-associated" antigens, (Shreffler *et al.*, 1974), although the possible relationship between these antigens and the functional properties of the *Ir* genes by which the *I* region was defined remains speculative.

The rapidity with which the field of Ia antigens has grown over the past 2 years has been made possible largely by the use of serological, genetic, and chemical methods developed for the study of the other regions of the *H-2* complex. For an appreciation of the enormous progress made over the past 10 years in the study of the structure and functions of products of the *H-2* complex, the reader is referred to the excellent review by Shreffler and David (1975) and the comprehensive text by Klein (1975). I shall limit the scope of the present chapter to the Ia antigens. I will attempt to review the historical development of the system of Ia antigens, then outline the present status of the nomenclature of these antigens and their current modes of detection, and finally present some experimental results bearing on the possible extent of the polymorphism of this antigenic system. There are already a variety of functional properties which have been associated with the Ia antigens. These include their probable role as stimulators of the MLC reactions (Lozner *et al.*, 1974; Fathman *et al.*, 1974; Meo *et al.*, 1975; Schwartz *et al.*, 1975), their presence on T-cell factors (Taussig *et al.*, 1974; Armerding *et al.*, 1976; Takemori and Tada, 1975), and their possible role in the phenomenon of enhancement (Staines *et al.*, 1974). Despite their undoubted relevance, I shall also consider these functional properties of Ia antigens as beyond the scope of this chapter, except as they bear on the genetic definition of the Ia antigens themselves.

II. DEFINITION OF THE Ia ANTIGENS

A. Historical

Until recently, the *I* region was defined by its functional properties rather than by structural cell surface antigenic products such as those determined by the *K* and *D* regions of the *H-2* complex. However, in an attempt to define the products of this region serologically, workers in several laboratories (David *et al.*, 1973; Hauptfeld *et al.*, 1973; Hämmerling *et al.*, 1974) carried out reciprocal immunizations between congenic strains of mice bearing the same K and D regions but differing in the I region. The strain combinations used and the serum reactivites obtained will be further described below. The antibodies produced were found to react in cytotoxic assays, causing lysis of lymphocytes in the presence of complement, but the reactivity was unusual in that only a subpopulation of lymphoid cells was killed as opposed to the complete killing generally observed with anti-H-2 reagents. Because the weight of evidence at that time indicated that Ir genes controlled T-cell immune functions (McDevitt and Benacerraf, 1969), it was proposed at first that the reactive subpopulation might be the T cells, and initial observations seemed to substantiate this hypothesis (Hauptfeld et al., 1973; Götze et al., 1973; David et al., 1973).

Simultaneous with these experiments, work in the author's laboratory was directed toward the production of antisera to genetically well-defined H-2K region antigens. During the examination of one such serum, an unexpected reactivity with a previously unrecognized antigen shared by B10 and B10.D2 was detected (Sachs and Cone, 1973). This reactivity was unusual both in that it was not predicted by the available H-2 chart and in that the antibodies appeared to kill only a subpopulation of splenic or lymph node lymphocytes, even if the globulin fraction from the antiserum was concentrated fourfold over its concentration in the immune serum. Cytotoxic tests and absorptions of cytotoxicity with congenic recombinant strains indicated that the genes determining this unexpected specificity were linked to H-2 and could be localized to the left of the I-B subregion. Subsequent tests showed that this specificity mapped to the right of the H-$2K$ region, indicating that it was indeed determined by a gene in the I-A subregion (Sachs et al., 1975a). A variety of criteria all indicated that this new antigenic specificity was expressed preferentially on B cells, thus accounting for the killing of only a subpopulation of splenic and lymph node lymphocytes.

Shortly thereafter, further characterization of the anti-I region antisera produced in other laboratories indicated that the subpopulation reacting with these sera was also predominantly B cells (Hämmerling et al., 1974; Hauptfeld, et al., 1974). It thus became apparent that the three nomenclatures devised to categorize these antigens, Lna (David et al., 1973), Ir-1.1 (Hauptfeld et al., 1973), and β (Sachs and Cone, 1973), were all similar systems of antigens determined by genes in the I region, and the name Ia (Ir-associated) antigens was proposed for this class of MHC determinants (Shreffler et al., 1974).

Over the following year, research on these Ia antigens expanded enormously, spurred in part by their possible usefulness as genetic markers and in part by the possibility that these cell surface antigens might themselves account for the important immune functions associated with the Ir region. Because this rapid expansion of interest brought with it a measure of confusion in terminology, a workshop on Ia antigens was held in November 1974 at the National Institutes

of Health as a forum for the exchange of ideas and for clarification of the definition and nomenclature of Ia antigens. The nomenclature adopted was essentially
that proposed by Shreffler and David (1975). The terminology and numerical
classification used throughout. this chapter will be those recommended by
consensus at this Ia Workshop. For a more complete description of the present
rules for nomenclature of Ia antigens, the reader is referred to the summary of
that workshop (Sachs *et al.*, 1975b).

B. Requirements for Defining Ia Antigens

In order to define a serum reactivity as an Ia specificity, the genes responsible for the antigen detected must be able to be mapped to the *I* region of the
H-2 complex. The availability of strains of mice bearing recombinant *H-2* haplotypes (Table I) has made this mapping possible for some 20 Ia antigens at
present. Most of the recombinant haplotypes arose during the production of
congenic resistant lines (Snell and Bunker, 1965; Stimpfling and Reichert, 1970)
or during purposeful breeding with the goal of selecting recombinants within the
H-2 region (Shreffler and David, 1972). The recombinant haplotypes were then
bred back onto a common background strain, providing a panel of animals differing from each other only in *H-2* and only to the left or to the right of the
point of crossover.

A hypothetical system of congenic recombinants is shown in Fig. 1. If a
serological reactivity suspected of detecting an Ia antigen is positive in one but

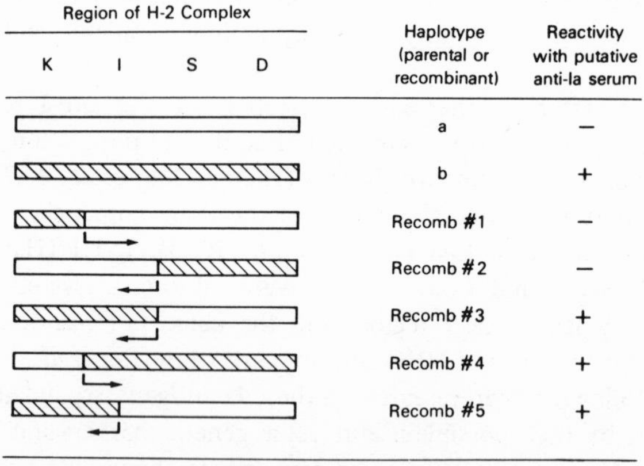

Figure 1. Hypothetical scheme for mapping of Ia antigen
specificity using congenic recombinant lines. Arrows beneath
informative recombinants indicate the position of the gene(s)
determining serological reactivity relative to the position of
crossover in the recombinant haplotype.

not in the other of two parental haplotypes which led to a series of recombinants, then the recombinants can often be used to define the left hand and the right hand boundaries of the genetic material which could conceivably determine the reactive antigen. As can be seen in Fig. 1, any of the pairs of recombinants 1 and 2, 1 and 3, 2 and 4, or 3 and 4 would suffice to define a serological specificity as Ia.

C. Subregions

In certain cases, Ia antisera have detected unexpected reactions when tested on recombinants in which the crossover position had previously been determined on the basis of K and D region specificities, Ss properties, and Ir function. The simplest interpretation of such reactions has been assumed to be that the recombinant event had in fact occurred within the *I* region. Such a hypothetical event is indicated by recombinant number 5, in Fig. 1. On this basis, several subregions have been defined within the *I* region. The expanded linear map thus produced is shown in Fig. 2, along with the specificities tentatively mapped within each subregion. Subregions *I-A* and *I-B* are defined by the same recombinant strains which led to the subdivision of the *Ir* region into *Ir-1A* and *Ir-1B* on the basis of immune responses to certain antigens (Lieberman *et al.*, 1972).

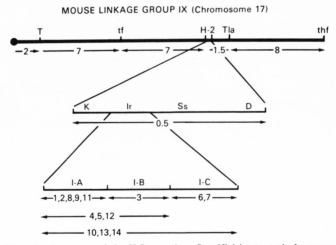

MOUSE LINKAGE GROUP IX (Chromosome 17)

Figure 2. Fine structure map of the H-2 complex: Specificities tentatively mapped to each of the I subregions are indicated beneath the expanded subregion in the figure (data from Shreffler and David, 1975; Sachs *et al.*, 1975b). Uncertainty in the mapping of some of the specificities is indicated by bars which span more than one subregion. The mapping of specificity Ia.3 to the I-B subregion has recently been questioned (Shreffler *et al.*, 1976a), opening the possibility that there may be no serological markers in the I-B region.

On the other hand, the subregion *I-C* has been defined only on the basis of unexpected Ia serological specificities. A fourth subregion, *I-E**(not shown), has recently been proposed on the basis of serologic reactivity with a product of the *H-2*^{k} haplotype which maps to the right of *I-B* and to the left of *I-C* when tested on available recombinant strains. This reactivity was found in a B10.A(4R) anti-B10.A(2R) antiserum which retained reactivity with B10.A and B10.A(2R) lymphocytes after absorption with B10.D2, and it was initially thought to represent an *I-B* subregion specificity on this basis (Sachs, 1976). Subsequent testing, however, indicates that this specificity is also positive on B10.A(5R) lymphocytes and is absorbed by B10.BR, suggesting that it defines a new subregion. The same specificity has also been detected in two other antisera, and has been assigned the number Ia.22, which tentatively defines the *I-E* subregion (Shreffler *et al.* 1976b; David *et al.* 1976).

D. The "Ia Chart"

The Ia antigens appear so far to exhibit the same type of extensive serological polymorphism that has previously been found for the H-2 system. That is, sequential absorption studies with available inbred strains continue to require splitting of serological reactivities, leading to an ever-increasing number of defined Ia specificities. At the time of the Ia Workshop some 15 specificities had been defined, and there were clear indications that further Ia specificities were present in some of the available antisera. Since the definition of Ia antigens requires the availability of recombinant haplotypes capable of mapping the reactivity, numerous other specificities must await the production of new recombinants before they will be definitively assigned numbers. The use of a prefix W has been adopted as a tentative notation for suspected Ia specificities awaiting definitive mapping studies. Including such WIa specificietes, the number of presently detectable Ia antigens is now over 20.

The distribution of H-2 serological specificities among available haplotypes has become known as the "H-2 chart," and by analogy the distribution of Ia specificities among available haplotypes (Fig. 3) might be termed the "Ia chart." Because of present uncertainty about the extent of Ia polymorphism, the Ia chart is far from complete. In addition to the fact that the system is new and only a fraction of possible anti-Ia antisera have been tested, there is the further restriction on this chart that it includes only those specificities which can be mapped. In fact, as will be described later, the experience in the author's laboratory has been that when a broadly specific anti-H-2 antiserum is rendered Ia specific by adsorption of anti-H-2K region and anti-H-2D region antibodies, and

---

*A decision was made at the Ia Workshop not to use letters already being used for regions of the H-2 complex for defining new I subregions.

IA SPECIFICITIES

H-2 Haplotype	1	2	3	4	5	6	7	8	9	10	11	12	13	14	15	16	17	18	19	W20	W21	22
b	−	−	3	−	−	−	−	8	9	−	−	−	−	−	15	−	−	−	−	W20	−	−
d	−	−	−	−	−	6	7	8	−	−	11	−	−	−	15	16	−	−	−	−	−	−
f	1	−	−	−	5	−	−	−	−	−	−	−	−	14	−	−	17	18	−	−	−	−
k	1	2	3	−	−	−	7	−	−	−	−	−	−	−	15	−	17	18	19	−	−	22
p	−	−	−	−	5	6	7	−	−	−	−	−	13	−	−	−	−	−	−	−	W21	−
q	−	−	3	−	5	−	−	−	9	10	−	−	13	−	−	16	−	−	−	−	−	−
r	1	−	3	−	5	−	7	−	−	−	−	12	−	−	−	−	17	−	19	−	−	−
s	−	−	−	4	5	−	−	−	9	−	−	12	−	−	−	−	17	18	−	−	−	−

Figure 3. The Ia chart. Distribution of Ia specificities among some of the common H-2 haplotypes of independent origin (Shreffler *et al.*, 1976a; David *et al.*, 1976).

is then further absorbed with cells bearing each of the defined Ia specificities it is thought to contain, residual anti-Ia antibodies reactive with the immunizing strain are always left behind. This indicates that the number of Ia antigenic specificities must be much greater than the number presently on the chart. It is therefore worth a note of caution to those who would use this chart to design or to analyze experiments that, while it may be helpful in identifying known or suspected Ia reactivities, it should not be used to predict the *absence* of Ia reactivity in a particular system.

III. PRODUCTION OF ANTI-Ia REAGENTS

A. Direct Immunization

The most straightforward way to produce anti-Ia antibodies, and the simplest to understand, is by immunization between congenic resistant strains of mice which differ only in the *I* region or in the *I* and *S* regions.* Presumably, if the animals are truly congenic, the only cell surface antigens against which they should produce antibodies should be products of the *I* region.

Unfortunately, the number of available strain combinations with which such

*The products of the S region have so far not been found on the cell surface, and differences in this region have therefore not been considered in defining Ia specificities (Shreffler and Passmore, 1971).

an approach may be employed is very limited, there at present being only three such reciprocal combinations of inbred strains (Fig. 4). The AQR strain is included in Fig. 4 even though the B10.AQR congenic line is not yet available (i.e., requires further backcross generations). To date, such antibodies can be produced in one direction [B10 × AQR anti-B10.T(6R)] by bringing the non-H-2 background of B10 into the responding strain, but in the reverse direction it is possible that the antibodies produced may include specificities for non-H-2 antigens.

In addition, there is a possible theoretical objection to defining the reactivities of such antisera as anti-Ia. Such a definition requires knowledge of the precise linear localization of the crossover events leading to the recombinant pairs used for immunization. Thus, for the first two combinations listed in Fig. 4, if the crossover event between the *K* and *I-A* regions in the AQR or the A.TL strains occurred within the *K* region rather than precisely between the *K* region and *I-A* subregion, then these strains might differ from their corresponding partners by limited H-2K region antigenic specificities as well as for Ia specificities. Since the number of genes in the *K* region, or in any of the regions for that matter, remains unclear, and since even intracistronic recombinations can occur, the likelihood of such intraregional recombination cannot be assessed. In addition, since the original determinations of recombination in these strains was done by H-2 typing, the possibility of detecting intraregional recombinants might depend on which reagents were used in the serological analyses. Conversely, if the recombinant event in these strains occurred within the *I-A* subregion, then certain combinations which had been though to be "*H-2K* region only" differences (A.TH–A.AL and AQR–B10.A) might also differ by limited Ia specificities. So far, however, there is no experimental evidence that these theoretical objections have caused any practical problems.

In the last recombinant pair listed in Fig. 4, the B10.A(4R)–B10.A(2R) combination, the recombinant event in the B10.A(4R) has been shown by functional

Donor-Recipient Pair	H-2 Haplotype					
	K	I-A	I-B	I-C	Ss	D
AQR	q	k	k	d	d	d
B10·T(6R)	q	q	q	q	q	d
A·TH	s	s	s	s	s	d
A·TL	s	k	k	k	k	d
B10·A(4R)	k	k	b	b	b	b
B10·A(2R)	k	k	k	d	d	b

Figure 4. Direct immunization. These three combinations have been used successfully to produce anti-Ia reagents in this laboratory and elsewhere. The origin of each subregion of the recombinant haplotypes is indicated by lowercase letters (see Table I). Within each pair, the K and D regions are derived from the same haplotype, leading therefore to the production of anti-Ia antibodies following reciprocal immunizations.

studies (Lieberman *et al.*, 1972) to have occurred within the *I* region. Antisera produced in this combination are therefore less likely to be contaminated with any anti-H-2K region specificities. However, the same theoretical objection could be raised for this combination with respect to recombination occurring within the *D* region of the B10.A(2R). It is interesting that in this combination skin grafts are accepted indefinitely in both directions, while skin grafts between A.TH and A.TL animals are rejected in 12–14 days (Sachs and Cone, unpublished results). Skin grafts in the AQR-B10.T(6R) system have variable fates, the basis for which is not yet fully understood (Elkins, personal communication). The reasons for these differences in rejection patterns with different Ia incompatibilities are not entirely clear, but may be a function of the different Ia antigens involved and/or the different *I* subregions involved. It has been postulated by Klein *et al.* (1974b) that there is a third histocompatibility locus within the *I-A* subregion of the *H-2* complex, but it is not clear whether the products of this locus are the same or different from the Ia antigens determined by that subregion.

While immunization of B10.A(4R) animals with lymphoid cells from B10.A(2R) was found to produce a reasonable titer of anti-Ia antibodies in about one-third of these animals, the reverse immunization did not produce detectable antibodies. In addition, it has been shown that a B10 anti-B10.A antiserum absorbed with B10.A(4R) cells still reacts against Ia antigens of the B10.A(2R) but a B10.A anti-B10 antiserum absorbed with B10.A(2R) cells does not have residual activity to Ia antigens of the B10.A(4R) (Lozner *et al.*, 1974). The basis for this discrepancy is not yet clear. There may be a differential immunogenicity of certain Ia antigens so that some are readily detected by the B10 or by the B10.A(4R) but the corresponding allele of these antigens possessed by the B10 and B10.A(4R) is not sufficiently antigenic to produce reasonable antibodies in the B10.A or the B10.A(2R) (David *et al.*, 1974). Alternatively, Lozner *et al.* (1974) have suggested that the recombinant event leading to the B10.A(4R) haplotype may have involved a deletion of a small amount of genetic material adjacent to the point of crossing over, leaving the B10.A(2R) with genetic information for which no corresponding alleles exist in the B10.A(4R). The one-way MLC reaction between these two strains might also be explained by such a deletion, and this correlation led to speculation by Lozner *et al.* (1974) that the Ia antigens might be the source of stimulation of the MLC reaction. In any event, even this combination may thus not represent "only an Ia difference."

B. Shared Ia Determinants

A second method for obtaining Ia-specific reactivity is to make use of an antiserum which contains both anti-H-2 and anti-Ia antibodies, but to test the serum on strains which share one or more Ia specificities with the immunizing strain and do not share any H-2 specificities detectable by the antiserum. This was the method used in our laboratory on the basis of which the Ia reactivity shared between B10 and B10.D2 was first determined (Sachs and Cone, 1973). The reaction pattern of a (B10.A × A)F$_1$ anti-B10 antiserum with B10 and with B10.D2 strains is shown in Fig. 5. This antiserum contains both anti-K-region and anti-D-region activity (anti-H-2.33 and anti-H-2.2) and, as expected, killed essentially all lymph node and spleen cells of the B10 strain to a titer of 1:128. The B10.D2 strain does not possess any H-2K region or H-2D region antigens in common with B10 which could be detected by this serum. However, it does possess Ia.8 in common with B10, and it is this specificity which accounts for the plateau killing at the 50% level seen in Fig. 5 when this serum was tested against B10.D2 splenic lymphocytes. This is, of course, the same reactivity which was originally called β when it was detected in the reverse direction (B10.A anti-B10.D2 tested on B10), as described above.

This method, however, has limitations on its usefulness. First of all, there are so many shared public H-2 specificities in both the H-2K and the H-2D regions that it is the exception rather than the rule for two strains not to share public H-2 specificities. In fact, H-2^b and H-2^d do share public specificities in

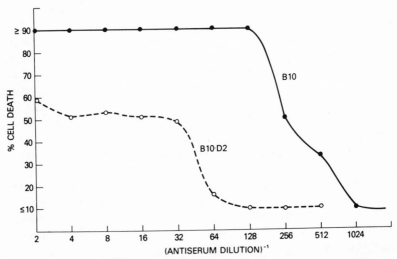

Figure 5. Shared Ia specificities. In this case, the (B10.A × A)F$_1$ anti-B10 antiserum reacts with multiple H-2 and Ia specificities when tested on H-2^b spleen cells, and thus causes killing of virtually all B10 target cells to a 1:128 dilution. However, the only shared specificity this serum reacts with on H-2^d spleen cells is Ia.8, and therefore a typical anti-Ia cytotoxicity curve is generated by titration on B10.D2 target cells.

the D region, but these are not detected by B10.A anti-B10 or B10.A anti-B10.D2 antisera because the $H-2^a$ and $H-2^d$ haplotypes share the same D region (Table I). Second, in order to be assured that the specificity detected is in fact an Ia specificity, one must have available recombinant strains between positive and negative parental types which permit one to map the specificity within the I region.

In addition, there is a possible theoretical objection to this method of defining Ia specificities. The fact that no known public H-2 specificities are shared between two strains is no assurance that such specificities do not exist. The definition of an H-2 specificity requires a strain which will react against that specificity in order to produce the reference reagent defining the specificity. Since there are known to be Ir genes, both $H-2$ linked and non-$H-2$ linked, which can participate in controlling the response to H-2 antigens (Lilly *et al.*, 1973; McKenzie, 1975), the failure to detect a shared H-2 specificity might very well depend on the strain used as the responder. During our attempts to produce

Table I. Haplotypes of Origin of Regions and Subregions of Selected H-2 Haplotypes^a

Haplotype	Representative strain	Origin of regions					
		K	I-A	I-B	I-C	S	D
a	A, B10.A	k	k	k	d	d	d
a1	A.AL	k	k	k	k	k	d
b	B6, B10	b	b	b	b	b	b
d	BALB/c DBA/2, B10.D2	d	d	d	d	d	d
g	HTG, B10.HTG	d	d	d	d	d	b
h2	B10.A(2R)	k	k	k	d	d	b
h4	B10.A(4R)	k	k	b	b	b	b
i5	B10.A(5R)	b	b	b	d	d	d
k	C3H, AKR, CBA, B10.BR	k	k	k	k	k	k
m	AKR.M, B10.AKM	k	k	k	k	k	q
o1	C3H.OL	d	d	d	d	k	k
o2	C3H.OH, C3H-H-2^0	d	d	d	d	d	k
s	A.SW	s	s	s	s	s	s
t1	A.TL	s	k	k	k	k	d
t2	A.TH	s	s	s	s	s	d
t3	B10.HTT	s	s	s	k	k	d
y1	AQR	q	k	k	d	d	d
y2	B10.T(6R)	q	q	q	q	q	d

^{a}Haplotypes of commonly used recombinants have been selected and certain haplotypes from which the recombinants arose are given for ease of reference in the text.

higher titers of anti-Ia antisera, we have prepared F_1 hybrids of responder strains with various other non-*H-2* backgrounds (such as A/J X B10.A and C3H X B10.A). The response to Ia antigens has indeed been increased by this procedure in several instances (e.g., see Fig. 4). However, we have also noted, on occasion, detection of either new or known public H-2 specificities not present in sera produced in the parental strains. The genetic basis of such responsiveness is presently being investigated in this laboratory (Hansen and Sachs, unpublished data). However, it is clear that at this time one should not assume from looking at the H-2 chart that a particular immunization combination will not produce antibodies against public H-2 specificities. Instead, each serum should be ana- lyzed individually to assure that only shared Ia specificities will be detected when this method is used.

C. Selective Absorptions

The third method by which anti-Ia reagents can be produced makes use of the difference in tissue distribution patterns of H-2 and Ia antigens. Since H-2 antigens are expressed rather ubiquitously on murine tissues, while Ia antigens are expressed preferentially on B lymphocytes, there are numerous cell types which can be used to remove H-2K and H-2D region specificities from H-2 allo- antisera while leaving the antibodies against Ia antigens relatively unaltered.

The effectiveness of this technique was demonstrated by Sachs and Cone (1975) using T-cell-derived tumor cells as well as thymocytes to remove anti-H-2 activity from several H-2 alloantisera. An example of the absorption patterns obtained is shown in Fig. 6. Shown in this figure are the cytotoxic curves ob- tained when a B10.D2 (H-2^d) anti-B10.BR (H-2^k) alloantiserum was absorbed with increasing numbers of RDM-4 tumor cells, a thymus-derived tumor of H-2^k type. At each stage of absorption the serum has been titered against B10.BR splenic lymphocytes as targets. It is apparent from the figures that absorption with 2 X 10^8 and 4 X 10^8 tumor cells/ml of serum produced marked changes in the cytotoxic pattern obtained but that two further doubling in- creases in numbers of cells used for absorption did not significantly alter the maximum percentage lysis of the target cell populations. The slight shift to the left in the cytotoxic curve obtained with serum absorbed at 16 X 10^8 cells/ml was attributed to a dilution artifact as established by the use of a radioactively labeled irrelevant protein (unpublished data). The antibodies remaining after such quantitative absorptions were shown to detect Ia antigens by tests on recombinant strains.

Similar results have been obtained by Columbani *et al.* (1976) with murine platelets as the absorbent. These authors used a quantitative microcomplement fixation test to assess the relative amounts of H-2 and Ia antigens on platelets and lymphocytes. They found that while 15–30 platelets were equivalent to one

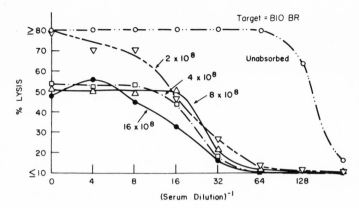

Figure 6. Selective absorptions. B10.D2 anti-B10.BR serum absorbed with RDM-4 (AKR) tumor cells. The cytotoxicity titration curves against B10.BR splenic target cells are plotted for each stage of absorption. The number of RDM-4 (AKR) tumor cells used for absorption per milliliter of B10.D2 anti-B10.BR serum is indicated for each curve.

splenic lymphocyte in absorptive capacity for H-2 antibodies, no absorption of anti-Ia antibodies could be detected using up to 40 times as many platelets as the number of lymphocytes necessary to absorb a similar amount of anti-Ia reactivity. Since platelets are readily available and do not require the establishment of a T-cell tumor line or a thymectomy, this procedure appears to be a versatile one and one which might readily be extended to other species. The results obtained by Columbani et al. (1976) have been confirmed in this laboratory, and the procedure has in fact been used successfully to demonstrate an Ia-like antibody in a human alloantiserum (Arbeit et al., 1975).

Still another tissue which has been successfully used to render H-2 antisera specific for Ia antigens is the red cell (Davies and Hess, 1974; Hauptfeld et al., 1975). The cytotoxicity curves obtained after absorption with red cells in both rat antisera and mouse alloantisera were very similar to the curves shown in Fig. 6. However, the amount of histocompatibility antigen present on red cells is very small relative to that on lymphocytes and platelets (Herberman and Stetson, 1965), and not all species express histocompatibility antigens on their peripheral red cells, limiting the applicability of this approach.

It is important to note that the absorption method for producing anti-Ia reagents does not require the availability of a cell type which is absolutely lacking in Ia antigens but requires, rather, an absorbing cell type which bears a much larger complement of H-2 antigens than of Ia antigens. Thus, for example, if an H-2 alloantiserum originally contains equal quantities of anti-H-2 and anti-Ia antibodies, it is clear that a cell type expressing 100 times as much H-2 antigen as Ia antigen would be capable of rendering the serum specific for Ia antigens at an absorbing cell concentration much too small to appreciably alter the titer of anti-Ia antibodies. Thus none of these absorption methods proves that the cells used for absorption are actually lacking in Ia antigens; they merely indicate the small amount of Ia antigen relative to the amount of H-2 antigen present on these cell surfaces. This is particularly apparent when one considers recent studies which have made use of the exquisite sensitivity of the "fluorescence-activated cell sorter" to demonstrate the presence of Ia antigens, in very small amounts, on thymocytes (Fathman *et al.*, 1975). As mentioned above, thymocytes have been successfully used to render H-2 alloantisera specific for Ia antigens (Sachs and Cone, 1975). Obviously, however, if the absorptions were carried to completion (2 orders of magnitude greater number of cells) such absorptions would have removed the Ia antibodies as well.

In addition, it is conceivable that certain but not all Ia antigens might be expressed on a particular cell type along with the H-2 antigens. In such a case, absorption might remove some Ia antibodies but would leave sufficient anti-Ia reactivity behind to give an indistinguishable pattern of cytotoxicity from that shown in Fig. 6. Thus, while absorption studies can indicate the relative absence of certain Ia specificities from cell populations, they do not necessarily indicate that all Ia specificities are lacking on those cell populations, and this must be tested independently.

IV. CORRELATIVE CRITERIA

Because of the limitations of all of the methods for defining Ia antigens enumerated above, it is clear that many more pairs of recombinant haplotypes will be necessary before definitive mapping can be performed for all of the existing Ia specificities. For this reason, several of the distinctive characteristics which have been associated with known Ia antigens provide attractive correlative criteria for the definition of new Ia specificities before recombinant strains are available for definitive mapping.

A. Tissue Distribution

As has been mentioned, one of the distinctive characteristics of the Ia antigens is their restricted tissue distribution. While anti-H-2 antibodies generally react with all mouse tissues and kill 100% of lymphoid populations, anti-Ia antibodies characteristically kill only a subpopulation of lymphoid cells. In our original description of a shared Ia antigen (Sachs and Cone, 1973), a variety of criteria were examined, all of which indicated that the subpopulations being killed correlated most closely with the B cells in the lymphoid preparations tested. Assays of the additivity of the killing of lymph node cells by this reagent and known B-cell (anti-κ) and T-cell (anti-θ) reagents were carried out by the chromium release method. Significant additivity was found when lymphoid cells were preincubated with the anti-θ reagent prior to treatment with the anti-Ia antibodies, but no significant increase in lysis was obtained when the cells were pretreated with the anti-κ reagent prior to treatment with anti-Ia. Using a fluoresceinated anti-κ reagent, no increase in the staining of lymph node or spleen cells was obtained by preincubation with the anti-Ia reagents (i.e., the B cells stained in both cases, although subjectively they were brighter after the preincubation with anti-Ia) while preincubation with an anti-H-2 reagent or an anti-θ reagent led to the subsequent staining of virtually all of the lymphoid cells by the fluoresceinated anti-κ reagent. Finally, cytotoxicity assays were performed on lymph node cells which were first separated into subpopulations enriched for either B or T cells. The anti-Ia reagent was found to kill a proportion of each of the populations consistent with the percentage of B cells as assessed independently by a fluoresceinated anti-immunoglobulin reagent.

This last method has proved to be a simple and reliable way to assess subsequent putative Ia antisera for subpopulation lysis. The method involves incubation of a lymphoid population with nylon wool which has first been preincubated with fetal calf serum as described by Julius *et al.* (1973). The majority of T cells do not adhere to such nylon and can be washed off with medium after a further 45-min incubation. Recovery of the B-cell-enriched fraction is then accomplished by vigorous mechanical agitation of the nylon, as described by Handwerger and Schwartz (1975). Aliquots of the starting lymphoid population and of each of the subpopulations thus produced are separately treated with a fluoresceinated anti-immunoglobulin reagent to assess the percentage of B cells in each population. Other aliquots are tested by a cytotoxicity assay for maximal percentage lysis obtainable with the anti-Ia reagent or an anti-H-2 control (which must always kill >90% of the cells to demonstrate adequacy of the assay conditions). As can be seen in Table II, antisera produced by each of the three methods for obtaining Ia antisera described above show patterns of cytotoxicity consistent with the killing of predominantly the B cells in each of the three populations tested. It should be noted, however, that any cells which adhere to these nylon columns and are not released by mechanical agitation would evade the assay. Such subpopulations of cells may exist (R. Schwartz, personal communication).

Interestingly, anti-Ia antisera produced in the A.TH–A.TL combination often show significant killing of both the adherent and nonadherent subpopulations produced by this nylon column fractionation. The killing of the T-cell-enriched subpopulations by such antisera is erratic and can be as high as 25% above complement backgrounds (Cone and Sachs, unpublished data). It was originally suspected that this killing of T cells might be due to the presence of anti-H-2K region specificity in the A.TH anti-A.TL antiserum. However,

Table II. Reactivity of Anti-Ia Antisera with Fractionated Lymphocytes

Method of anti-Ia production	Antiserum	Cells fractionated	Fraction	Percent Ig+	Complement control	Percent lysis
Direct	B10.A(4R)	B10.A	Pre	54	<10	69
anti-I	anti-	spleen	Nonadherent	10	21	36
immunization	B10.A(2R)		Adherent	85	<10	>90
Shared Ia	B10.A anti-	B10 lymph	Pre	32	<10	48
specificity	B10.D2	node	Nonadherent	7	37	43
			Adherent	68	17	77
Absorbed H-2	B10.D2 anti-	B10.BR	Pre	46	10	59
antiserum	B10.BR	spleen	Nonadherent	12	27	37
	absorbed		Adherent	75	11	87
	with					
	RDM-4					

absorption of this serum with B10.A platelets was incapable of reducing the T-cell killing or the staining of T cells by this antiserum (Sachs, Dickler, and Cone, unpublished data). It thus appears that Ia antigens on T cells may be more readily detected by this immunization combination than by others. Alternatively, some Ia specificities may be expressed on T cells to a greater extent than others, and this particular immunization combination may involve more such Ia specificities.

It is thus apparent that predominant expression of an MHC-linked antigen on the B-cell subpopulation of lymphoid cells suggests that the antigen is likely to be determined by genes in the *I* region. In fact, the third approach described above for the production of anti-Ia reagents depends on this distinction in tissue distribution, since the absorption of an anti-H-2 antiserum with thymocytes, T-cell-derived tumors, or platelets removes the anti-H-2K and H-2D region activities at absorbing cell concentrations which leave the anti-Ia reactivity relatively unaltered. Thus predominant B-cell reactivity can be considered a correlative criterion for the Ia antigens. In fact, several authors have already suggested that B-cell reactivities in certain human alloantisera may be detecting "Ia-like" antigens of man (Jones *et al.*, 1975; Arbeit *et al.*, 1975; Winchester *et al.*, 1975; Mann *et al.*, 1975; van Rood *et al.*, 1975). A note of caution is necessary, however; the studies in the mouse which have shown predominant B-cell expression of Ia antigens have employed antisera produced in congenic strains of mice which differ only at the *H-2* complex. Within such antisera it has been shown that the Ia antibodies detect antigens predominantly expressed on B cells while the H-2K and H-2D region antibodies detect antigens distributed ubiquitously on mouse tissues. However, if the antisera are produced between strains differing at non-*H-2* loci, it is possible that other B-cell reactivities such as Ly-4 (McKenzie and Snell, 1975) could be obtained which would not necessarily be directed toward antigens determined by the *I* region. It is thus necessary in using such a correlative criterion in an outbred species to show independently that the reactivity is with an antigen, the genes for which segregate with the MHC of that species.

Ia antigens have also been detected on macrophages, sperm cells, and epidermal cells (Hämmerling *et al.*, 1975), although the amount of these antigens present relative to the amount on B cells was not precisely assessed. In addition, Ia antigens have been demonstrated on thymocytes by two independent methods (Fathman *et al.*, 1975; Goding *et al.*, 1975), both of which employ much higher levels of sensitivity than the methods of cytotoxicity or visual immunofluorescence which were first used to assess the tissue distribution of Ia antigens. The amount of Ia antigens on thymocytes was found to be very small relative to that on peripheral B cells. Finally, a recent report by David *et al.* (1975) indicates that Ia antigens are much more readily detected on mitogen-stimulated T cells than on ordinary nonstimulated T cells. If confirmed, this finding may explain the discrepancy between many previous studies showing presence or absence of the Ia antigens on T cells, since the levels of stimulation of the cells examined may have differed between different studies.

B. Chemistry

A great deal of effort has been expended over the past 12 years on the isolation and characterization of cell surface antigens determined by the MHC. One of the main reasons for this effort has been the hope that purified histocompatibility antigens might be used to induce tolerance to transplantation. While this approach has met with only very limited success, much has been learned about the purification and characterization of these antigens. A variety of methods have been employed, including hypotonic lysis, sonication, enzymatic digestion, and solubilization with nonionic detergents (for reviews, see Nathenson and Cullen, 1974; Ferrone *et al.*, 1975). The use of nonionic detergents which are sufficiently nondenaturing to permit antigen–antibody reactions to occur, such as NP-40 (Schwartz and Nathenson, 1971), has led to major steps forward over the past 5 years.

The current sequence of procedures used for isolation of MHC antigens using specific precipitation in nonionic detergents is listed in Table III. Step 3 in Table III, the affinity chromatography on a lectin column, has been shown to greatly simplify the gel pattern obtained by this method (Hayman and Crumpton, 1972; Cullen *et al.*, 1975a). Fortunately, both H-2 and Ia antigens bind to such a lectin column and can be eluted by α-methylmannoside, giving a purification of about twentyfold over the starting solubilized membrane preparations. Figure 7

Table III. Isolation of Mouse MHC Antigens

1. Spleen cells labeled *in vitro* with [^{3}H] leucine
2. Membranes solubilized with NP-40[a]
3. Preparation purified by affinity chromatography on lentil lectin column, eluted by α-methylmannoside
4. Specific antibodies added
5. Precipitation with goat anti-mouse Ig
6. Precipitate dissolved in SDS[b] with mercaptoethanol
7. Electrophoresis of preparation on 10% disc. PAGE[c] in SDS
8. Gels cut and fractions counted

[a] Nonidet P-40 (Shell trademark).
[b] Sodium dodecylsulfate.
[c] Discontinuous polyacrylamide gel electrophoresis.

shows the pattern of peaks obtained on SDS gels by this method for known products of the major histocompatibility complex. The arrows in each panel indicate the positions of migrations of heavy and light chains of immunoglobulin, labeled with a different radioisotope and run along with the precipitate being analyzed to yield molecular weight references. As can be seen from this figure, both H-2K and H-2D region antigens yield peaks on these gels with an apparent molecular weight of approximately 45,000. On the other hand, anti-Ia antibodies lead to the precipitation of two peaks with molecular weights of approximately 28,000 and 35,000. The resolution of these Ia peaks has been improved by the introduction of a discontinuous gel system. Thus, while early studies describing gel patterns for Ia antigens showed only one broad, poorly defined peak covering the range 28,000–35,000 (Cullen *et al.*, 1974), more recent studies (Cullen *et al.*, 1975a, b) have shown predominantly two major peaks as indicated in Fig. 7. In some cases, a third small peak has been seen between the two major peaks using the discontinuous gel system. The basis for these multiple peaks is not clear. They could conceivably be artifactually produced from a single molecular species during preparation of the antigen or during electrophoresis. On the other hand, they may indicate a true heterogeneity in the Ia molecules, or perhaps a subunit structure, the two major peaks representing the two major subunits.

As a correlative criterion, the molecular size and gel pattern of the Ia antigens require a rather specialized technology compared to the assessment of tissue distribution. However, if that technology is available, this method provides an elegant and sensitive way to detect new or suspected Ia antigens, in particular antiserum–strain combinations (Delovitch and McDevitt, 1975; Silver *et al.*, 1975; Vitetta *et al.*, 1974). In addition, the method provides one of the few possible correlative criteria which can indicate that an antiserum detects only H-2K or H-2D and not Ia antigens. This becomes important in many functional studies requiring H-2 controls for the effects of anti-Ia antibodies.

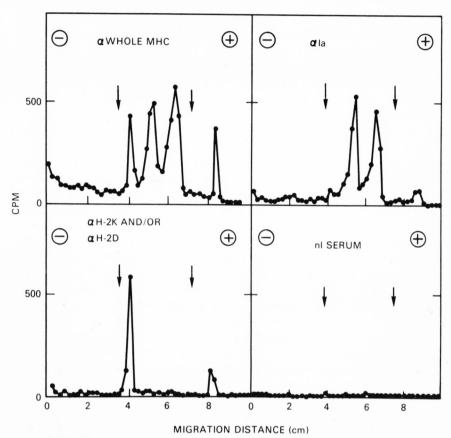

MIGRATION DISTANCE (cm)

Figure 7. Representative gel patterns obtained with antisera of known specificity. Under the electrophoretic conditions (in SDS), all protein species have a net negative charge and therefore run from cathode (–) to anode (+). Migration distance is related to size, and the arrows show position of heavy (50,000) and light (25,000) chains of γG for reference. When the serum tested has specificity for H-2K or H-2D region antigens only (lower left), a peak at approximately 45,000 daltons is obtained. When the serum detects only Ia antigens (upper right), two peaks at approximately 28,000 and 35,000 daltons are obtained. When both types of specificity are present (upper left) all three peaks are obtained, and when normal control serum is used (lower right) no appreciable peaks are found. A low molecular weight peak (approximately 15,000 daltons) is usually also found when anti-H-2K or anti-H-2D region antigens are precipitated, and this may be murine β_2-microglobulin.

C. Blocking of the Fc Receptor

The B lymphocytes of a variety of species have been shown to possess a cell surface receptor, termed the "Fc receptor," which binds antigen–antibody com-

plexes and heat-aggregated immunoglobulin through the Fc portion of the complexed immunoglobulin molecule (Basten *et al.*, 1972; Dickler and Kunkel,
1972). Using an assay for the Fc receptor involving fluorescein-labeled heat-
aggregated immunoglobulin, Dickler and Sachs (1974) have reported that the
binding of such complexes to the murine B-cell Fc receptors was inhibited
specifically by anti-Ia antibodies. Table IV shows representative data from these
experiments.

As can be seen in Table IV, murine splenic lymphocytes when tested either
with a fluoresceinated rabbit anti-mouse immunoglobulin (FRMIG) or with
fluoresceinated aggregates (F-Agg) show approximately 50% positive lymphocytes. Independent studies using two different fluorescent labels have shown
that principally the same population of cells (i.e., the B cells) stain with both
reagents (Dickler and Sachs, 1974). When the splenic lymphocytes were preincubated with an antiserum containing antibodies against the whole H-2 complex
(Experiments 1 and 2, Table IV), the percent cells staining with FRMIG increased to > 96%, indicating that mouse alloantibodies had bound to essentially
all of the cells, causing both B cells and T cells to stain with this reagent. On the
other hand, the percentage of splenic lymphocytes staining with F-Agg was
markedly inhibited to 6.5 and 7.5% in the examples shown.

It was thus clear that antibodies against the products of one or more regions
of the *H-2* complex were capable of inhibiting binding of complexed immuno-

**Table IV. Effect of Pretreatment with Alloantisera on Detection of the Fc
Receptor**

Expt.	Strain	Serum used for preincubation	Relevant specificity	Surface[a] Ig	Aggregate[b] positive
1	B10	Normal B10.A	–	52.5	52.0
		B10.A anti-B10	K, I, S, D	96.0	6.5
2	B10.A	Normal B10	–	49.5	47.0
		B10 anti-B10.A	K, I, S, D	>99.5	7.5
3	B10	Normal B10.A	–	53.0	53.5
		B10.A anti-B10.D2	I	53.5	9.5
4	B10.BR	Normal B10.D2	–	48.5	46.5
		B10.D2 anti-B10.BR absorbed with RDM-4	I	48.0	9.5
5	B10.A	Normal B10.A(4R)	–	53.0	50.5
		B10.A(4R) anti-B10.A(2R)	I	51.0	15.0
6	A.TL	Normal A/J	–	55.0	53.5
		A/J anti A.SW	K	>99.5	54.0
7	B10.A(2R)	Normal B10.A	–	49.0	50.5
		B10.A anti-B10	D	81.0	49.0

[a] Detected by fluoresceinated rabbit anti-mouse Ig (FRMIG).
[b] Detected by fluoresceinated aggregated human Ig (F-Agg).

globulin to the B-cell Fc receptor. In order to assess further which regions were involved, antisera against Ia antigens prepared by each of the three methods outlined in Section III were used for the same kind of inhibition assay (Experiments 3, 4, 5; Table IV). The results indicated that all of these anti-Ia reagents were capable of producing the same levels of inhibition of aggregate binding as did antisera directed against products of the whole *H-2* complex. In this case, however, the staining with FRMIG did not increase significantly over the staining obtained with this reagent after preincubation with medium alone or with normal serum, presumably because the anti-Ia antibodies bound to the same subpopulation of lymphoid cells which stain due to their own surface immunoglobulin (i.e., the B-cell subpopulation). Antisera against Ia antigens determined by at least two I subregions were capable of causing this type of inhibition (Dickler *et al.*, 1975b).

While these studies indicated that the anti-Ia antibodies in an anti-H-2 antiserum were sufficient to block the Fc receptor of B cells, they did not imply necessarily that only anti-Ia antibodies in these sera were capable of producing such blocking. Experiments 6 and 7 in Table IV provide evidence that antibodies against products of the *H-2K* region and *H-2D* region alone are incapable of inhibiting the B-lymphocyte Fc receptor. These examples make use of the recombinant *H-2* haplotypes of the A.TL and B10.A(2R) strains (Table I). The A/J anti-A.SW antiserum reacted with essentially all splenic lymphocytes of the A.TL animal, as would be expected, since the antiserum contains antibodies against products of the *H-2K*s region. Thus the serum killed essentially all splenic lymphocytes of the A.TL strain and caused surface immunoglobulin staining of all A.TL lymphocytes. However, since the remainder of the *H-2* complex (except for the K region) of the A.TL derives from the A.AL strain, this antiserum would be expected to be genetically incapable of reacting with I region specificities or specificities in the H-2D region. As can be seen in Table IV, despite reactivity with the H-2K region antigens, no blocking of uptake of F-Agg could be detected after preincubation of the A.TL cells with this antiserum. Controls indicated that the Fc receptor of these cells could be blocked if the antiserum used for pretreatment contained appropriate anti-Ia antibodies (such as a B10 anti-B10.A antiserum, reactive with the products of the I^k and D^d subregions) and that the A/J anti-A.SW antiserum was capable of causing inhibition of the Fc receptor of B cells possessing Ia antigens with which the serum could react (A.SW). Similarly, use of the B10.A(2R) recombinant strain showed that antibodies against products of the *H-2D* region are incapable of blocking the Fc receptor despite binding to a large percentage of the B lymphocytes. Again, controls indicated that the B10.A(2R) B-cell Fc receptors could be blocked by antibodies against the appropriate Ia antigens (B10 anti-B10.A antiserum) and that the H-2 antiserum which failed to block Fc receptors of the B10.A(2R) was capable of blocking the Fc receptor of B10 cells against the Ia antigens of which it could react.

Additional studies indicating the specificity of this inhibition of the Fc receptor (Dickler and Sachs, 1974: Dickler *et al.*, 1975b) included the following: (1) antisera against mouse immunoglobulin, which also binds to B lymphocytes, did not block the Fc receptor; (2) the same antisera which were capable of inhibiting B-cell Fc receptors did not inhibit complement rosettes, another receptor of splenic B lymphocytes; (3) Fab$'_2$ fragments of anti-Ia antibodies contained within an anti-H-2 serum produced comparable inhibition of the B-cell Fc receptor to the whole immunoglobulin from which they were prepared; and (4) mixtures of splenic lymphocytes from two different strains, one of which could and the other of which could not react with a particular anti-H-2 antiserum, showed only inhibition of the Fc receptors on a fraction of the B cells in the preparaion consistent with the number of B cells of the reactive strain. Thus, by all of these criteria, the ability of an anti-H-2 antiserum to inhibit the Fc receptor of B lymphocytes would appear to be a reasonable correlative criterion to indicate that the antiserum contains antibodies against Ia antigens. Conversely, an anti-H-2 antiserum which can be shown to bind to B lymphocytes but which does not inhibit aggregate binding to the Fc receptor may be judged by these criteria to be free of anti-Ia antibodies. The specificity of this method has subsequently been confirmed (Krammer and Pernis, 1975) with assays using either fluoresceinated antibody–antigen complexes or antibody–coated bovine erythrocytes.

There are, however, several important caveats for the use of Fc receptor blocking as a correlative criterion for detecting Ia antigens. First, one must be sure that the antiserum being tested contains antibodies only against products of the MHC. In all of the cases described above, the antisera were produced between congenic resistant lines, differing only in their *H-2* complex or in parts thereof. However, it is clear from subsequent studies that at least one other antigen system exists in the mouse which is also associated with the Fc receptor (Dickler *et al.*, 1975a). Thus, while blocking of the Fc receptor is capable of distinguishing between K and D region antigens and the Ia antigens, it is not capable of distinguishing between Ia antigens and antigens determined by this other locus. It is thus important, in using this assay in a species in which congenic resistant animals are not available, to show independently that the antigen being studied segregates with the MHC.

A second caveat involves the sensitivity of the assay used to detect B-cell Fc receptors. It has been reported by Schirrmacher *et al.* (1975) that Fc receptors of B lymphocytes as detected by sensitized chicken red blood (Crbc) cell rosettes (EA rosettes) can be inhibited by antibodies and Fab$'_2$ fragments of antibodies against any of a variety of cell surface antigens. These include anti-immunoglobulin and anti-H-2K and anti-H-2D region antibodies, all of which were shown to be negative controls in the studies by Dickler and Sachs (1974). There are no negative controls in the studies by these authors, however, and antibodies against any component of the B lymphocyte surface were found capable of blocking this type of EA rosette. It would thus appear that this rosetting assay using Crbc for detecting the Fc receptor is much more susceptible to nonspecific inhibition by reagents which can disturb the B lymphocyte surface than is the Fc receptor assay employing binding of aggregated immunoglobulin, antigen–antibody complexes, or bovine EA rosettes. For use as a correlative criterion for detecting Ia antigens, the inhibition of F-Agg and not the inhibition of chicken EA rosettes would thus be recommended.

Interestingly, even by use of the chicken EA rosette inhibition assay, antibodies to H-2K region and H-2D antigens show much less inhibitory capacity for similar amounts of antibody than do antibodies to Ia antigens (R. Schirrmacher and P. Halloran, personal communication). In addition, recent studies in this laboratory employing high-titered anti-H-2K region antibodies (A.TL anti-A.AL of a cytotoxic titer approximately 2 orders of magnitude higher than that of the antisera used in the original studies) have shown some inhibition of F-Agg binding to B lymphocytes when the sera were used in high concentrations. When the sera were diluted, however, they continued to stain essentially all of the splenic lymphocytes at dilutions which caused no inhibition of the Fc receptor. It is not clear yet whether this inhibition is an indication of a lack of specificity when a very large amount of anti-H-2 antibody is used or indicates that there are low concentrations of anti-Ia antibodies even in these "anti-H-2K region controls." In any case, these findings indicate that the discrepancy between inhibition studies using aggregate binding and using chicken EA rosetting may be a question of the relative sensitivity of the two assays rather than a difference in the actual Fc receptors being assessed. Thus, while anti-Ia antibodies are the best inhibitors of Fc receptors in both assays, nonspecificity due to peturbation of the B-cell surface by anti-H-2K or anti-H-2D region antibodies may occur with a much lower concentration of antibodies using the rosetting technique than using the aggregate binding technique.

Third, it is important to note that these inhibition studies refer only to inhibition of the B-cell Fc receptor. There are other Fc receptors, such as those found on macrophages (Berken and Benacerraf, 1966) and killer cells in antibody-mediated cellular cytotoxicity (Schirrmacher et al., 1975), neither of which can be inhibited by anti-Ia antibodies in our hands (Henkart et al., unpublished data; Dickler et al., unpublished data) or in the hands of others (Schirrmacher et al., 1975). These may therefore be separate entities from the B-cell Fc receptor.

The mechanism of inhibition of Fc receptors by anti-Ia antibodies remains unclear. Interestingly, antibodies against individual Ia antigens produce just as marked inhibition of aggregate binding as do antibodies against multiple Ia antigens on the same B-lymphocyte population. In addition, antibodies against the Ia antigens of one parental strain of an F_1 hybrid cause inhibition of aggregate binding which is just as complete as that obtained if the antibodies are tested on parental B lymphocytes rather than F_1. Both of these findings indicate that the mechanism of inhibition is steric rather than direct, and that the Ia antigens must be found clustered together in small patches on the surface of the B lymphocyte such that antibodies against some of the antigens in the patch are capable of inhibiting aggregate binding to the entire patch. Steric inhibition would be possible both if the Ia antigens themselves function to bind the Fc portion of complexed immunoglobulin (i.e., identity between Ia antigens and the Fc receptor) or if the Ia antigens were clustered together in association with a separate molecule which serves Fc receptor function (i.e., close association). Recent cocapping studies tend to favor the latter interpretation (Basten *et al.*, 1975), but these studies are not yet conclusive. We have recently used this patch concept as the basis of an hypothesis concerning the possible function of Ia antigens in the immune response (Sachs and Dickler, 1975).

D. Other Methods

An additional method of distinguishing Ia reactivity from H-2 reactivity has been reported by Hauptfeld *et al.* (1975). The method is essentially that described by Cullen *et al.* (1973) to show serological independence of certain HL-A antigens. A lymphoid cell suspension was first treated with an antiserum detecting the products of one *H-2* region and then exposed to an anti-immunoglobulin reagent to induce resistance to further complement-mediated killing by the same reagent. The cells were then treated with antibodies to the products of a different H-2 region and assessed for an increase in complement-mediated lysis. The authors proposed that if a serum specificity expected to detect an Ia antigen can be shown to behave independently from known H-2K and H-2D region specific reagents in such an assay, it is then probably an Ia specificity. The method thus depends on the cell surface separability of the products of *H-2K*, *H-2D*, and *I* regions of the *H-2* complex. The general usefulness of this method may be limited by its requirement for reagents which, by other criteria, react with only K or D region products or only Ia antigens.

The role of Ia antigens in a variety of functional properties associated with the *I* region has been the subject of intensive investigation in a variety of laboratories. At least two cell factors capable of inducing B cells to produce antibody have been shown to be removed by anti-Ia antibodies (Taussig *et al.*, 1974; Armerding *et al.*, 1974). In addition, anti-Ia antibodies have been demonstrated to specifically inhibit stimulator cells in the MLC reaction, presumably because the Ia antigens are a major source of MLC stimulation (Meo *et al.*, 1975; Schwartz *et al.*, 1976). Obviously as these systems become better understood and as the differences in effect between anti-Ia antibodies and antibodies to H-2K and H-2D region antigens are documented, the functional assays will themselves provide new correlative criteria for the presence of anti-Ia activity in alloantisera.

V. EXTENT OF THE POLYMORPHISM

It should be clear from the preceding four sections that the field of Ia antigens is a new and rapidly developing one. New specificities and even new subregions continue to be described, and it is clear that mistakes will be made and that changes in present tables will probably be necessary. Thus any review at the present time is bound to be incomplete in the near future.

How incomplete the present description will be, however, is to some extent a function of the extent of polymorphism of the Ia antigens, and I would therefore like to conclude with two sets of experimental studies from which some predictions about the extent of the Ia polymorphism can be made. The two aspects of polymorphism I would like to address are, first, an estimate of the number of subregions of the I region which one may expect to define by further recombinant strains, and, second, the degree of polymorphism at each subregion, that is, the number of different alleles which one may expect to define.

A. Number of Subregions

The first chemical isolation studies of Ia antigens employed antisera which detected antigens determined by different I subregions. Cullen *et al.* (1974) reported SDS gel patterns of an antigen preparation from B10.HTT tested in a sequential precipitation analysis with normal serum, A.TH anti-A.TL antiserum, and A.TL anti-A.TH antiserum. Since the B10.HTT appears to represent an H-2 haplotype in which a recombinant event has led to I-A and I-B subregions of H-2^s origin (like the A.TH) and an I-C subregion of H-2^k origin (like the A.TL), this analysis was a means of assessing the dependence or independence of precipitation of Ia antigens encoded by these different I subregions. The series of steps employed in a sequential precipitation analysis is indicated in Table V. Studies on the B10.HTT indicated that the I-A and I-C subregion antigens were found on independently precipitable molecules.

Similarly, Sachs *et al.* (1975a) showed that two Ia antigens present in the recombinant strain B10.A(5R) precipitated independently in a sequential precipitation analysis. In this case, one of the antigens was Ia.9, which is an Ia antigen of the I^b haplotype which has been mapped serologically to the I-A subregion and the other was Ia.7, which has been mapped serologically to the I-C subregion. Thus, in both of these analyses, Ia antigens encoded by different I

Table V. Steps in the Sequential Precipitation Analysis

1. Labeled antigen prepared as in Table III
2. Antigen mixed with each antiserum or normal serum being compared
3. Precipitation induced with goat anti-mouse Ig
4. Supernatant saved for second precipitation step
5. Aliquots of each supernatant mixed with each antiserum or normal serum being compared
6. Precipitation induced with goat anti-mouse Ig
7. Precipitates dissolved and assayed as in Table III

subregions were found to be precipitable on different molecules, as might be expected if these antigens were the products of different genes.

If the number of genes in the I region determining Ia antigens were very large, then the definition of subregion might depend to a large extent on the number of recombinants available capable of separating certain of the Ia specificities serologically, and would continue to increase as further recombinants are found. In such a case, it would be unlikely for two Ia specificities to coprecipitate on the same molecule even if they happened to map to the same I subregion with the recombinant strains presently available. On the other hand, if the number of genes determining Ia antigens were not very large, one might expect that different antigenic specificities might be found which would coprecipitate on the same molecule, as has been described for individual H-2K region and H-2D region specificities (Cullen and Nathenson, 1971). It was thus of interest ot examine combinations of Ia specificities which mapped in the same subregion by a similar sequential precipitation analysis.

Cullen *et al.* (1975b) performed such an analysis for several Ia specificities mapping within the *I-A* subregion. An example of the results obtained, using reagents detecting Ia.8 and Ia.9, is shown in Fig. 8. In contrast to the results previously obtained when specificities mapping in different subregions were assessed, both of the Ia reagents tested in this analysis were found to cause complete coprecipitation of the alternate specificity. Thus, as seen in Fig. 8, preprecipitation of a B10 antigen preparation with anti-Ia.8 produced a failure to detect Ia.8 and Ia.9 in the supernatant, and preprecipitation with anti-Ia.9 caused failure to detect further Ia.9 or Ia.8. The independence of H-2.33, an H-2K region private specificity of B10 detected by only one of the antisera, serves as an internal control on the sequential precipitation method and is also a nice example of the independence of these cell surface products.

Very similar results were obtained for specificities Ia.8 and Ia.11 on an antigen preparation from the strain B10.D2. As seen from Fig. 2, these two Ia specificities have also been mapped to the *I-A* subregion. Thus, for two separate sets of I-A subregion specificities, coprecipitation was found, in contrast to the independent precipitation obtained for specificities mapping in different sub-

TEST ANTISERA

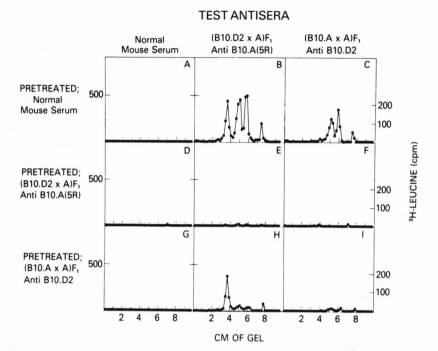

Figure 8. Sequential precipitation analysis on a B10 spleen cell antigen preparation. The three sera used were (1) normal mouse serum; (2) (B10.D2 X A)F$_1$ anti-B10.A(5R), which detects Ia.9 and H-2.33 when tested on B10; and (3) (B10.A X A)F$_1$ anti-B10.D2, which detects Ia.8 when tested on B10. After initial precipitation with each reagent (shown on left side of figure), the supernatants were subjected to a second precipitation with each reagent (shown on top of figure as "test antisera"). It is clear from the results that anti-Ia.8 clears for both Ia.8 and Ia.9 and that anti-Ia.9 similarly clears for both antigens. As expected, the anti-Ia.8 reagent does not clear for H-2.33 since this is present on a different molecule.

regions. The simplest interpretation of these results appears to us to be that antigens determined by the same subregion (at least for the *I-A* subregion) are carried on the same molecule. If this were not the case, the chances seem small that the first two sets of specificities in the same subregion which we examined would have been coprecipitated. These results leave open the possibility, however, that the products of the *I-A* subregion may be associated at the stage of precipitation with anti-Ia reagents, but that they are really on separate molecules. For this reason, a similar set of coprecipitation studies were carried out on an antigen preparation from an F$_1$ between *H-2*[b] and *H-2*[d] haplotypes, the (B10 X DBA/2)F$_1$. In this case, antigens Ia.8 and Ia.11 are encoded by one parental genome and Ia.8 and Ia.9 are encoded by the other. Cullen *et al.* (1975b) found in this case that anti-Ia.11 did not remove all of the Ia.9 from the preparation, nor did anti-Ia.9 remove all of the Ia.11. Thus association of I-A subregion molecules at the stage of precipitation cannot be the whole explanation for the coprecipitation of I-A subregion specificities obtained in the case of homozygotes. Because the Ia molecules are complex (multiple peaks), even this study of the F_1 antigen does not rule out the possibility that different I-A subregion specificities may be carried on different polypeptide chains which are associated in the same molecule. However, these studies do suggest that the number of genes coding for Ia antigens is probably much smaller than the number of Ia specificities which have so far been identified. They indicate, therefore, that the number of subregions (? Ia genes) may not be as great as would have been suggested by the serological analysis alone.

B. Number of Alternative Serological Specificities

The weight of present biochemical evidence indicates that the antigenic specificities of both H-2 and Ia antigens are determined by the primary sequence of the protein portion of these molecules (Nathenson and Cullen, 1974; Cullen et al., 1975a). Since single amino acid substitutions are known in many instances to be detectable serologically, the maximum degree of polymorphism of a polypeptide antigen theoretically possible is given by n^{20}, where n is the number of amino acids making up the polypeptide portion of the molecule. Clearly, for molecules such as H-2 and Ia antigens, this theoretical maximum is astronomical. However, the functional properties of any cell surface constituent will obviously place major restraints on possible amino acid substitutions, since only amino acid substitutions which will not destroy that function can be permitted. One of the distinguishing characteristics of MHC antigens as opposed to most other protein systems is the high degree of polymorphism which is tolerated. This has in fact led to the speculation that the polymorphism itself may constitute one of the functions of the MHC antigens. In any case, it is clear that the number of antigens detectable in both the H-2 and the Ia systems is very large and will continue to expand as presently defined specificities are further subdivided by absorption with new strains.

In this regard, it is conceptually important that analyses of the H-2K and H-2D region antigens by transplantation and serology indicate that certain haplotypes have been found in an indistinguishable form in multiple strains which have been inbred separately for at least 100 generations. For example, the strains C3H, CBA, AKR, and C57BR have all been determined to have the $H-2^k$ haplotype (Snell and Stimpfling, 1966). It remains possible that these strains had a common origin more than 60 years ago. However, the fact that the H-2 antigens of these haplotypes have remained indistinguishable indicates that, despite the high degree of polymorphism of the K and D region antigens, the system is not so subject to genetic drift as to permit major serological alterations during the hundreds of generations that the strains are known to have been apart.

Since the Ia antigens were not included in the serological typing which indicated that these strains bore the same *H-2* haplotype, it would appear possible that Ia antigenic differences might be found between strains which otherwise have been thought to share the same *H-2* haplotypes. Thus, although we can not at present assess the full degree of polymorphism of either the H-2 or the Ia antigens, it would seem possible to assess relative susceptibility to genetic drift of these two systems by determining whether or not Ia antigenic differences can be discerned between strains previously determined to share the same H-2K region and H-2D region specificities. To this end, we have absorbed a B10.D2 (*H-2^d*) anti-B.10.BR (*H-2^k*) antiserum sequentially with increasing numbers of lymphoid cells of four different *H-2^k* strains. The results are illustrated in Fig. 9. Unlike the results shown in Fig. 6, in which absorption of this same antiserum with a tumor cell lacking Ia antigens was performed, all of these absorptions led to clearing of cytotoxic activity against B10.BR from this serum.

Similar results were obtained for the reciprocal antiserum, B10.BR (*H-2^k*) anti-B10.D2 (*H-2^d*), absorbed with B10.D2, DBA/2, or BALB/c, all *H-2^d* strains. If B10.BR and B10.D2 differed by Ia antigens which were not shared by the other strains used for absorption, one might have expected that anti-Ia activity

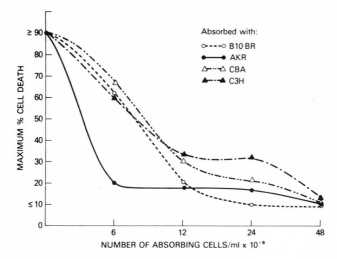

Figure 9. Quantitative absorptions. Cytotoxicity on B10.BR targets of B10.D2 anti-B10.BR. It is clear from the cytotoxicity absorption curves that all four H-2^k spleen cell preparations were capable of clearing cytotoxic activity toward B10.BR target cells. While this indicates no major qualitative differences in the Ia antigens present on the cells from different strains, the differences in shape among the absorption curves may indicate minor quantitative differences between antigens present in the different strains. This may indicate a small amount of genetic drift (Klein *et al.*, 1974a).

would have remained in the absorbed antisera, as was seen in Fig. 6. Of course, it is possible that not all Ia antigens are equally immunogenic to different hosts. If differences in Ia antigens did exist among strains of the same *H-2* haplotypes but no corresponding antibodies were present in the sera which we absorbed, this experiment would have failed to detect such differences. However, within these experimental limitations it would appear from these results that the susceptibility to polymorphism of the Ia antigens is at least no greater than that of the H-2K and H-2D region antigens.

Both of these experimental methods of assessing the extent of polymorphism of the Ia antigen system provide us with encouragement that the system is not hopelessly complex and that the polymorphism will be amenable to further definition by presently available methods. On the other hand, a great deal more effort and perhaps some new techniques will be needed before the structural and functional basis of this polymorphism is fully understood.

VI. SUMMARY

The Ia antigens constitute a polymorphic series of cell surface determinants. At present, their definition is mainly a genetic one, and thus any cell surface antigen which can be demonstrated to be encoded by a gene in the *Ir* region of the *H-2* complex may be classified as an Ia antigen. There are presently three subregions of the *I* region defined on the basis of available recombinant haplotypes, and designated at *I-A, I-B,* and *I-C.* Mapping of individual Ia specificities indicates that numerous specificities are determined by genes in the *I-A* subregion, several in the *I-C* subregion, and few, if any, in the *I-B* subregion. This may be a reflection of the state of the art, however, rather than an accurate assessment of the extent of polymorphism.

The Ia antigens appear to be expressed preferentially on the B-cell subpopulation of lymphoid cells. However, with the use of sensitive techniques they have also been demonstrated on some T cells, on macrophages, on sperm cells, and on epidermal cells. The Ia antigens have also been demonstrated on several T-cell factors which appear to be involved in the immune response. Whether or not all of the Ia antigens thus localized are identical or represent overlapping specificities within the same sera remains in many cases to be determined.

There are presently three ways of defining Ia specificities serologically: (1) by direct immunization between strains differing only in the *I* region; (2) by detection of shared Ia determinants using polyspecific sera which contain H-2K region and H-2D region antibodies but which are nevertheless specific only for Ia antigens when tested on target cells of other strains; and (3) by selective absorption of H-2K region and H-2D region antibodies from an H-2 antiserum by cells bearing these antigens but lacking (or relatively lacking) Ia antigens. All three of these methods produce anti-Ia reagents of reasonable titer for use in both serological and functional experimentation. The definition of the specificity as an Ia specificity in each case requires the availability of appropriate recombinant strains to map the specificity to the *I* region.

In addition, there are several correlative criteria which have been developed in order to detect Ia activity in alloantisera in the absence of the availability of appropriate recombinants for mapping of the specificity. These include the tissue distribution of the Ia antigens (namely, their predominant expression on the B-cell subpopulation), their characteristics molecular size, their association on the B-cell surface with the Fc receptor, and their lack of association with other products of the major histocompatibility complex as distinguished either chemically or by cocapping studies. These correlative criteria make it possible to distinguish probable anti-Ia reactivity in a variety of serological reactions, but the results must still be interpreted with caution until appropriate recombinants have been obtained which can map the specificities to the *I* region.

The Ia antigens have already been implicated in a variety of functional properties associated with the *I* region of the MHC, including T cell–B cell interactions in the immune response. If, in fact, the Ia antigens are responsible for the T cell–B cell interaction leading to immune responses, then defects in such interactions might indeed lead to the failure of particular immune responses. Such failures would constitute, by definition, "*Ir* genes." Since the cell surface products responsible for such failures would thus map in the *I* region, the Ia antigens themselves may explain the existence of an *Ir* region in the MHC. It is clear that the functional properties of Ia antigens will provide exciting avenues of research in the next few years. It is hoped that an understanding of the genetic and serological aspects of the Ia antigens described in this chapter may help to clarify interpretations of such functional properties.

VII. REFERENCES

Arbeit, R.D., Sachs, D.H., Amos, D.B., and Dickler, H.B., 1975, *J. Immunol.* **115**:1173.
Armerding, D., Sachs, D.H., and Katz, D.H., 1974, *J. Exp. Med.* **140**:1717.
Bach, F.H., 1973, *Transplant. Proc.* **5**:23.
Bailey, D.W., and Mobraaten, L.E., 1969, *Transplantation* **7**:394.
Basten, A., Miller, J.F.A.P., Sprent, J., and Pye, J., 1972, *J. Exp. Med.* **135**:610.
Basten, A., Miller, J.F.A.P., Abraham, R., Gamble, J., and Chia, E., 1975, *Int. Arch. Allergy Immunol.* **50**:309.
Berken, A., and Benacerraf, B., 1966, *J. Exp. Med.* **123**:119.
Columbani, J., Columbani, M., Shreffler, D.C., and David, C.S., 1976, *Tissue Antigens* **7**:74.
Cullen, S.E., and Nathenson, S.G., 1971, *J. Immunol.* **107**:563.
Cullen S.E., Bernoco, D., Carbonara, A.O., Jacot-Guillarmed, H., Trinchieri, G., and Cepellini, R., 1973, *Transplant. Proc.* **5**:1835.

Cullen, S.E., David, C.S., Shreffler, D.C., and Nathenson, S.G., 1974, *Proc. Natl. Acad. Sci. USA* **71**:648.

Cullen, S.E., Freed, J.H., Atkinson, P.H., and Nathenson, S.G., 1975a, *Transplant. Proc.* **7**:237.

Cullen, S.E., David, C.S., Cone, J., and Sachs, D.H., 1975b, *J. Immunol.* **116**:549.

David, C.S., 1975, *Mouse News Letter* **53**:17.

David, C.S., and Shreffler, D.C., 1974, *Transplantation* **18**:313.

David, C.S., Shreffler, D.C., and Frelinger, J.A., 1973, *Proc. Natl. Acad. Sci. USA* **70**:2509.

David, C.S., Frelinger, J.A., and Shreffler, D.C., 1974, *Transplantation* **17**:122.

David, C.S., Meo, T., McCormick, J., and Shreffler, D., 1976, *J. Exp. Med.* **143**:218.

David, C.S., Sachs, D.H., Cullen, S.E. and Shreffler, D.C., 1976 (in preparation).

Davies, D.A.L., and Hess, M., 1974, *Nature (London)* **250**:228.

Delovitch, T.L., and McDevitt, H.L., 1975, *Immunogenetics* **2**:39.

Dickler, H.B., and Kunkel, H.G., 1972, *J. Exp. Med.* **138**:191.

Dickler, H.B., and Sachs, D.H., 1974, *J. Exp. Med.* **140**:779.

Dickler, H.B., Cone, J.L., Kubicek, M.T., and Sachs, D.H., 1975a, *J. Exp. Med.* **142**:796.

Dickler, H.B., Arbeit, R.D., and Sachs, D.H., 1975b, in: *Membrane Receptors of Lymphocytes* (M. Seligmann, ed.), p. 259, North-Holland, Amsterdam.

Fathman, C.G., Handwerger, B.S., and Sachs, D.H., 1974, *J. Exp. Med.* **140**:853.

Fathman, C.G., Cone, J.L., Sharrow, S.O., Tyrer, H., and Sachs, D.H., 1975, *J. Immunol.* **115**:584.

Ferrone, S., Pellegrino, M.A., and Reisfeld, R.A., 1975, in: *The Antigens*, Vol. III (M. Sela, ed.), p. 362, Academic Press, New York.

Goding, J.W., White, E., and Marchalonis, J.J., 1975, *Nature* **257**:230.

Götze, D., Reisfeld, R.A., and Klein, J.J., 1973, *J. Exp. Med.* **138**:1003.

Hämmerling, G.J., Deak, B.D., Mauve, G., Hammerling, U., and McDevitt, H.L., 1974, *Immunogenetics* **1**:68.

Hämmerling, G., Mauve, G., Goldberg, E., and McDevitt, H.L., 1975, *Immunogenetics* **1**:428.

Handwerger, B.S., and Schwartz, R.H., 1975, *Transplantation* **18**:545.

Hauptfeld, M., Hauptfeld, V., and Klein, J., 1975, *J. Immunol.* **115**:351.

Hauptfeld, V., Klein, D., and Klein, J., 1973, *Science* **181**:167.

Hauptfeld, V., Hauptfeld, M., and Klein, J., 1974, *J. Immunol.* **113**:181.

Hayman, J.J., and Crumpton, J.M., 1972, *Biochem Biophys. Res. Commun.* **47**:923.

Herberman, R., and Stetson, C.A., 1965, *J. Exp. Med.* **121**:533.

Jones, E.A., Goodfellow, P.N., Bodmer, J.G., and Bodmer, W.F., 1975, *Nature (London)* **256**:650.

Julius, M.H., Simpson, E., and Herzenberg, L.A., 1973, *Eur. J. Immunol.* **3**:645.

Klein, J., 1970, *Genetics* **64**:s35.

Klein, J., 1975, *Biology of the Mouse Histocompatibility-2 Complex*, Springer-Verlag, New York.

Klein, J., Hauptfeld, M. and Hauptfeld, V., 1974a, *J. Exp. Med.* **140**:1127.

Klein, J., Hauptfeld, M., and Hauptfeld, V., 1974b, *Immunogenetics* **1**:45.

Krammer, P.H., and Pernis, B., 1975, *Scand. J. Immunol.* (in press).

Lieberman, R., Paul, W. E., Humphrey, W., and Stimpfling, J.H., 1972. *J. Exp. Med.* **136**:1231.

Lilly, F., Graham, H., and Coley, R., 1973, *Transplant. Proc.* **5**:193.

Lozner, E.C., Sachs, D.H., Shearer, G.M., and Terry, W.D., 1974, *Science* **183**:757.

Mann, D.L., Abelson, L., Harris, S., and Amos, D.B., 1975, *J. Exp. Med.* **142**:84.

McDevitt, H.O., and Benacerraf, B., 1969, *Adv. Immunol.* **11**:31.

McDevitt, H.O., Deak, B.D., Shreffler, D.C., Klein, J., Stimpfling, J.H., and Snell, G.D., 1972, *J. Exp. Med.* **135**:1259.

McKenzie, I.F.C., 1975, *Immunogenetics* **1**:511.

McKenzie, I.F.C., and Snell, G.D., 1975, *J. Immunol.* **114**:848.

Meo, T., David, C.S., Rijnbeek, A.M., Nabholz, M., Miggiano, B.C., and Shreffler, D.C., 1975, *Transplant. Proc.* **7**:127.

Nathenson, S.G., and Cullen, S.E., 1974, *Biochim. Biophys. Acta* **334**:1.

Sachs, D.H., 1976, in: *The Role of the Histocompatibility Gene Complex in Immune Responses* (Katz and Benacerraf, eds.), p. 731, Academic Press, New York.

Sachs, D.H., and Cone, J.L., 1973, *J. Exp. Med.* **138**:1289.

Sachs, D.H., and Cone, J.L., 1975, *J. Immunol.* **114**:165.

Sachs, D.H., and Dickler, H.B., 1975, *Transplant. Rev.* **23**:159.

Sachs, D.H., Cullen, S.E., and David, C.S., 1975a, *Transplantation* **19**:388.

Sachs, D.H., David, C.S., Shreffler, D.C., Nathenson, S.G., and McDevitt, H.O., 1975, *Immunogenetics* **2**:301.

Schirrmacher, V., Halloran, P., and David, C.S., 1975, *J. Exp. Med.* **141**:1201.

Schwartz, B.D., and Nathenson, S.G., 1971, *J. Immunol.* **107**:1363.

Schwartz, R.H., Fathman, C.G., and Sachs, D.H., 1976, *J. Immunol.* **116**:929.

Shreffler, D.C., and David, C.S., 1972, *Tissue Antigens* **2**:232.

Shreffler, D.C., and David, C.S., 1975, *Adv. Immunol.* **20**:125.

Shreffler, D.C., and Passmore, H.C., 1971, *Immunogenetics of the H-2 System*, p. 58, Karger, Basel.

Shreffler, D., David, C., Gotze, D., Klein, J., McDevitt, H., and Sachs, D., 1974, *Immunogenetics* **1**:189.

Shreffler, D.C., Meo, T. and David, C.S. 1976a, in: *The Role of the Histocompatibility Gene Complex in Immune Responses* (Katz and Benacerraf, eds.), p. 3, Academic Press, New York.

Shreffler, D.C., David, C.S., Cullen, S.E., Neiderhuber, J.E. and Frelinger, J.A., 1976b, in: *Origins of Lymphocyte Diversity* (XLI Cold Spring Harbor Symposium on Quantitative Biology), Cold Spring Harbor Laboratory, New York.

Silver, J., Sibley, C., Morand, P., and Hood, L., 1975, *Transplant. Proc.* **7**:201.

Snell, G.D., and Bunker, H.P., 1965, *Transplantation* **3**:235.

Snell, G.D., and Stimpfling, J.H., 1966, in: *Biology of the Laboratory Mouse* (E. Green, ed.), p. 457, McGraw-Hill, New York.

Staines, N.A., Guy, K., and Davies, D.A.L., 1974, *Transplantation* **18**:192.

Stimpfling, J.H., and Reichert, A.E., 1970, *Transplant Proc.* **2**:39.

Takemori, T., and Tada, T. 1975, *J. Exp. Med.* **142**:1241.

Taussig, M.J., Mozes, E., and Isac, R., 1974, *J. Exp. Med.* **140**:301.

van Rood, J. J., van Hooff, J.P., and Keuning, J.J., 1975, *Transplant. Rev.* **22**:75.

Vitetta, E.S., Klein, J., and Uhr, J.W., 1974, *Immunogenetics* **1**:82.

Winchester, R.J., Fu, S.M., Wernet, P., Kunkel, H.G., Dupont, B., and Jersild, C., 1975, *J. Exp. Med.* **141**:924.

Preliminary Amino Acid Sequences of Transplantation Antigens: Genetic and Evolutionary Implications

J. Silver and L. Hood

Division of Biology
California Institute of Technology
Pasadena, California

I. INTRODUCTION

The major histocompatibility complex of the mouse (H-2 complex) is a multigenic chromosomal region which was originally defined on the basis of eliciting rapid graft rejection (Gorer, 1937; Amos *et al.*, 1955). Individuals that differ solely at this region rapidly reject tumor and skin grafts from one another (Counce *et al.*, 1956). More recently, the major histocompatibility complex has occupied a central role in modern immunological research because of the variety of important immunologically related functions coded by this region (Shreffler and David, 1975; Klein, 1976). These include (1) genes determining specific immune responsiveness to a wide variety of antigens (the Ir genes) (Benacerraf and McDevitt, 1972; McDevitt *et al.*, 1974a), (2) genes regulating T lymphocyte-B lymphocyte interactions that lead to specific immune responses (Katz *et al.*, 1975), and (3) genes controlling the levels and/or structures of complement components (Goldman and Goldman, 1975). In addition, susceptibility to viral carcinogenesis also maps in this region (Lilly and Pincus, 1973).

Apart from those associated with the complement system, the gene products coded by the H-2 complex appear to be hydrophobic cell surface proteins including the classical major transplantation antigens (H-2K and H-2D molecules) and the I-region-associated (Ia) antigens (David *et al.*, 1973; Götze *et al.*, 1973; Hämmerling *et al.*, 1974; Hauptfeld *et al.*, 1973; Sachs and Cone, 1973). In the past few years, techniques have been developed for the isolation of these cell surface polypeptides (Cullen *et al.*, 1974; McDevitt *et al.*, 1974b; Vitetta *et al.*, 1974; Silver *et al.*, 1975). Even more recently, microsequencing techniques have been developed which permit the analysis of subnanomole quantities of polypeptides (Schecter, 1973; Jacobs *et al.*, 1974; Silver and Hood, 1975). These microsequencing techniques have been employed on the *N*-terminus of the H-2K and H-2D antigens by four different laboratories (Ewenstein *et al.*, 1976; Henning *et al.*, 1976; Silver and Hood, 1976; Vitetta *et al.*, 1976). Comparable data on the classical transplantation antigens of man are also available (Terhorst *et al.*, 1976). These preliminary amino acid sequence data place important genetic and evolutionary constraints on our understanding of the H-2 complex, much as the initial immunoglobulin sequences placed constraints on our understanding of the "antibody problem" some 10 years ago (Hilschmann and Craig, 1965). For the mouse transplantation antigens, homology relationships are evident; the nature of amino acid differences among homologous gene products is becoming apparent; and, perhaps most important, provocative new hypotheses about the genetics and evolution of the genes coded by this complex and multigenic region are being raised (Silver and Hood, 1976).

We will review briefly the nature of the H-2 complex of the mouse, as well as methods for the chemical isolation and characterization of the H-2 gene products. (More detailed reviews on the biology, genetics, chemistry, and serology of the H-2 complex have been written by Nathenson and Cullen, 1974, Klein, 1975a, and Shreffler and David, 1975.) We will then discuss the genetic and evolutionary implications of the preliminary amino acid sequence data on the classical transplantation antigens. In some cases, our discussions will be somewhat speculative because of the very limited data available. In spite of this, we feel it important to raise clearly the intriguing genetic and evolutionary paradoxes these preliminary data pose. Finally, we will discuss briefly the possible evolutionary relationships among the H-2 molecules and other cell surface molecules coded by chromosome 17 of the mouse.

II. THE H-2 COMPLEX OF THE MOUSE

A. Genetics (Shreffler and David, 1975)

The H-2 complex is the most thoroughly analyzed major histocompatibility complex of those studied among vertebrates. It is located on chromosome 17 of the mouse and can be divided into four major regions, termed K, I, S, and D, marked by the *H-2K*, *Ir-1*, *Ss-Slp*, and *H-2D* genes, respectively (Fig. 1). The boundaries of each region are determined by intra-H-2 recombinations between these traits. Whenever two traits are clearly separated by a crossover and are unaltered by the recombination event, one can assume that the traits are controlled

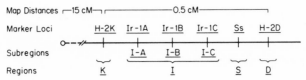

Figure 1. Fine structure genetic map for the H-2 gene complex of mouse chromosome 17. Map distances (centimorgans), marker loci, regions, and subregions are indicated. Circle represents the centromere. Adapted from McDevitt (1976).

by distinct genes. In a similar manner, the I region has been subdivided into at least three subregions, designated I-A, I-B, and I-C (Shreffler and David, 1975; Sachs *et al.*, 1975). Alternate genes at defined loci are termed *alleles*. A unique combination of alleles at the loci within the H-2 complex is termed a *haplotype*, denoted by H-2 with a letter superscript. Many different inbred strains of mice carry distinct haplotypes. The recombinational frequency between the *H-2K* and *H-2D* loci is 0.5 cM, enough DNA to code for up to 2000 polypeptides about 200 amino acids in length (Klein, 1975).

B. Function (Klein, 1975)

The various kinds of traits under control of the H-2 complex are listed in Table I. The K and D regions code for serologically detectable cell surface antigens which have classically been defined as the *transplantation antigens*. Although the function of these molecules is unknown, recent studies suggest that the K and D antigens may function in the discrimination of altered self antigens, e.g., in distinguishing normal cells from virally infected or hapten-modified cells (Zinkernagel and Doherty, 1974; Shearer, 1974). Accordingly, the K and D antigens may be signposts for immune surveillance. The S region includes genes determining the structures and/or levels of the first four components of complement (McDevitt, 1976; Goldman and Goldman, 1975). The I region contains the immune response genes that determine an individual's ability to respond to a variety of synthetic and natural antigens (Benacerraf and McDevitt, 1972; McDevitt *et al.*, 1974a). The I region also codes for cell surface (Ia) antigens which may act as transplantation antigens comparable to the K and D antigens (Shreffler and David, 1975; Klein, 1976) as well as for cell surface molecules that permit T and B cells to cooperate in the induction of specific immune responses (Munro and Taussig, 1975; Mozes, 1975).

One question is of paramount interest regarding the organization of genes in the H-2 complex. Namely, how many functional genes are coded by each of the regions and subregions of this complex? It is apparent that some of the traits in Table I may be ascribed to a single gene product [e.g., the K (or D) antigen is

Table I. Genetic Traits Controlled by the H-2 Complex[a]

Trait	Gene symbol	Controlling region
Cell surface antigens		
Serologically detected cellular antigens (all tissues)	*H-2K, H-2D*	K, D
I-region differentiation antigens	*Ia*	I
Biological assays		
Transplantation antigens	*H-2K, H-2D, H-2I*	K, I, D
Cell-mediated lympholysis target antigens	*H-2K, H-2D*	K, D
Hybrid resistance	*Hh*	K or D
Mixed leukocyte reaction	*Lad*	K, I, D
Graft vs. host reaction	*Lad*	K, I, D
Immune-related functions		
Tumor virus susceptibility	*Rgv-I*	K or I
Immune responses	*Ir-IA, Ir-IB*, etc.	I
T cell–B cell interactions	−	I
Complement levels	*Ss*	S

[a]Adapted from Shreffler and David (1975).

serologically detectable on all tissues, is a transplantation antigen, and does serve as a target for cell-mediated lympholysis]. Other traits appear to be coded by multiple genes (e.g., immune response genes). The genetic and serological evidence currently available is compatible with the supposition that the K and D antigens are each coded by a single gene. The sequences of transplantation antigens that we will discuss shortly raise some intriguing questions about this assumption. In contrast, more than 30 immune response genes have been described (Schreffler and David, 1975). Indeed, recombinational studies suggest that the I region encodes at least three distinct genes (Sachs *et al.*, 1975); it may contain many more. The S region appears to encode a variety of traits related to the complement system and may also constitute yet another multigenic family (gene cluster) (McDevitt, 1976). The structural analysis of these gene products will provide information as to the multiplicity of genes in each of these genetic regions.

C. Evolution (van Rood *et al.*, 1976)

The general structure and function of the major histocompatibility complex are remarkably similar in all mammals that have been studied to date (i.e., man, mouse, rhesus monkey, dog, and guinea pig) (Fig. 2). All of these animals have two or more serologically detectable (SD) antigens which mediate the transplantation rejection process and are presumably analogous to the K and D antigens of the mouse. All have a genetic region which elicits a strong mixed leukocyte reaction (MLR), presumably analogous to that elicited by the I region of the H-2 complex. Indeed, immune response genes have been mapped to the major histocompatibility complex in the guinea pig and rhesus monkey (Dorf *et al.*, 1974; Balner and Toth, 1973), and have been tentatively localized in man (Marsh *et al.*, 1973). Moreover, the human HL-A complex, the most thoroughly analyzed major histocompatibility complex apart from that of the mouse, codes for a properdin component on the alternative activation pathway of complement (Bf) (van Rood *et al.*, 1976). Furthermore, the structures and/or levels of complement components $C'2$, $C'4$, and $C'8$ appear to be encoded in or near the HL-A complex (van Rood *et al.*, 1976). A variety of diseases characterized by abnormal immune responses also appear to be associated with certain HL-A haplotypes (McDevitt and Bodmer, 1974, Möller, 1975). Accordingly, this constellation of traits encoded by the major histocompatibility locus appears to be highly conserved throughout mammalian evolution—fundamental testimony to the vital role this gene complex plays in a variety of immune-related functions in various mammalian lines.

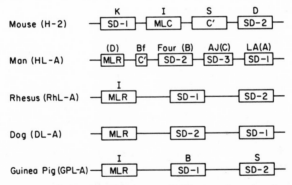

Figure 2. Genetic map of the major histocompatibility complex of various mammals. SD denotes the region coding for *serologically detectable* antigens (classical transplantation antigens). MLC denotes the region coding for antigens that evoke strong *mixed leukocyte reactions*. In some cases, immune response (I) genes appear to be coded in the MLC region. C' denotes the region coding for complement levels and/or components. For mouse, man, and guinea pig, the specific nomenclature of each region is given above the general designations. For man, the old and new (parentheses) nomenclature is given (van Rood *et al.*, 1976). Bf denotes the gene coding for a properdin component on the alternative pathway of complement activation. The precise linkage relationships of regions in the rhesus monkey, dog, and guinea pig MHC are uncertain. In the guinea pig, two SD genes have been deduced on the basis of chemical studies. Information for this figure was drawn from the following sources: mouse (Shreffler and David, 1975), man (van Rood *et al.*, 1976; Bach and van Rood, 1976), rhesus monkey (Bach and van Rood, 1976; Dorf *et al.*, 1974; Balner and Toth, 1973), dog (Bach and van Rood, 1976), and guinea pig (W. Paul, personal communication).

D. The K and D Transplantation Antigens

By appropriate genetic manipulation (described in the next section), mice can be bred which may be used for the preparation of antisera directed specifically against allelic alternatives of the K, I, S, and D gene products. These antisera fall into a category termed *alloantisera* and have been extremely useful in delineating the general properties of the K and D molecules (Klein, 1975). Three characteristics are of particular interest. First, the K and D gene products are found on almost all cells and tissues, although lymphoid cells appear to have a higher concentration of these molecules than most other tissues (Medawar, 1956/1957). This ubiquitous tissue distribution almost certainly reflects the functional role, as yet uncertain, of these widely distributed molecules. Second, most K and D gene products possess at least one unique, or *private*, antigenic specificity and multiple common, or *public*, antigenic specificities (Shreffler and David, 1975; Klein, 1975) (Table II). The cross-reactivity of certain of the public antigenic specificities among the K and D alleles suggests that they diverged from a common ancestral gene (Shreffler et al., 1971). Third, the K and D genes exhibit extensive genetic polymorphism. Among the standard inbred strains of mice there are 11 alleles at the K locus and ten alleles at the D locus (Klein, 1974), resulting in more than 25 chromosomal combinations, or haplotypes, of the K and D alleles (Shreffler and David, 1975). Moreover, when wild mice from different areas are examined, each small breeding unit has a new private K (and D) antigenic specificity distinct from all known private specificities and from those of mice in nearby breeding units (Klein, 1974). Given the worldwide distribution of mice, the potential polymorphism of the system is enormous. Presumably, the extensive polymorphism of the K and D genes in the mouse population reflects some fundamental functional requirement for extreme diversity among individuals of the mouse species.

The K and D molecules have the following general chemical properties (see Nathenson and Cullen, 1974): (1) They are hydrophobic glycoproteins about 45,000 daltons in molecular weight. (2) The antigenic specificities (public and

Table II. Private and Public Specificities for Selected K and D Gene Products[a]

Gene product	Private specificities	Public specificities																				
K^k	23	1	3	5		8	11		25											45		47	
K^b	33			5						27	28	29	35	36	39						46		
D^b	2				6					27	28	29											
D^d	4		3		6			13		27	28	29	35	36		41	42	43	44				49

[a]Taken from Klein (1975). Boxes indicate positions of homology.

private) appear to reside in the protein and not the carbohydrate portion of this molecule. (3) One-dimensional tryptic fingerprints on ion exchange columns demonstrate peptide differences of 80% between the K^d and D^d gene products and peptide differences of 60–70% between the D^d and D^k gene products. The earlier hypothesis of a common ancestral gene for the K and D transplantation antigens which was based on serological cross-reactivities is supported by these data. The differences in the peptide profiles of two D alleles suggest that these gene products differ from one another at multiple amino acid positions. These multiple residue differences have important genetic implications that will be discussed subsequently. (4) Mild proteolytic digestion of lymphocytes with papain releases a 37,000-dalton fragment that retains the antigenic activity of the native K or D gene product. The amino acid sequence analysis of the N-terminus of this enzymatic fragment is identical to that carried out on the intact detergent-solubilized fragment (Ewenstein et al., 1976; Henning et al., 1976), implying that the N-terminal portion of these molecules is exposed to the solvent whereas the C-terminal portion is embedded in the membrane (Fig. 3). Glycophorin, a cell surface protein of red blood cells, and membrane-bound immunoglobulins, perhaps the only other well-studied membrane proteins, have similar membrane orientations (Marchesi, 1975; Uhr, 1975). Thus membrane proteins may generally be fixed to membranes via their C-terminal regions with their N-terminal regions exposed to the solvent. (5) The K or D gene products are noncovalently associated with β_2-microglobulin on the cell surface (Silver and Hood, 1974). The β_2-microglobulin, a polypeptide of about 100 residues, shows significant homology with the constant-region homology units of immunoglobulins (Smithies and Poulik, 1972; Peterson et al., 1972). The association of the K and D gene products with a free immunoglobulinlike domain has been cited as support for the hypothesis that the immunoglobulin and H-2 genes were derived from a common ancestor (Strominger et al., 1974; Peterson et al., 1975). The 45,000 dalton K or D gene product has been designated the heavy (H) chain and the 12,000 dalton β_2-microglobulin has been designated the light (L) chain (Fig. 3). (6) On the cell surface, the K and D molecules and β_2-microglobulin are found as a H-L monomer (Henning et al., 1976) (Fig. 3).

A variety of interesting questions can be approached by the amino acid sequence analysis of the H-2K and H-2D gene products: (1) Are the K and D gene products homologous to one another? (2) Are the K and D gene products

Figure 3. A model of the K or D (H) gene product associated with β_2-microglobulin (L) on the cell surface.

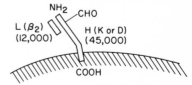

homologous to their LA and four counterparts from the major histocompatibility complex of man (see Fig. 2)? (3) Are the K and D gene products homologous to other gene products coded by the H-2 complex? (4) Are the K and D gene products homologous to those of other complex genetic loci such as the three immunoglobulin families? (5) Is there any special regional distribution of the private as opposed to public specificities (e.g., are private specificities localized in hypervariable regions or do the K and D gene products exhibit variable and constant regions similar to immunoglobulins)? (6) How is the extensive polymorphism of the K and D genes distributed throughout the corresponding polypeptides? Some of these questions have been answered in a tentative fashion by the preliminary amino acid sequence on the K and D molecules which will be discussed subsequently.

III. THE ISOLATION AND CHEMICAL CHARACTERIZATION OF H-2 MOLECULES

A. Overview

Three properties of the cell surface antigens coded by the H-2 complex dictate the types of approaches that can be employed in the isolation of these molecules: (1) they are hydrophobic glycoproteins, (2) they are intermingled with many other cell surface molecules, and (3) they are present in limited quantities even on those cells with the highest concentration of these molecules. The basic approach employed for the isolation of cell surface antigens has been to (1) radiolabel the cell surface molecules of lymphocytes (e.g., spleen cells), (2) dissolve lymphocytes and their membranes in a nonionic detergent, (3) precipitate the H-2 gene products with highly specific alloantisera, and (4) fractionate and isolate these molecules by molecular weight sieving in SDS polyacrylamide gels. Microsequencing techniques have been developed for subsequent chemical analysis of protein isolated by this method.

B. Preparation of Specific Alloantisera

The mouse offers several advantages for studying the biology and chemistry of the major histocompatibility complex. First, highly inbred strains are available and can readily be produced from outbred mice. Thus genetically identical individuals are available for the production of antisera, the preparation of H-2 gene products, and the numerous bioassays employed in the study of the H-2 complex (Table I). Second, strains that are recombinants at various points within the H-2 complex have permitted the delineation of the regions and subregions of the H-2 complex. Finally, strains of mice can be bred that are genetically identical except for one region of the H-2 complex. These strains are said to be *congenic*. Thus the H-2 complex of a B-strain mouse may be placed on an A-strain chromosomal background, resulting in a congenic strain designated A.B. Accordingly, when lymphocytes from the A.B strain are injected into A-strain mice, specific antibodies (alloantisera) are raised against the cell surface H-2 gene products of the B-strain mouse. This mode of analysis can be rendered even more precise by constructing congenic strains from mice with recombinant H-2 chromosomes. For example, congenic strain A.TH ($H-2^{t2}$) is an H-2 recombinant strain which was derived from two inbred strains carrying, respectively, the $H-2^a$ and $H-2^s$ haplotypes by a crossover event that occurred between the S and D regions (Fig. 4). Therefore, the A.TH strain carries the K, I, and S regions from the $H-2^s$ haplotype and the D region from the $H-2^a$ haplotype. Immunization of A.TH mice with A.SW lymphocytes would produce a specific antiserum only directed against the D-region gene products of the A.SW strain which are expressed on the lymphocyte cell surface. In this manner, specific antisera can be generated against each of the gene products coded by various regions and subregions of the H-2 complex.

Several precautions must be considered when defining the specificities of antisera produced in such a manner. First, the number of genes in the H-2 complex almost certainly exceeds the number of available genetic markers. This means that independently derived recombinants which appear identical by the limited number of genetic markers currently available may differ in genes for which no genetic markers are available. This is shown in Fig. 5a, where Y is a hypothetical gene located within the H-2 complex with no known genetic marker. Accordingly, the antiserum raised against the lymphocytes of one recombinant may have antibodies directed against cell surface molecules that are absent in a second apparently identical recombinant strain (Fig. 5a). Second, congenic strains may retain genes that are outside the H-2 complex, but closely linked to it, and for which there are no genetic markers. This is shown in Fig. 5b, where Z is such

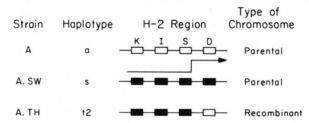

Figure 4. Schematic diagram of the H-2 complex of parental and recombinant strains. The A and A.SW strains are parental and the A.TH is a recombinant strain derived as indicated by the arrow.

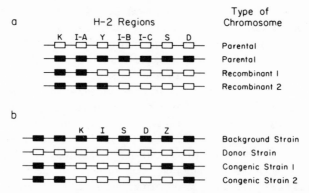

Figure 5. Schematic diagrams of hypothetical genes in or near the H-2 complex. (a) Two independent recombinant mice (1 and 2) that differ at a hypothetical gene (Y) within the H-2 complex. (b) Two congenic strains of mice (1 and 2) that differ at a hypothetical gene (Z) closely linked to the H-2 complex.

a hypothetical gene. Therefore, the use of lymphocytes from such a strain may result in antisera which are directed against the products of a non-H-2 gene.

C. Isolation of Cell Surface Molecules

The method routinely employed for the isolation of H-2-region cell surface products from spleen or tumor lymphocytes using specific antisera is termed *indirect immunoprecipitation* (Fig. 6) and is described below (Schwartz and Nathenson, 1971).

1. Radiolabeling Cell Surface Proteins

Because the products of the H-2 complex are present on the cell in minute quantities ($\leqslant 10^5$ molecules/cell), they are radiolabeled before isolation with either [^{3}H] amino acids or ^{125}I, which acts as an identification tag in the subsequent isolation and chemical characterizations. The ^{125}I-labeling of cell surface proteins on lymphocytes is catalyzed by lactoperoxidase and has the advantages of being rapid, convenient (since it requires little sample preparation), and very sensitive (because of the high specific activity of the label). Radioiodination is restricted primarily to tyrosine residues and therefore limits the types of chemical procedures that may be used in subsequent structural analysis. An alternative method for labeling cell surface proteins is the *in vitro* incubation of lymphocytes in the presence of [^{3}H] amino acids for 4–6 h. This procedure labels cell surface as well as internal proteins. However, it does require that the proteins of interest have a relatively high turnover rate in order to be efficiently labeled.

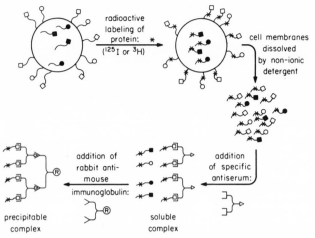

Figure 6. Schematic diagram for indirect immunoprecipitation (see text).

The major advantage of this procedure is that it permits a more detailed structural analysis of the H-2 proteins, since, in theory, every amino acid residue may be labeled.

2. Membrane Solubilization

The cell membrane and all of its constituent proteins are solubilized with a nonionic detergent (e.g., Triton X-100). The H-2 proteins retain their antigenicity in the solution and the detergent does not significantly interfere with the subsequent antigen–antibody precipitation reactions.

3. Immunoprecipitation

A mouse alloantiserum directed against the products of specific regions of the H-2 complex is added to the solution of radioactively labeled cell surface proteins. This permits the formation of soluble antigen–antibody complexes which may be precipitated by the addition of rabbit anti-mouse immunoglobulin (rabbit antibody directed against mouse antibody).

4. Molecular Weight Sieving

After extensive washing of the immunoprecipitate, the complexed radioactively labeled proteins are further purified by sodium dodecylsulfate (SDS) polyacrylamide gel electrophoresis. The radioactively labeled products of the H-2 complex may be eluted from the gels with approximately 90% yield. Protein

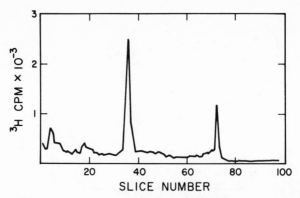

Figure 7. SDS-polyacrylamide gel electrophoresis pattern of the immunoprecipitate from B10.A (5R) spleen cells and alloantiserum D-4, which is directed against the D^d product. The larger peak (H-2D^d molecule) is approximately 45,000 daltons in molecular weight and the smaller peak (β_2-microglobulin) is about 12,000 daltons.

purified in this manner may now be subjected to a wide variety of chemical procedures, including microsequence analysis.

When specific alloantisera directed against different K (or D) alleles are employed in the above procedure, the SDS polyacrylamide pattern of the immunoprecipitate under reducing conditions yields two peaks, 45,000 and 12,000 daltons in molecular weight (Fig. 7). These two peaks are noncovalently associated since the low molecular weight component is isolated even in the absence of reducing agent. Indirect immunoprecipitation yields identical results when the LA and four gene products of the human HL-A complex are analyzed by similar techniques (Springer and Strominger, 1973). In the human system, the low molecular weight component has been identified serologically as β_2-microglobulin, a molecule which is homologous to the heavy-chain constant-region domains of immunoglobulins (Peterson *et al.*, 1972). In the mouse, both of these components have been subjected to microsequence analysis.

D. Microsequence Analysis

A mouse spleen has approximately 10^8 cells. A spleen lymphocyte may have as many as 5×10^5 K and D molecules on its cell surface (Hämmerling and Eggers, 1970). Accordingly, a single spleen should theoretically yield 5×10^{13} molecules or about 100 pmol of K or D gene product. This estimate is high because the yield will not be 100%, nor are all the cells in the spleen lymphocytes. Conventional amino acid sequence analysis on the automated sequenator employs 100–800 nmol of sample. Since we are dealing with 1000 times less material, the need to employ microsequencing techniques is obvious.

The microsequencing technique we employ is diagrammed in Fig. 8. Spleens from individual mice are removed and the cells are cultured *in vitro* for 4-6 h with groups of tritiated amino acids. The K and D gene products and β_2-microglobulin are isolated by indirect immunoprecipitation, eluted from SDS polyacrylamide gels, and concentrated and sequenced in the presence of carrier ovalbumin (which has a blocked *N*-terminal group) as previously described (Silver and Hood, 1975). The tritiated phenylthiohydantoin (PTH) amino acid residues are resolved by thin-layer chromatography in the presence of the appropriate unlabeled PTH-amino acids and counted.

The sequence data obtained for the β_2-microglobulin and one typical D gene product are presented in Fig. 9. The data display several characteristics typical of conventional automated sequence analysis. There is a gradually rising background due to random hydrolysis of the protein. Sequence residues are characterized by a sharp rise in radioactivity associated with a particular amino acid

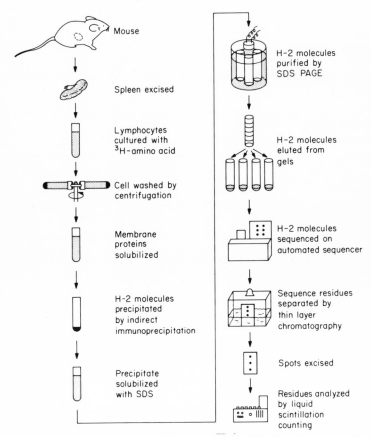

Figure 8. Schematic diagram of the procedures used for the microsequencing technique (see text).

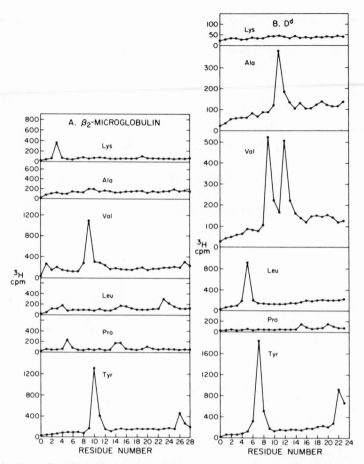

Figure 9. (A) Amino acid sequence data from the β_2-microglobulin of mouse. (B) Amino acid sequence data from the D^d gene product. The amount of radioactivity associated with each of the six incorporated amino acids is plotted against residue number (see text).

followed by a more gradual decline. The latter phenomenon, known as "lag," is the result of an incomplete Edman reaction and tends to increase throughout the run. We believe the amino acid residue present in lowest yield, lysine at position 19, is real in that three separate analyses of the β_2-microglobulin molecule have each given this residue with virtually no background noise in preceding or successive residues. Since each amino acid is incorporated to a different extent, the data for each amino acid must be treated independently. For those residues that appear two or more times (e.g., tyrosine, valine, proline), an average repetitive yield can be calculated. The repetitive yields for these three residues ranged between 89 and 94%, which is similar to the repetitive yields obtained from conventional runs. Furthermore, these high repetitive yields suggest that a single major component is being sequenced. We should be able to detect a 10-20% minor contaminant. Obviously, this statement is qualified by our inability to detect polypeptides with a blocked N-terminus or heterogeneity in residues that were not labeled.

Let us now consider the genetic and evolutionary implications of the partial amino acid sequence data that have been obtained on gene products coded by the major histocompatibility locus of mouse and man.

IV. N-TERMINAL AMINO ACID SEQUENCES OF THE TRANSPLANTATION ANTIGENS

A. The Light Chain (12,000 Daltons): Mouse β_2-Microglobulin

The partial sequence of the 12,000-dalton component of mouse is compared to the known sequences of β_2-microglobulins isolated in large quantities from the urine of other species in Fig. 10. The dashes, as well as the identified residues in the mouse H-2-associated polypeptide, represent important data. Since only six amino acids were labeled (alanine, leucine, lysine, proline, tyrosine, and valine), a dash indicates that the corresponding residue is *not* one of the six labeled residues. Residue positions represented by dashes have information and can be used in homology comparisons. For example, at position 1 the mouse H-2-associated polypeptide is *not* valine, and hence it is distinct from its rabbit counterpart at this position even though we cannot make a positive identification of the mouse residue at this position.

All 11 residues that we were able to identify are identical to residues at homologous positions in the known sequences of other β_2-microglobulin molecules (Fig. 10). This extensive homology demonstrates unequivocally that the small polypeptide associated with the 45,000 molecular weight components is the mouse β_2-microglobulin. More important, the analysis of this partial amino acid sequence at the level of 100 pmol or less demonstrates the feasibility and reliability of extending these microsequencing methods to the analysis of other cell surface molecules available in limited quantities.

B. The Heavy Chain (45,000 Daltons): An H-2K or H-2D Gene Product

The heavy chain can no longer react with specific alloantisera after isolation from SDS polyacrylamide gels, presumably because the SDS has denatured the polypeptide. However, three lines of evidence convince us that this component

	1	2	3	4	5	6	7	8	9	10
Human	Ile	Gln	Arg	Thr	Pro	Lys	Ile	Gln	Val	Tyr
Dog	Val	Gln	His	Pro	Pro	Lys	Ile	Gln	Val	Tyr
Rabbit	Val	Gln	Arg	Ala	Pro	Asn	Val	Gln	Val	Tyr
H-2 associated polypeptide	-	-	Lys	-	Pro	-	-	-	Val	Tyr

	11	12	13	14	15	16	17	18	19	20
Human	Ser	Arg	His	Pro	Ala	Glu	Asn	Gly	Lys	Ser
Dog	Ser	Arg	His	Pro	Ala	Glu	Asn	Gly	Lys	Pro
Rabbit	Ser	Arg	His	Pro	Ala	Glu	Asn	Gly	Lys	Asp
H-2 associated polypeptide	-	-	-	Pro	Pro	-	-	-	Lys	Pro

	21	22	23	24	25	26	27
Human	Asn	Phe	Leu	Asn	Cys	Tyr	Val
Dog	Asn	Phe	Leu	Asn	Cys	Tyr	Val
Rabbit	Asn	Phe	Leu	Asn	Cys	Tyr	Val
H-2 associated polypeptide	-	-	Leu	-	-	Tyr	Val

Figure 10. Partial amino acid sequences of β_2-microglobulins from man, dog, and rabbit compared with the H-2-associated (12,000 dalton) polypeptide of mouse. A dash indicates that no one of six labeled amino acids (alanine, leucine, lysine, proline, tyrosine, and valine) is present at that position. The rat β_2-microglobulin has lysine at position 3 and proline at position 15 (M. D. Poulik, C. Shinnick, and O. Smithies, personal communication). The lysine at position 3 in the mouse β_2-microglobulin has been confirmed by other investigators (B. T. Ballou, D. McKean, and O. Smithies, personal communication). Boxes indicate that the corresponding residues are identical to their mouse counterparts. The β_2-microglobulin sequences were obtained from the following sources: human (Cunningham et al., 1973), dog (Smithies and Poulik, 1972), and rabbit (Cunningham and Berggard, 1975).

is the K or D gene product. First, the papain fragment 37,000 daltons in molecular weight does retain the serological reactivity of the native molecule (Shimada and Nathenson, 1969). As previously mentioned, the N-terminal sequence of the papain fragment is identical to that of the SDS-purified component from the same cells (Henning et al., 1976; Ewenstein et al., 1976). If this serological activity is contained in a minor component, the component must cleave with papain in a fashion identical to the putative major non-H-2 component. We feel that this possibility is unlikely. Second, control indirect immunoprecipitation experiments using specific alloantisera and radioactively labeled lymphocytes that lack the corresponding H-2K or H-2D specificities yield very little [3H] protein in the 45,000 molecular weight range (Nathenson and Cullen, 1974; Silver et al., 1975). Thus very little radiolabeled protein in the 45,000 molecular weight range is isolated by this procedure unless the specific antigen is present in the immunoprecipitation mixture. Finally, it is possible that a small contaminant is being picked up by this procedure and sequenced by our sensitive techniques. This possibility is unlikely because each of the two K and two D gene products is different from all the rest. Therefore, if a contaminant is present, it must vary in accordance with the different allelic gene products. In addition, there is a remarkable degree of concordance obtained from four different laboratories which are sequencing the K and D gene products. Furthermore, the mouse and human transplantation antigens, isolated by completely different procedures, are homologous, as will be discussed subsequently. Thus the serological controls and the presence of amino acid sequence variability correlated with the differing alleles provide strong support for the supposition that the heavy (45,000 dalton) polypeptides are the H-2k or H-2D gene products.

C. The K and D Gene Products: Homologous to One Another and Probably Descended from a Common Ancestral Gene

The preliminary amino acid sequence results from four different laboratories on various K and D gene products are presented in Fig. 11 (Ewenstein *et al.*, 1976; Henning *et al.*, 1976; Silver and Hood, 1976; Vitetta *et al.*, 1976). Also given in Fig. 11 are data obtained from the LA and four gene products of the human HL-A system (Terhorst *et al.*, 1976). Two technical comments are in order. First, there is reasonable agreement among the laboratories on the sequences of the K and D gene products.* Since these laboratories are using similar microsequencing techniques, this provides added confidence in the microsequencing methodology. Second, the HL-A gene products were isolated from transformed human lymphoid lines which express 10-50 times more HL-A antigens than normal cells. These molecules were isolated in ⩾ 10 mg quantities and conventional amino acid sequence techniques were used.

Of the 12-16 residue positions that are identifiable in each K or D molecule (Fig. 11), six are identical in all four proteins (residues 6, 7, 8, 11, 12, 15). In addition, the K and D molecules share residues at several other positions (e.g., positions 1, 2, 3, 5, 9, 14, 17, 21, 22). Individual K and D molecules show 63-85% homology with one another over the positions that can be compared (Table III). Once again, a dash (in Fig. 11) indicates an unidentified amino acid that is different from those identified in other chains at that position. A blank

---

*A single sequence disagreement has been noted. A tentative proline at position 2 in the D^d gene product (Henning *et al.*, 1976) was not observed by us (Silver and Hood, 1976). There are two possible explanations for this negative discrepancy. This particular sample may have been lost at some stage of processing or different strains of mice with serologically identical alleles may have gene products that differ in sequence. This discrepancy stresses the need to be extremely conservative in interpreting the microsequence data as these techniques are actively in the process of being perfected.

Position

Position	1*	2*	3	4	5*	6	7	8	9*	10	11	12	13	14	15	16	17	18	19	20	21	22
Mouse transplantation antigens																						
K^k	Met	Pro	His		Leu	Arg	Tyr	Phe	His		Ala	Val	Ile		Pro		Leu	Lys		Pro	Phe	Ala
K^b	-	Pro	His		Leu	Arg	Tyr	Phe	Val		Ala	Val		Arg	Pro		Leu		-		Arg	Tyr
D^d	Met		His		Leu	Arg	Tyr	Phe	Val		Ala	Val		Arg	Pro		-		-	Pro		Tyr
D^b		Pro			-	Arg	Tyr		-		Ala	Val		Arg	Pro		Leu		-	Pro	Arg	Tyr
Human transplantation antigens																						
2	Gly	Ser		Ser	Met	Arg	Tyr	Phe	Thr	Ser	Val	Ser			Pro	Gly		Gly	Glu			
7, 12	Gly	Ser		Ser	Met	Val (Arg)	Tyr	Phe	Tyr	Thr	Ala	Val	Ser	Arg	(Pro)	Gly	(Pro)	Gly	Glu			

Figure 11. Partial *N*-terminal sequences of mouse and human transplantation antigens. An asterisk indicates species-associated residues. A dash indicates the *absence* of a particular residue found at that position in other mouse chains. The plus sign indicates that position 9 in the D^b molecule is *not* valine (histidine was not tested). A blank indicates that no sequence information is available at that position. Boxes around the mouse residues indicate positions of identity. Boxes around the human residues indicate identity with their mouse counterparts. Parentheses indicate an uncertainty in residue assignment. The 2 and 7, 12 specificities are gene products from the human four and LA regions, respectively. The 7 and 12 molecules could not be separated from one another and were sequenced as a mixture. See footnote in Section IVC for comment on a minor sequence discrepancy. The mouse data are taken from Ewenstein *et al.* (1976), Henning *et al.* (1976), Silver and Hood (1976), and Vitetta *et al.* (1976). The human data are from Terhorst *et al.* (1976).

Table III. Amino Acid Similarity Matrix
of Mouse Transplantation Antigens[a]

	K^k	K^b	D^d	D^b
K^k		63	63	64
K^b	10/16		79	85
D^d	10/16	11/14		69
D^b	9/14	11/13	9/13	

[a]In the lower (left) triangle, the first number indicates the number of identities and the second the number of residues that can be compared. In the upper (right) triangle, the percentage of identity is given.

indicates that no information is available on the residue at that position. These observations strongly support earlier suppositions that the K and D loci are homologous to one another and must have come from a common ancestral gene (Shreffler *et al.*, 1971; Klein and Shreffler, 1971; Brown *et al.*, 1974; Murphy and Shreffler, 1975).

D. The K and D Products of the H-2 Complex: Homologous to the LA and Four Gene Products of the HL-A Complex

The *N*-terminal sequences of the human transplantation antigens from the LA (2) and four (7 and 12) regions are also depicted in Fig. 11. The gene products from the four regions were isolated from a human cell line heterozygous (i.e., 7 and 12) at this locus. These allelic products could not be separated and were sequenced together as a mixture. One allelic product from the four locus (e.g., 7) differs from a second (e.g., 12) by a single valine–arginine interchange at position 7. The LA gene product has identical residues at 13/16 and 14/16 residues (81-88% homology) when compared with the two "four" gene products. Hence the four and LA gene products are homologous to one another and their corresponding genes must have descended from a common ancestral gene.

Of the 13 amino acid sequence residues that can be compared among the mouse H-2 and human HL-A gene products, four positions are identical (positions 7, 11, 12, and 15) and three positions share at least one residue (positions 6, 11, and 14) (Fig. 11). Thus the three human HL-A gene products demonstrate 44–67% homology with their mouse counterparts over those positions that can be compared. This homology strongly supports the supposition that the human and murine transplantation antigens have descended from a common ancestral gene. This indicates that the major histocompatibility complexes of the mouse and man are homologous to one another in structure and presumably should exhibit a similar spectrum of biological functions as well as employ similar genetic and evolutionary strategies.

E. The K and D Gene Products: Apparently Not Homologous to Immunoglobulins Based on Limited Sequence Comparisons

It has been proposed that the immunoglobulin gene families descended from the major transplantation complex. This postulated evolutionary relationship is based on several general features both systems share—their extreme polymorphism, their cell surface location, and their role in regulating the immune response (Bodmer, 1972; Gally and Edelman, 1972). In addition, the K and D gene products are noncovalently associated with β_2-microglobulin, a molecule homologous to the constant domains of immunoglobulins (see Smithies and Poulik, 1972), and preliminary structural studies have suggested the presence of immunoglobulinlike domains in the K and D molecules (Peterson et al., 1975). The limited sequence data presented in Fig. 11 show questionable, if any, sequence homology with the various immunoglobulin domains or the β_2-microglobulins.* There are a number of possible explanations for this apparent lack of homology: (1) The amino acid sequence data are insufficient to determine sequence homology. (2) The K and D genes are not evolutionarily related to immunoglobulin genes. (3) The N-terminal portions of the K and D molecules may be particularly variable, perhaps reflecting some important associated function; other portions of these molecules may show homologies with immunoglobulins. (4) The transplantation antigens did share a common ancestor with immunoglobulins; however, they have diverged sufficiently from immunoglobulins to mask any obvious sequence relationships. This is true of the V and C regions of immunoglobulins (Poljak et al., 1973). The association of the K and D products with an immunoglobulin-like molecule suggests that conformational homology may exist. Perhaps the contact residues between the two chains will be structurally homologous to their immunoglobulin counterparts from V_L and V_H domains. Indeed, the six contact residues for the V_L regions (positions 35, 37, 42, 43, 86, and 99) are strikingly conserved in all light chains as are their seven

*Vitetta and her co-workers feel that the K^k gene product shows limited homology (~ 20%) with immunoglobulins (Vitetta et al., 1976). This homology is obtained by placing two sequence gaps (insertions or deletions) in the homology comparisons—a procedure which raises statistical questions as to the validity of the homology produced because of the very limited regions examined and the diversity of the immunoglobulin homology units (see Needleman and Wunsch, 1970).

V_H region counterparts (positions 37, 39, 43, 45, 47, 95, and 108) (Poljak *et al.*, 1975). These postulated homologies can be tested by additional sequence data. Whatever the case may be, the data currently available do not reveal any striking homology relationship between the transplantation antigens and immunoglobulins at the level of primary amino acid sequence.

F. Exhibition of Species-Associated Residues by the H-2 and HL-A Transplantation Antigens

Both the K and D transplantation antigens exhibit common amino acid residues at certain positions which distinguish these polypeptides from the LA and four transplantation antigens of man. These are termed *species-associated* residues.* For example, at positions 1, 2, 5, and 9, two or three of the mouse transplantation antigens share residues that are different from those of the human transplantation antigens at the corresponding positions (Fig. 11).† In this regard, it will be important to examine additional human and mouse transplantation antigens, particularly some from wild mice, to verify the presence of extensive species-associated residues. However, the fact that four gene products from the mouse and three from two unrelated humans exhibit species-associated residues suggests to us that they will be found in most human and mouse transplantation antigens. Indeed, preliminary sequence data on a fifth mouse transplantation antigen (K^b) support the presence of species-associated residues at positions 2 and 5 (the other two positions were not examined) (Henning *et al.*, 1976).

The presence of species-associated residues for *both* the K and D gene products of the mouse on the one hand and the LA and four gene products of man on the other suggests that these two loci arose in the mouse and human evolutionary lines *after* their divergence (Fig. 12a). The alternative hypothesis, that gene duplication occurred in the common ancestor *before* speciation, as suggested by the observation that most vertebrate species analyzed to date have multiple transplantation antigens, would require extensive identical (parallel) mutations in two pairs of genes (i.e., K and D on the one hand and LA and four

---

*A species-associated residue need not be present in every member of a polymorphic population. For example, if the heterogeneous immunoglobulin V_κ regions of the guinea pig had aspartic acid and glutamic acid in a 9:1 ratio at position 1 and the rabbit had alanine and isoleucine in a 9.5:1 ratio, then aspartic acid–glutamic acid and alanine-isoleucine would, respectively, be species-associated residues for guinea pigs and rabbits.

†The fact that most mouse alloantisera show extensive cross-reactivity among molecules sharing public antigens while not reacting at all with human cells (or presumably their transplantation antigens) (D. Shreffler, personal communication) also suggests that many antigenic determinants are shared by mouse transplantation antigens that are not found on the human transplantation antigens. However, this simplistic interpretation of serological results obviously has many limitations (Klein, 1975b).

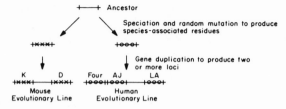

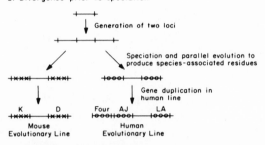

Figure 12. Schematic diagram of two hypotheses for the evolution of genes for the mammalian transplantation antigens (see text). (a) Duplication *after* speciation. (b) Duplication *before* speciation. The ×'s and ○'s designate species-associated residues in the mouse and human evolutionary lines, respectively.

on the other) to generate the mouse and human species-associated residues (Fig. 12b). Indeed, duplication of some genes coding for the transplantation antigens *after* speciation is already required to explain the observation that the HL-A complex of man contains three regions coding for transplantation antigens (LA, four, AJ) (van Rood *et al.*, 1976), whereas the H-2 complex appears to contain only two (K and D) (Fig. 2). Thus different species may have undergone different numbers of gene duplication events to produce one, two, three, or more loci coding for classical transplantation antigens. Accordingly, these genetic loci may be part of a multigenic system that can undergo gene expansion and contraction, presumably by homologous-but-unequal crossing over (see Hood *et al.*, 1975). An alternative explanation would be that the K and D genes have exchanged information with one another, presumably by gene conversion or crossing over.

G. Difference of the Two K Allelic Products from One Another by Multiple Amino Acid Residues and Difference of the Two D Allelic Products by Multiple Residues

The K gene products differ by six out of 16 residues and the D products by four of 14 residues (residues 1, 9, 14, 19, 21, 22 and 2, 5, 9, 17, respectively; see

Fig. 11 and Table III). These constitute 29–38% sequence differences over the limited regions examined. Furthermore, two of the three K substitutions with identified residue alternatives (e.g., positions 9, 14, and 21) differ by two base substitutions in the genetic code dictionary—further emphasizing the evolutionary separation of these "alleles." These differences are consistent with the multiple serological specificities which differentiate the K (and D) alleles from one another (Table II) and with the multiple differences noted in peptide maps. To our knowledge, these amino acid differences constitute some of the largest ever reported for two "alleles," if, indeed, differences of this magnitude are found throughout the entire molecule.

We have suggested that alleles (or allotypes) can be divided into two categories (Gutman *et al.*, 1975). Alternative forms of *simple allotypes* segregate in a Mendelian fashion in mating studies and differ by one or a few amino acid substitutions (e.g., the Inv marker of the human κ-chain; Terry *et al.*, 1969). In contrast, alternative forms of *complex allotypes* differ by multiple amino acid residues and generally segregate in a Mendelian fashion (e.g., the group a and group b allotypes of the rabbit; see Mage *et al.*, 1973). By these definitions, the K and D alleles, based on limited sequence data, are complex allotypes. The importance of the distinction between simple and complex allotypes lies in the very different types of genetic or evolutionary mechanisms implied (see Gutman *et al.*, 1975). Simple allotypes are probably coded by alternative alleles at a single structural locus. In contrast, complex allotypes may be explained by one of three general genetic models (Fig. 13).

1. Classical Allelic Model

The K (or D) alleles may have evolved by the divergence of alleles at a single genetic locus (Fig. 13a). Because of the extensive differences among these alleles, it is tempting to postulate that when mice evolved as a species, multiple alleles already differing significantly in sequence were incorporated into the new evolutionary line. However, this does not appear to be the case, at least with the gene products examined to date, because the presence of species-associated residues suggests that the genes coding for the mouse and human transplantation antigens diverged from common ancestral genes after speciation (so as to avoid multiple identical or parallel mutations; see Fig. 12). If these allelic gene products differ by 30–40% of their amino acid sequence throughout their entire length, then these polypeptides may differ by as many as approximately 100 residues. The allelic model assumes that a variant (single base substitution) gene arises by mutation and is fixed in the population. This new gene must then incur a second mutation that is once again fixed and this entire process must be repeated 100 times.

The structure of the wild mouse population may favor the rapid divergence of alleles (Klein, 1974). Wild mice breed in small demes (groups) with a single

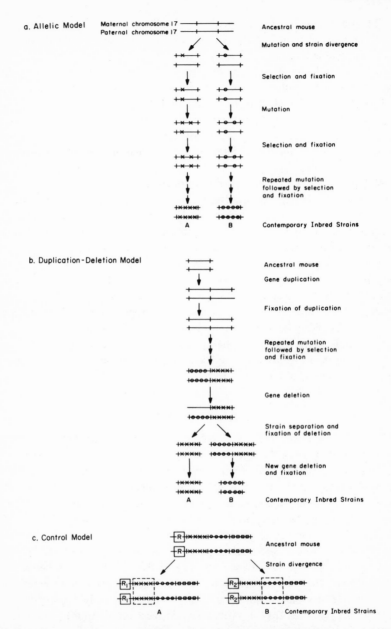

Figure 13. Three genetic and evolutionary models for complex allotypes (see text). X's and O's designate the divergence of genes that exhibit Mendelian behavior in contemporary inbred strains of mice, A and B. In the control model, the dotted boxes indicate distinct genes that are expressed in different inbred strains, regulated by control mechanisms R_1 and R_2.

dominant male and sharp geographical boundaries. There is little, if any, migration among demes. However, young mice are continually migrating from the old deme to establish new and subsequently independent demes. In these small isolated populations, variants can be fixed either by natural selection or by nonrandom fluctuations in a very limited pool of chromosomes. Since the fluctuations in gene frequencies are extreme in small populations, the chances for fixation (or elimination) of an allele are greatly enhanced over the chances in a large population (Hood et al., 1975a). However, alleles of gene products for other systems in the mouse (e.g., cytochrome c and the hemoglobins) do not show the same degree of diversity exhibited by the transplantation antigens (Dayhoff, 1972). Hence one must assume that natural selection plays an important role in generating this diversity.

The question arises as to whether mice as a species have had sufficient evolutionary time for their K (and D) alleles to have evolved to be so different. In this regard, it will be interesting to determine whether the transplantation antigens of guinea pigs and rats have species-associated residues when compared to those of mice. If they do, the time span over which the allelic differences can be produced is further reduced. For example, if the rat and mouse transplantation antigens have species-associated residues, their corresponding "alleles" must have arisen after speciation some 10 million years ago. In contrast, the C_κ immunoglobulin regions of man and mouse, two species which diverged about 75 million years ago, differ by only 40% of their amino acid sequence (Dayhoff, 1972). Finally, it should be pointed out that there is no precedent for alleles that differ by as much as 30–40% of their amino acid sequence (Gutman et al., 1975).

2. Duplication–Deletion Model

The duplication–deletion model suggests that the transplantation genes of the mouse were duplicated and that many differences were fixed in these duplicated genes (Fig. 13b). Later in the evolution of the mouse line, crossing-over events deleted most of these genes so that individual H-2 chromosomes of mice had just a single K (and D) gene. The presence of species-associated residues suggests that this gene expansion and contraction process must have occurred after the divergence of man and mouse. This model would permit many more mutations to be fixed as opposed to the allelic model since it would ease the requirements for stringent natural selection. That is, one K gene may be freed to accept many substitutions while the second is temporarily the functional transplantation antigen. Indeed, this is presumably how one gene of a duplicated pair evolves to assume a new function (Ohno, 1970). There are precedents for the evolution, via a crossing-over event, of alleles that differ by multiple substitutions (Gilman, 1972; Huisman, 1975).

3. Control Model

The transplantation "alleles" may be closely linked duplicated genes with a control mechanism that permits the duplicated genes to be expressed so as to mimic a Mendelian pattern of genetic segregation (Fig. 13c). This model suggests that each mouse chromosome 17 has genes coding for many of the K and D "alleles" the mouse species can express. The genetic polymorphism may reflect a control mechanism which operates at the chromosomal level to determine which of the K and which of the D alleles is expressed by a particular chromosome 17. This theory postulates that the chromosomal mechanism for commitment (to the expression of one K and one D allele) is transmitted through the germ line and is very stable. Perhaps this mechanism is mediated by the translocation of a genetic element, as may occur in maize (McKlintock, 1956) and immunoglobulin genes (Galley and Edelman, 1972). The high rate of mutation at the K locus ($\sim 5 \times 10^{-4}$ mutations/generation) in contrast to other mammalian genetic systems (Klein, 1976) may be a reflection of an alteration in this control mechanism so that different K (or D) genes are expressed. Thus the "mutant" K (or D) genes may reflect a switch in the control mechanism to express another closely linked gene rather than the actual mutation of a structural gene. In this regard, it will be extremely important to determine whether the "mutant" gene product differs from its "parental" gene product by one or by multiple amino acid substitutions. The former would be consistent with the mutation of a structural gene, whereas the latter would favor the control mechanism concept.*

There are possible precedents for this type of control mechanism. The group a and b allotypes of rabbit immunoglobulins are complex allotypes of the V_H and C_κ regions, respectively (i.e., their allelic products exhibit multiple amino acid differences). Some individual rabbits can express at low levels a "wrong" V_H allotype—one that should not be present in the individual according to the genotype of his parents (Mudgett et al., 1975). Indeed, one unusual rabbit expressed three group a and three group b allotypes (Strosberg et al., 1974). Both these observations suggest that the complex allotypes of the rabbit are, at least in part, closely linked genes regulated by a control mechanism that generally permits the complex allotypes to be expressed in a Mendelian fashion (see Farnsworth et al., 1976, for a discussion of this point). Accordingly, the complex allotypes of the rabbit may employ a control gene mechanism similar to that depicted in Figure 13c. This model has also been elegantly discussed by Bodmer (1973).

There are several distinctions and similarities among these three models that

---

*Preliminary peptide map analyses suggest that two H-2 mutants differ from their corresponding wild-type gene products by one or a few peptide differences (Nathenson et al., 1976). Indeed, some "mutants" may be true single base substitution of a particular structural gene whereas others may reflect a "switch" of the control mechanism. Accordingly, the important unanswered question is whether the mutant and wild-type alleles differ by one or by multiple base substitutions.

need to be emphasized. The duplication–deletion model and the control model view the K (and D) alleles as having evolved as duplicated and closely linked genes, while the classical allelic model assumes that these alleles evolved as alternative forms of a single structural gene. However, the duplication–deletion model and the classical allelic model contend that a single structural gene with multiple allelic forms encodes the contemporary K (and D) gene products.

The classical allelic model would be eliminated as an explanation for the complex K (and D) allotypes if it is unequivocally demonstrated (e.g., by structural analysis) that a mouse can produce H-2 alleles it should not have inherited from its parents (i.e., "wrong" alleles). This model would also find it difficult to explain K (or D) mutants that differed by multiple amino acid residues from the wild-type gene product. The control gene model could be verified if it could be demonstrated (e.g., by nucleic acid hybridization) that each mouse has many genes coding for the K (or D) gene products. Furthermore, if this model is correct, perhaps experimental conditions could be found which might cause the control mechanism to "switch" to the expression of different gene products [e.g., certain *in vitro* conditions (Rivat *et al.*, 1973) and stress states (Bosma and Bosma, 1974) appear to cause "wrong" complex allotypes of immunoglobulins to be expressed]. The duplication–deletion model would predict that occasional mice may have chromosomes with "hybrid" K (or D) genes or with multiple K (or D) genes. Because of the species-associated residues which distinguish the mouse K and D gene products from their human counterparts, each of these theories must assume that the K and D genes (or clusters of genes) arose subsequent to the human–mouse speciation.

It is intriguing to note that the only two allelic products of a single human HL-A region examined, 7 and 12, differ far less from one another than do their mouse counterparts (e.g., $\sim$ 5% vs. $\sim$ 35%; see Fig. 11). Indeed, these human alleles will still differ from one another by multiple residues, but it is not apparent why there should be such a striking difference in the apparent extent of diversity among the polymorphic forms of the human and mouse transplantation systems.

H. Indistinguishability of the K Products as a Class from the D Products as a Class on the Basis of Limited Sequence Data

The K gene products do not appear to be significantly more closely related to one another than to the D gene products. For example, the D^d gene product shows 79% homology with K^b, 63% homology with K^k, and 69% homology with its allelic counterpart, the D^b gene product (Fig. 11 and Table III). Likewise, no amino acids are restricted to only the K or the D gene products (Fig. 11). This lack of "D-ness" or "K-ness" is perhaps the most surprising observation in these data.

These amino acid sequence observations are in apparent conflict with the serological data on the K and D gene products. In general, multiple public sero-

Table IV. H-2 Chart of the K and D Antigens[a,b]

H-2 haplotype	Antigens of the K series — Public																				K Private	Antigens of the D series — Public															D Private
	1	3	5	7	8	11	25	27	28	29	34	35	36	37	38	39	42	45	46	47	Private	1	3	5	6	13	27	28	29	35	36	41	42	43	44	49	Private
b	—	—	5	—	—	—	—	—	28	29	—	35	36	—	—	—	—	—	46	—	33	—	—	—	6	—	27	28	29	—	—	—	—	—	—	—	2
d	—	3	5	7	8	—	—	—	28	29	34	—	—	37	—	39	—	—	46	47	31	—	3	—	6	13	27	28	29	35	36	41	42	43	44	49	4
f	—	—	c	7	8	—	—	—	28	29	—	—	—	—	—	39	—	—	46	—	?	—	—	—	6	—	27	—?	—?	—	—	—	—	—	—	—	9
j	1?	—	5	—	—	11	—	—	—	—	—	35	—	37	38	—	—	45	—	—	15	—	—	—	6	—	—	28	29	35	—	41	—	—	44	—	2
k	1	3	5	7	8	11	25	—	—	—	—	—	—	—	—	—	—	45	—	47	23	1	3	5	6	—	—	—	—	—	—	—	—	—	—	49	32
p	1	3	5	7	8	—	—	—	—	—	34	—	—	37	38	—	—	—	46?	·	16	1	3	5	—	13	—	—	29	—	—	41	42	—	—	49	?
q	1	3	5	7	8	11	—	—	—	—	—	—	—	—	—	—	—	45	—	—	17	1	3	5	6	—	—	—	—	c	c	—	42	43	—	49	30
r	1	3	5	7	8	11	25	—	—	—	—	—	—	—	—	—	—	45	—	47	·	1	—	5	6	—	—	—	—	c	c	—	—	—	—	49	18?
s	1	—	5	7	8?	—	—	—	—	—	—	35	36	—	—	—	42	45	—	—	19	1	3	—	6	—	—	28	29	—	36	—	42	43	—	49	12
u	c	—	5	—	8?	—	—	—	—	—	—	35	36	—	—	—	—	45	·	·	20	c	3	—	6	13?	27?	28	29	—	c	41	42	—	—	49	4
v	1	3	5	—	—	—	—	—	—	—	—	—	—	—	—	—	—	45?	—	—	21	1	3	—	6	—?	—?	28?	·	—	—	—	—?	43	—	49	30
z	—	5	—	—	—	—	—	27	—	29	—	—	—	—	—	—	—	—	46	47	·	—	—	—	6	—	—	28?	·	·	·	—	—	—	—	·	·

[a]From Klein (1975).
[b]Symbols: —, absence of an antigen; ·, unknown; ?, presence or absence of antigen is uncertain; c, some antisera cross-react with the indicated H-2 haplotype.

logical specificities are shared by gene products of a single region (K or D) (Table IV). For example, public specificities 7, 8, 11, 25, 37, 38, 39, 45, 46, and 47 are found only on K molecules, whereas specificities 6, 13, 41, 43, 44, and 49 are found only on D molecules (Table IV). Thus the serological data suggest that there is "K-ness" and "D-ness" in the respective molecules.*

How can the apparent paradox posed by the serological and sequence data be resolved? There are three general explanations, the first two of which are trivial: (1) Our limited partial sequence data may be misleading in this regard; this may be the most likely possibility. (2) The N-terminal regions of these molecules may not have any important function, or they may have a function compatible with great variability. Thus they are capable of accepting many mutations. Other regions of these molecules may show "K-ness" and "D-ness." These trival explanations can be tested by additional amino acid sequence data.

Let us consider, however, the genetic and evolutionary implications of possibility (3), namely, that subsequent amino acid sequence data will demonstrate a lack of "K-ness" or "D-ness" in at least a portion of these molecules. This observation coupled with two others, species-associated residues and the shared public specificities of allelic gene products, places severe constraints on possible genetic and evolutionary models of these regions. None of the models for complex allotypes discussed above can easily explain the lack of "K-ness" or "D-ness." In the allelic model, if the allelic forms of the K or D genes arose subsequent to the divergence of man and mouse, the alleles of one region should be more closely related to one another than to those of the second region and, accordingly, display "K-ness" and "D-ness" (Fig. 13a). The duplication–deletion model would require that the K and D genes form a single gene (or cluster) before reduction to a series of alleles at two structural loci in order to explain the lack of "D-ness" or "K-ness" (Fig. 13b). The same would be true of the control gene model (Fig. 9c). However, even if the K and D genes formed a single gene family, this would be inconsistent with the fact that many public specificities are found only on K (or D) gene products (Table IV).

One possible resolution of the paradox caused by the amino acid sequence and serological data would be the possibility that the K and D proteins are actually coded by two genes, analogous to the V and C genes of immunoglobulins. The two C genes (C_D and C_K) might contain the public (shared) specificities, whereas the V genes for both K and D molecules might be drawn from a common gene family (cluster). Thus the family of V genes could evolve to have species-associated residues by crossing over just as appears to be the case with the families of antibody V genes (Hood et al., 1975b). Each V gene would have its own private specificity (analogous to an idiotype). There would be a lack of

---

*Recent studies suggest that there is much cross reactivity among the K and D public specificities (Klein, personal communication). If there is no serological "K-ness" or "D-ness," obviously there would be no need to postulate C regions for the transplantation antigens.

"K-ness" or "D-ness" among the V genes since they are evolving in a common multigene family. Accordingly, if subsequent sequence data confirm the lack of "K-ness" or "D-ness" in a major portion of the transplantation antigens, an explanation formally analogous to that given above will be necessary.

V. CELL SURFACE MOLECULES CONTROLLED
BY CHROMOSOME 17 OF THE MOUSE

Chromosome 17 has three gene clusters (T/t, H-2, and Tla) that code for at least five different types of cell surface molecules: the T/t antigens, the K antigens, the Ia antigens, the D antigens, and the TL antigens. Mutations at the T/t locus affect specific points in the embryonic development of the notochord, axial skeleton, and the neural tube through the specification of cell surface molecules found only on embryonic cells (and sperm) (Bennett and Dunn, 1964; Artzt and Bennett, 1975). These mutants fall into six complementation groups and their corresponding defects appear to lie in abnormal cell–cell interactions that occur at reproducible and precise stages of development. The H-2 locus codes for two and possibly more distinct multigene families (McDevitt, 1976): (1) The I region contains multiple immune response genes which have been separated into at least three subregions: I-A, I-B, and I-C (Fig. 1). The I-A and I-C subregions code for distinct Ia molecules whose precise function is as yet unknown. The Ia molecules coded by the I-A and I-C subregions can cross-react serologically (Murphy, 1975), implying that they descended from a common ancestral gene. (2) The S region definitely controls the levels of one complement component (C$'$4) (Meo et al., 1975; Lachman et al., 1975; Curman et al., 1975) and appears to control the levels of several others (C$'$1, C$'$2, and C$'$3) (Goldman and Goldman, 1975). In addition, several other components of similar structure and function (C$'$2 from the classical pathway and C$'$3 proactivator from the alternative complement pathway) appear to be regulated by genes in the HL-A complex of man (Fig. 2) (Fearon et al., 1973; Allen, 1974). Whether the S-region genes are regulatory or structural in nature is unknown. In either case, it appears likely that this region will constitute yet another example of a multigene family. (3) The possibility has been raised in preceding sections that the K and D antigens are actually coded by multigene families. Finally, the Tla region contains at least several genes which control the expression of thymocyte differentiation antigens (TL antigens) (Boyse and Old, 1969).

Recently it has been suggested that the T/t (Vitetta et al., 1975a) and TL (Vitetta et al., 1975b; Anundi et al., 1975) antigens are homologous to the K and D gene products on the basis of similar molecular weights and their association with β_2-microglobulin. If confirmed by structural studies, this suggests that the corresponding genes may have diverged from a common ancestor and that, indeed, chromosome 17 of the mouse may code for a series of evolutionarily related multigene families.

Structural studies on these membrane proteins in the future will be directed at discerning the nature and extent, if any, of homology that may exist among these multigene families. It will also be interesting to determine whether these multigene families share strategies for information storage, information expression, and information evolution similar to those seen in the antibody gene families (see Hood *et al.*, 1975a,b).

VI. SUMMARY

Preliminary amino acid sequence data on the transplantation antigens of mouse and man have led to provocative hypotheses about the genetic organization and evolution of genes coded by the major histocompatibility complex of mammals. New microsequencing techniques should permit a detailed analysis of these gene products and an eventual choice among the alternative hypotheses now posed. These data have made it apparent that the H-2 complex is a fascinating and complicated chromosomal region which will continue for some time to intrigue immunologists, geneticists, biochemists, and cell biologists.

NOTE ADDED IN PRESS

A second paper on the partial sequence of HLA antigens has recently appeared in *Nature* by Crumpton and Bodmer and their colleagues Bridgen *et al.*, 1976, *Nature (London)* **261**:200.

ACKNOWLEDGMENTS

This work was supported by grants from the National Science Foundation and the National Institutes of Health. J. S. has an Established Investigatorship Award from the American Heart Association. L. H. has an NIH Research Career Development Award. We thank Drs. Capra, Cunningham, Edelman, Nathenson, Strominger, and Vitetta for sending us preprints prior to their publication. Portions of this chapter were adapted from Silver and Hood (1976).

VII. REFERENCES

Allen, F.H., Jr., 1974, *Vox Sang.* 27:382.
Amos, D.B., Gorer, P.A., and Mikulska, Z.B., 1955, *Proc. Roy. Soc. London Ser. B* 144:369.
Anundi, H., Rask, L., Östberg, L., and Peterson, P.A., 1975, *Biochemistry* 14:5046.

Artzt, K., and Bennett, D., 1975, *Nature (London)* **256**:545.
Bach, F.H., and van Rood, J.J., 1976, *N. Engl. J. Med.* (in press).
Balner, H., and Toth, E.K., 1973, *Tissue Antigens* **3**:273.
Benacerraf, B., and McDevitt, H.O., 1972, *Science* **175**:273.
Bennett, D., and Dunn, L.C., 1964, *Science* **144**:260.
Bodmer, W., 1972, *Nature (London)* **237**:139.
Bodmer, W.F., 1973, *Transplant. Proc.* **5**:1471.
Bosma, M.J., and Bosma, G., 1974, *J. Exp. Med.* **139**:512.
Boyse, E.A., and Old, L.J., 1969, *Annu. Rev. Genet.* **3**:269.
Brown, J.L., Kato, K., Silver, J., and Nathenson, S.G., 1974, *Biochemistry* **13**:3174.
Counce, S., Smith, P., Barth, R., and Snell, G.D., 1956, *Ann. Surg.* **144**:198.
Cullen, S.E., David, C.S., Shreffler, D.C., and Nathenson, S.G., 1974, *Proc. Natl. Acad. Sci. USA* **71**:648.
Cunningham, B.A., and Berggard, I., 1975, *Science* **187**:1079.
Cunningham, B.A., Wang, J.L., Berggard, I., and Peterson, P.A., 1973, *Biochemistry* **12**:4811.
Curman, B., Östberg, L., Sandberg, L., Malmheden-Eriksson, I., Stalenheim, G., Rask, L., and Peterson, P.A., 1975, *Nature (London)* **258**:243.
David, C.S., Shreffler, D.C., and Frelinger, J.A., 1973, *Proc. Natl. Acad. Sci. USA* **70**:2509.
Dayhoff, M., 1972, *The Atlas of Protein Sequence and Structure*, National Biomedical Research Foundation, Silver Spring, Md.
Dorf, M.E., Balner, H., deGroot, M.L., and Benecerraf, B., 1974, *Transplant. Proc.* **VI**:119.
Ewenstein, B.M., Freed, J.H., Mole, L.E., and Nathenson, S.G., 1976, *Proc. Natl. Acad. Sci. USA* **73**:915.
Farnsworth, V., Fleishman, R., Rodbey, S., and Hood, L., 1976, *Proc. Natl. Acad. Sci. USA* **73**:923.
Fearon, D.T., Austen, K.F., and Ruddy, S., 1973, *J. Exp. Med.* **138**:1305.
Gally, J., and Edelman, G.M., 1972, *Annu. Rev. Genet.* **6**:1.
Gilman, J.G., 1972, *Science* **178**:873.
Goldman, M.G., and Goldman, J.N., 1975, *Fed. Proc.* **34**:979.
Gorer, P.A., 1937, *J. Pathol. Bacteriol.* **44**:691.
Götze, D., Reisfeld, R.A., and Klein, J., 1973, *J. Exp. Med.* **138**:1003.
Gutman, G., Loh, E., and Hood, L., 1975, *Proc. Natl. Acad. Sci. USA* **72**:4046.
Hämmerling, G.J., Deak, B.D., Mauve, G., Hämmerling, U., and McDevitt, H.O., 1974, *Immunogenetics* **1**:68.
Hämmerling, U., and Eggers, H.J., 1970, *Eur. J. Biochem.* **17**:95.
Hauptfeld, V., Klein, D., and Klein, J., 1973, *Science* **181**:167.
Henning, R., Milner, R.J., Reske, K., Cunningham, B.A., and Edelman, G.M., 1976, *Proc. Natl. Acad. Sci. USA* **73**:118.
Hilschmann, N., and Craig, L.C., 1965, *Proc. Natl. Acad. Sci. USA* **53**:1403.
Hood, L., Campbell, J.H., and Elgin, S.R.C., 1975a, *Annu. Rev. Genet.* **9**:305.
Hood, L., Wilson, J., and Wood, W.B., 1975b, *Molecular Biology of Eucaryotic Cells*, Chap. 7, W.A. Benjamin, Menlo Park, Calif.
Huisman, T.H.J., 1975, *Ann. N.Y. Acad. Sci.* **241**:549.
Jacobs, J.W., Kemper, B., Niall, H.D., Habener, J.F., and Potts, J.T., Jr., 1974, *Nature (London)* **249**:155.
Katz, D.H., Graves, M., Dorf, M.E., Dimuzio, H., and Benacerraf, B., 1975, *J. Exp. Med.* **141**:263.
Klein, J., 1974, *Annu. Rev. Genet.* **8**:63.
Klein, J., 1975, *Biology of the Mouse Histocompatibility-2 Complex: Principles of Immunogenetics Applied to a Single System*, Springer-Verlag, New York.
Klein, J., 1976, in: *Contemporary Topics in Immunobiology*, Vol. 5 (W. O. Weigle, ed.), Plenum, New York.

Klein, J., and Shreffler, D.C., 1971, *Transplant. Rev.* **6**:3.

Lachman, P.J., Grennan, D., Martin, A., and Demant, P., 1975, *Nature (London)* **258**:242.

Lilly, F., and Pincus, T., 1973, *Adv. Cancer Res.* **17**:231.

Mage, R., Lieberman, R., Potter, M., and Terry, W.D., 1973, in: *The Antigens*, Vol. 1 (M. Sela, ed.), p. 300, Academic Press, New York.

Marchesi, U., 1975, in: *Cell Membranes: Biochemistry, Cell Biology and Pathology* (G. Wrissmann and R. Claiborne, eds.), p. 45, H.P. Publishing Co., New York.

Marsh, D.G., Bias, W.B., Hsu, S. H., and Goodfriend, L., 1973, *Science* **179**:691.

McDevitt, H.O., 1976, *Fed. Proc.* (in press).

McDevitt, H.O., and Bodmer, W.F., 1974, *Lancet* **I**:1269.

McDevitt, H.O., Bechtol, K.B., and Hämmerling, G.J., 1974a, in: *Cellular Selection and Regulation in the Immune Response* (G.M. Edelman, ed.), p. 101, Raven Press, New York.

McDevitt, H.O., Bechtol, K.B., Hämmerling, G.J., Lonai, P., and Delovitch, T.L., 1974b, in: *The Immune System: Genes, Receptors, Signals* (E. Sercarz, A.R. Williamson, and C.F. Fox, eds.), p. 597, Academic Press, New York.

McKlintock, B., 1956, *Cold Spring Harbor Symp. Quant. Biol.* **21**:197.

Medawar, P.B., 1956/1957, *Harvey Lect.* **52**:144.

Meo, T., Krasteff, T., and Shreffler, D., 1975, *Proc. Natl. Acad. Sci. USA* **72**:4536.

Möller, G. (ed.), 1975, *Transplant. Rev.* **22**:1.

Mozes, E., 1975, *Immunogenetics* **2**:397.

Mudgett, M., Fraser, B.A., and Kindt, T.J., 1975, *J. Exp. Med.* **141**:1448.

Munro, A.J., and Taussig, M.J., 1975, *Nature (London)* **256**:103.

Murphy, D., and Shreffler, D.C., 1975, *J. Exp. Med.* **141**:374.

Murphy, D.B., 1975, *Fed. Proc.* **34**:1016.

Nathenson, S.G., and Cullen, S.E., 1974, *Biochim. Biophys. Acta* **344**:1.

Nathenson, S.G., Brown, J.K., Ewenstein, D.M., Rajan, T.V., Freed, T.H., Sears, D.W., Mole, L.E., and Scharff, M.D., 1976, in: *The Role of Products of the Histocompatibility Gene Complex in Immune Responses* (D.H. Katz and B. Benacerraf) Academic Press, New York.

Needleman, S., and Wunsch, C., 1970, *J. Mol. Biol.* **48**:443.

Ohno, S., 1970, *Evolution by Gene Duplication*, Springer, New York.

Peterson, P.A., Cunningham, B.A., Berggard, I., and Edelman, G.M., 1972, *Proc. Natl. Acad. Sci. USA* **69**:1697.

Peterson, P.A., Rask, L., Sege, K., Klaresky, L., Anundi, H., and Östberg, L. 1975, *Proc. Natl. Acad. Sci. USA* **72**:1612.

Poljak, R., Amzel, L., Avey, H., Chen, B., Phizackerley, R., and Saul, F., 1973, *Proc. Natl. Acad. Sci. USA* **70**:3305.

Poljak, R.J., Amzel, L.M., Chen, B.L., Phizackerley, R.P., and Saul, F., 1975, *Immunogenetics* **2**:393.

Rivat, L., Gilbert, D., and Ropartz, C., 1973, *Immunology* **24**:1041.

Sachs, D.H., and Cone, J.L., 1973, *J. Exp. Med.* **138**:1289.

Sachs, D.H., David, C.S., Shreffler, D.C., Nathenson, S.G., and McDevitt, H.O., 1975, *Immunogenetics* **2**:1.

Schecter, I., 1973, *Proc. Natl. Acad. Sci. USA* **70**:2256.

Schwartz, B.D., and Nathenson, S.G., 1971, *J. Immunol.* **107**:1363.

Shearer, G.M., 1974, *Eur. J. Immunol.* **4**:527.

Shimada, A., and Nathenson, S.G., 1969, *Biochemistry* **8**:4048.

Shreffler, D.C., and David, C.S., 1975, *Adv. Immunol.* **20**:125.

Shreffler, D.C., David, C.S., Passmore, H.C., and Klein, J., 1971, *Transplant. Proc.* **3**:176.

Silver, J., and Hood, L., 1974, *Nature (London)* **249**:764.

Silver, J., and Hood, L., 1975, *Nature (London)* **256**:63.

Silver, J., and Hood, L. E., 1976, *Proc. Natl. Acad. Sci. USA* **73**:599.

Silver, J., Sibley, C., Morand, P., and Hood, L., 1975, *Transplant. Proc.* **7**:201.

Smithies, O., and Poulik, M.D., 1972, *Proc. Natl. Acad. Sci. USA* **69**:2914.

Springer, T., and Storminger, J.L., 1973, *Fed. Proc.* **32**:1018.

Strominger, J.L., Cresswell, P., Grey, H., Humphreys, R.H., Mann, D., McCune, J., Parham, P., Robb, R., Sanderson, A.R., Springer, T.A., Terhorst, C., and Turner, M.J., 1974, *Transplant. Rev.* **21**:126.

Strosberg, A.D., Hamers-Casterman, C., Van der Lou, W., and Hamers, R., 1974, *J. Immunol.* **113**:1313.

Terhorst, C., Parham, P., Mann, D.L., and Strominger, J.L., 1976, *Proc. Natl. Acad. Sci. USA* **73**:910.

Terry, W.D., Hood, L., and Steinberg, A.G., 1969, *Proc. Natl. Acad. Sci. USA* **63**:71.

Uhr, J., 1975, in: *Cell Membranes: Biochemistry, Cell Biology and Pathology* (G. Weissmann and R. Claiborne, eds.), p. 223, H.P. Publishing Co., New York.

van Rood, J.J., van Leeuwen, A., Termijtelen, A., and Keuuing, J.J., 1976, in: *The Role of Products of the Histocompatibility Gene Complex in Immune Responses* (D.H. Katz and B. Benacerraf, eds.), Academic Press, New York.

Vitetta, E.S., Klein, J., and Uhr, J.W., 1974, *Immunogenetics* **1**:82.

Vitetta, E.S., Uhr, J.W., and Boyse, E.A., 1975a, *J. Immunol.* **114**: 252.

Vitetta, E.S., Artzt, K., Bennett, D., Boyse, E.A., and Jacob, F., 1975b, *Proc. Natl. Acad. Sci. USA* **72**:3215.

Vitetta, E.S., Capra, J.D., Klapper, D.G., Klein, J., and Uhr, J.W., 1976, *Proc. Natl. Acad. Sci. USA* **73**:905.

Zinkernagel, R.M., and Doherty, P.C., 1974, *Nature (London)* **251**:547.

Biological and Biochemical Properties of Solubilized Histocompatibility-2 (H-2) Alloantigens

Lloyd W. Law and Ettore Appella

Laboratory of Cell Biology
National Cancer Institute
Bethesda, Maryland

I. INTRODUCTION

Glycoproteins form a major part of the cell surface. Included among these glycoproteins are the important histocompatibility antigens—the major systems being H-2 in the mouse and HL-A in man—principally involved in tissue rejection.

H-2 is known to be present on all adult cells except possibly sperm. The H-2 complex (MAC) comprises a large region of chromosome 17—of approximately 0.4 cM. This gene complex may be divided into several regions as shown in Fig. 1 based on recombination studies. The two major genes concerned with tissue rejection are termed *H-2K* and *H-2D*, located at either end of the complex and separated by a considerable amount of genetic material; a third major locus governing tissue rejection, termed *H-2I*, has recently been described (Klein *et al.*, 1974) and maps near H-2K. Independent determinants (hybrid resistance determinants) of cell surface components phenotypically expressed only on blood-forming and leukemic cells have been defined as primarily due to *Hh* genes (Cudkowicz, 1968); these have been mapped either within or near the two ends of the MHC. The *Ss-Slp* region and a region of immune response genes designated *Ir-1A*, *Ir-1B*, and *Ia-3* have been found through the use of serological methods and genetic recombinants to map between the two extreme H-2K and H-2D regions. Antigens coded by the Ir region appear to be MLR-stimulating determinants. Those serologically defined specificities determined only by either the *H-2K* or the *H-2D* gene are called "private" specificities,

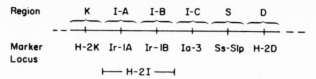

Figure 1. Map of H-2 gene complex in the IXth linkage group of the mouse. See text for discussion of regions. Adapted from Murphy and Shreffler (1975).

whereas those that belong to either the K or D end or both, are termed "public" specificities. This cross-reactivity has been demonstrated by serological methods and more than 40 distinct alleles have been detected in these H-2 loci.

II. BIOLOGICAL PROPERTIES OF SOLUBLE H-2 ANTIGENS

Our starting material for solubilization and purification of H-2^a antigen was A/J spleen cells. Table I lists the private and public specificities of the H-2^a haplotype compared, for example, with the H-2^d haplotype. Fractionation of our papain-solubilized material on a Sephadex G150 column yielded, in addition to an F1 peak in the excluded volume, two peaks in the included volume, namely, fractions F2 and F3. Through the use of an assay of inhibition of antibody-mediated cytotoxicity (^{51}Cr release), activity of the specificities H-2.1,3 and H-2.11 and of H-2.4, H-2.5, H-2.23, and H-2.3,28 was found to be confined entirely to the F2 fraction and peaked in the same tube. The H-2^a antigen in the F2 fraction is known to consist of a large component and a small β_2-microglobulin as described later. The molecular weight is estimated to be close to 50,000. F1 and F3 fractions did not show alloantigenic activity. The F2 fraction was shown to have alloantigenic specificity since H-2.22 activity, not present in H-2^a haplotype mice, was not detected in separate preparations of the

Table I. H-2 Determinants of Strains A and B10.A (H-2^a Haplotypes) and B10.D2 (H-2^d Haplotype)

Haplotype	Genotype	Public determinants	Private determinants	
			H-2K	H-2D
H-2^a	H-2K^k, H-2D^d	1,3,5,6,8,10,13,14,25,27, 28,29,35,36	23	4
H-2^d	H-2K^d, H-2D^d	3,6,13,27,28,29,35,36, 41,42,43	31	4

pooled F2 fractions (Strober *et al.*, 1970). The fact that the activity of H-2 specificities assayed was confined to a single peak in the F2 fraction suggests strongly that these are on separate molecules of similar molecular weight or that they are all on the same molecule.

The three fractions of chromatographed material partially purified were assayed for their capacity to elicit transplantation immunity both in noncongenic strains of mice, A/J donor to CBA (H-2^k) recipients, and in congenic strains which differ only at the H-2 locus, B10.A donor to B10.B (H-2^b) or B10.D2 (H-2^d) recipients. All three fractions induced transplantation immunity in doses of 10-100 μg in noncongenic strains, whereas only the F2 fraction produced significant skin graft rejection in the congenic combination B10.A→B10.B (Strober *et al.*, 1970). These results indicate that the transplantation antigens present in fractions F1 and F3 are controlled by *non*-H-2 loci since the activity of these materials was markedly diminished in the congenic strain combination. The transplantation antigens present in the F2 fraction are therefore controlled by the H-2 locus since only F2 activity, and not F1 and F3, was seen in the congenic strain combination. This striking association of alloantigenic specificities and transplantation antigens controlled by the H-2 locus in fraction F2 strongly suggests that both are present on the same molecules.

Graff and Nathenson (1971) also have reported second-set skin graft responses in donor–host combinations that presented only an H-2 difference without non-H-2 differences. Their papain-solubilized antigens subjected to CM-Sephadex chromatography were derived from tissues of the H-2^d and H-2^b haplotypes. These authors describe two different sized fragments (classes I and II) and these classes must apparently be combined to obtain biological activity. We have not observed the existence of such classes of material in our papain-digested spleen cell membranes of H-2^a haplotype.

There are reports of immunogenic activity of solubilized H-2 antigens, principally of H-2^d haplotype origin, by other investigators (Rosenberg *et al.*, 1971; Graff *et al.*, 1970; Ranney *et al.*, 1973; McKenzie *et al.*, 1970); in many instances, however, congenic donor–recipient mice were not used. Skin graft prolongation and accelerated rejection were observed depending on the schedule of immunization. Although prolongation was ascribed to immunological enhancement, adequate specificity controls were not always included in these studies. Hilgert (1974) gives a survey of data in the literature from 1962 through 1973 dealing with the biological effects, principally of skin rejection, employing particulate H antigens or those solubilized by various procedures.

Further biological assays of our solubilized H-2 antigens were pursued since the presence of all of the expected alloantigenic specificities cannot be used alone as a test of completeness of transplantation antigens; the activity of these specificities was measured by an inhibition assay that presumably detects haptens as well as complete antigens.

III. SPECIFIC IMMUNOLOGICAL ENHANCEMENT

Present evidence suggests strongly that in order to obtain specific immunological enhancement, achieved most effectively with allogeneic tumor grafting, appropriate alloantibodies must combine with all the determinants of the H-2 transplantation antigens of the graft donor. Thus the induction of immunological enhancement is presumed to be a test for completeness of antigen.

We have assayed the biological capacities of our solubilized A/J (H-2^a) membrane materials to prolong the growth and survival of two A/J strain tumors: YAA-Cl grafted on CBA (H-2^k) mice and sarcoma I grafted on mice of the B10.D2 (H-2^d) strain (Law et al., 1971). Specific immunological enhancement was achieved on the basis of the following criteria:

1. Active enhancement was noted in both systems studied with crude membrane material or fraction 2 but not with fraction 3; both crude membrane preparation and fraction 2 are known to contain H-2 antigens. The soluble fraction 3 was shown to be immunogenic in causing strain A (H-2^a) skin graft rejection in CBA (H-2^k) recipients, but was not immunogenic when congenic recipients, differing only at the H-2 locus, were used (Strober et al., 1970). This observation suggested that the transplantation antigens in this fraction were controlled by loci other than H-2. The absence of enhancing capacity in fraction 3 further confirms this conclusion and reemphasizes the major role of H-2 antigens in immunological enhancement. Cytotoxic and/or hemagglutinating antibodies were detected in relatively high titers in the sera of those recipients of the cell membrane (CM) preparation or of fraction 2 (see Table II).
2. Passively transferred antisera from recipients of the cell membrane material or fraction 2, but not from recipients of fraction 3, enhanced the growth of YAA-C1 and sarcoma 1 tumors in CBA and B10.D2 mice, respectively; passive immunization was more effective in enhancement of the growth of sarcoma I.
3. Enhancement by solubilized H-2^a antigens was specific. Passive transfer of antisera from mice immunized with fraction 2 did not enhance tumor Py 89 of C57BL (H-2^b) origin, yet the tumor was readily enhanced by antisera produced by H-2^b antigens in suitable recipients.

Although these results demonstrate that all important H-2^a antigenic determinants have been recovered and show biological activity, this does not imply that these molecules are identical to those present in situ on the intact cell. Fragmentation may have occurred despite the maintenance of immunogenicity. A further critical test for completeness of the molecule is the induction of tolerance.

Table II. Cytotoxic (Cy) and Hemagglutinating (H) Antibodies Induced in B10.D2 Mice by Soluble H-2^a Antigens

	Log$_2$ titers^a	
Inoculum	H-ab	Cy-ab
CM fraction	512	32
Fraction 2	512	32
Fraction 3	0	2
Saline	0	2

^{a}Reciprocals of titers on day 27; cytotoxic titers increased in groups 1 and 2 to 128 on day 37. Fifty micrograms of the antigen preparation in buffered saline was inoculated intraperitoneally twice a week for 3 wk. Sarcoma I was inoculated subcutaneously in these mice 28 days after the last injection and increased growth with delayed rejection was seen only in groups 1 and 2. Antisera from a similar set was used for passive transfer of enhancement and a striking enhancement was observed only with sera of groups 1 and 2 (Law *et al.*, 1971, 1974b).

IV. INDUCTION OF CELLULAR AND HUMORAL TOLERANCE WITH SOLUBILIZED H-2 ANTIGENS

The papain-solubilized, G150 Sephadex-chromatographed F2 fraction of H-2^a antigens was studied for its capacity to induce immunological tolerance in B10.D2 mice. Total deletion of cytotoxic, hemagglutinating, and classical enhancing antibodies was observed in the majority of B10.D2 mice inoculated at birth thence daily, or every other day, over a 30-day period (Law *et al.*, 1972). However, complete tolerance, i.e., cellular and humoral tolerance, was not achieved in these mice; B10.A skin grafts and neonatal hearts were rejected in the usual time and manner. Our findings to date may be summarized as follows:

1. This regularly induced unresponsiveness was found to be specific and not the result of a nonspecific suppression sometimes observed with protein antigens. B10.D2 mice humorally tolerant to H-2^a antigens were quite capable of producing cytotoxic antibodies to B10 (H-2^b) antigen.
2. The usual regimen for induction of tolerance was i.v. inoculation of 40 or 80 μg of F2 fraction at birth followed by daily i.p. inoculations of 40 μg. A similar schedule of inoculation of 0.4 μg at birth followed by daily 0.4 μg inoculations for 30 days also induced levels of unresponsiveness comparable to that induced by the higher dose. In contrast, B10.D2

Table III. Induction of Humoral Tolerance in B10.D2 Mice
with the F2 Fraction of H-2^a Antigen

Antigen dose (μg)	Number of mice	Mean cytotoxic titers (reciprocal of log$_2$)	Unresponders
40^a	58	1.4^{b,c}	62%
None	49	7.3	–
4	10	5.0	None
None	11	5.0	–
0.4	20	2.2^c	45%
None	19	6.2	–

[a] All inoculations of soluble antigen were done i.v. at birth thence daily × 30, i.p.
[b] All mice were skin-grafted at 30–40 days of age with B10.A skin, then inoculated × 2 with 60 × 10^6 (B10.A × B10.D2)F$_1$ spleen cells; cytotoxic titers were determined 2 wk after the last immunization.
[c] Difference between soluble H-2^a antigen-treated mice and controls was 7.0 ± 1.03 vs. 1.5 ± 0.43 ($P<0.001$).

recipients of the 4 μg dose did not differ from their matched controls as measured by complement-dependent cytotoxic antibody (Table III). A single treatment at birth with soluble antigen did not induce unresponsiveness; this reflects a difference with results using several disaggregated heterologous protein antigens (Law et al., 1974a).

3. Humoral tolerance was relatively long lasting. B10.D2 mice rendered unresponsive to H-2^a soluble antigen remained unresponsive for at least 16 wk after cessation of antigen treatment. These results suggest that H-2^a soluble antigen is not cleared rapidly from tissues.

4. Assays of lymphoid cells from humorally tolerant mice for certain cell-mediated functions such as GVH, MLR, and CML revealed that these functions were preserved, in contrast to a lack of activity in tolerant mice exhibiting cell-mediated unresponsiveness (Law et al., 1973).

5. Sera from our humorally tolerant mice did not "block" the cytostatic effect of specifically sensitized lymphocytes, in contrast to sera from allograft-tolerant mice, in an in vitro microcytotoxicity assay (Wright et al., 1974). Thus it is possible that cell-mediated immune responses in humorally tolerant mice are not impaired because humorally tolerant mice are unable to produce specific "blocking" factors. However, employing a short-term ^{51}Cr-release assay, it was observed that neither sera from humorally tolerant nor sera from completely tolerant mice had the capacity to "block." Only sera from B10.D2 mice that had high levels of cytoxic antibodies against lymphoid cells bearing H-2^a antigens were

capable of "blocking" *in vitro* or inducing enhancement *in vivo* (Law *et al.*, 1974b).

The dissociation of humoral and cell-mediated immunity detailed here using H-2^a solubilized and partially purified antigens has no immediate explanation. It is conceivable that some determinants may be lost as a result of fragmentation with papain. A primary requirement for complete tolerogenicity, presumably, is a full set of determinants. The change in physical conformation of the H-2^a molecule may indeed affect the presentation of antigen. The absence of a small (10,000 daltons) hydrophobic piece of the molecule could influence conformation. This piece necessary for membrane integration is apparently free, however, of antigenic determinants. Chemical manipulation of an antigen has been shown (Parish, 1971) to modulate the class of immune response and the type of tolerance which it will evoke. Even if the form of the antigen presented remains constant, various factors are known, from studies of the induction of tolerance with intact lymphoid cells or with particulate material, to influence the outcome of the response (see Hilgert, 1974). Table IV summarizes the biological activities of H-2^a soluble antigen.

The tolerance-inducing dose of allogeneic lymphoid cells for newborn mice is directly related to the strength of the immune reaction provoked by the same antigens administered to adults (Howard *et al.*, 1961). Complete tolerance (cell-mediated as well as humoral) is difficult to achieve in the congenic combination B10.A (donor) → B10.D2 (recipient). A total of 7–10 × 10^6 (B10.A × B10.D2)F$_1$ cells induce tolerance in only 20% or less of recipients, whereas in the reciprocal donor–host combination B10.D2 → B10.A approximately 80% of the newborn recipients are rendered operationally tolerant by the i.v. inocula-

Table IV. Biological Characterization of F2 Fraction (H-2^a Antigen)

Yield: 65% crude membrane material (CM); specific activity 32× of CM

Specific activities confined to this fraction and peaked in same tube

Activity of public and *private* allogeneic specificities: H-2.1,3,*4,5*,11,*23*,25,28 (immunologically specific)

Transplantation immunity (skin graft and neonatal heart rejection) elicited in *congenic mice* by F2 and not by F1 and F3 fractions

Cytotoxic and hemagglutinating antibodies induced by F2 in congenic B10.D2 and B10.B mice

Specific immunological enhancement induced by F2 fraction (A strain tumors in congenic mice)

Humoral tolerance induced in congenic newborn and adult B10.D2 mice (specific and long lasting)

Migration inhibition of peritoneal exudate cells (PEC) by crude soluble (CS) and F2 fractions (specific)

β_2-Microglobulin activity detected in our H-2^a preparation

tion of only $1-5 \times 10^6$ F_1 cells. Multiple antigenic specificities are operative in B10.A → B10.D2, whereas principally H-2.31 (and 34) is responsible for immunological reactivity in B10.D2 → B10.A. Passive enhancement is reported to be easily achieved in this latter combination (McKenzie and Snell, 1973), and several investigators (McKenzie et al., 1970; Rosenberg et al., 1971; Ranney et al., 1973) including our group have observed enhancing activity on skin graft or neonatal heart grafting with soluble H-2^d antigen using multiple injections of antigen with proper timing.

In contrast to our inability to achieve complete tolerance in B10.D2 mice with H-2^a antigens (within the limits of the regimens and doses employed), complete tolerance and partial tolerance of the cell-mediated form were induced in B10.A newborn mice with papain-solubilized B10.D2 (H-2^d) spleen cell antigens (see Table V). The biological activity of an F2 fraction and of further purified fractions has not yet been studied. That tolerance rather than enhancement is the explanation for the above results is seen in the failure to transfer unresponsiveness by pooled sera from our tolerized B10.A mice using as assays both skin grafts and enhanceable tumors.

Heterologous serum proteins that are highly immunogenic do not easily induce tolerance without an additional immunosuppressive factor; attempts are now being made to induce complete tolerance (both cell mediated and humoral) in B10.D2 mice with soluble H-2^a antigen and immunosuppression (see Brent et al., 1972).

Table V. Induction of Tolerance by Soluble H-2^d Antigen in
B10.A Newborn Mice[a]

| Group | B10.D2 skin graft survival in days (number of mice in group) | | | |
	No tolerance	Partial tolerance	Complete tolerance	Controls
I[b]	–	43.0(3)	>150(2)	20.5(5)
II[c]	18.0(2)	30.0(5)	>150(2)	17.0(5)
III	17.2(18)	–	>150(4)	13.5(5)
IV	–	$\left\{ \begin{array}{l} 21.7(7)^d \\ 50.0(2) \end{array} \right\}$	–	14.7(5)

[a] Unpublished results of L. W. Law, E. Appella, and S. Strober.
[b] Papain-solubilized antigen from B10.D2 spleen cells inoculated i.v. at birth (40 μg), then 20 μg daily i.p. × 30 in groups I, II, II; inoculations in group IV 40 μg at birth, then 20 μg × 15.
[c] Cytotoxic antibodies against B10.D2 lymphoid cells were assayed in group II after three weekly inoculations of antigen in the form of 60×10^6 (B10.A × B10.D2)F_1 spleen cells: mean $\log_2$ titers were 4.2 in controls, 5.1 in partially tolerant mice, and 0 in completely tolerant mice.
[d] B10.D2 skin grafts persisted for 26 days in four mice; B10.B skin grafts on partially tolerant and tolerant mice were rejected at the same time as controls.

We have studied the mechanism underlying the induction of humoral tolerance with our soluble H-2^a antigen by repopulating neonatally thymectomized hosts with thymus cell and lymph node cells from tolerant mice and lethally irradiated hosts with bone marrow and spleen cells (S. Strober, L. W. Law and E. Appella, to be published). Thymocytes and lymph node cells from tolerant donors were found capable of partially restoring humoral immunity in neonatally thymectomized hosts. Humoral immunity in tolerant animals was not broken by IV injection of nontolerant host strain lymphoid cells. Reactivity of irradiated hosts, however, completely returned to normal levels following transfer of spleen and bone marrow cells from tolerant donors. This "masking" phenomenon or reversible suppression of putatively tolerant B cells resembles the unresponsiveness in mice induced by the polysaccharide SIII (Howard, 1973).

The ultimate application of transplantation tolerance in man using soluble, purified transplantation antigens would appear reasonable and warranted since (1) large quantities of antigen are not necessary for induction, and (2) complete tolerance that is cell mediated as well as humoral can be achieved across major histocompatibility barriers with certain allelic differences.

V. OTHER BIOLOGICAL EFFECTS OF SOLUBILIZED H-2 ANTIGENS

Tissue grafting is time consuming and rather cumbersome. Thus the activity of solubilized H-2 antigens has been studied utilizing several *in vitro* assays. A major concern, however, is what *in vivo* event a particular *in vitro* assay reflects.

Inhibition of peritoneal cell (PEC) migration was observed when PEC from B10.D2 mice, immunized with congenic B10.A tissues, were incubated with our solubilized F2 fraction antigen from A strain (H-2^a haplotype) mice. This preparation had no effect on the migration of PEC from nonimmunized mice or on PEC sensitized by B10.B (H-2^b) congenic mice. This specificity was also rigidly maintained when using intact cells rather than F2 antigen. As low a concentration of antigen as 2 μg/ml (0.7 μg/chamber) using a micro-agarose assay was effective and a good dose–response relationship was observed (Maurer *et al.*, 1976). Similar findings have been reported by Maehara and McIvor (1975) and by Likhite and Sehon (1972). These investigators used relatively crude extracts, however.

In contrast to the effectiveness of our F2 fraction in migration inhibition, lymphocyte stimulation (LS) has not been achieved in the MLR assay using either the CS or F2 fraction (unpublished observations of J. H. Dean, E. Appella, and L. W. Law) despite the fact that intact, sensitized B10.D2 cells stimulate B10.A cells exceedingly well and in a specific manner.

Recently, Engers *et al.* (1975, and personal communication) have studied the capacity of particulate and soluble alloantigenic preparations to induce cytolytic thymus-derived effector cells (CTL) *in vitro*. Particulate antigen stimulated CTL when sensitized cells but not when nonsensitized cells were used as responding cells; solubilized antigen in contrast did not stimulate.

Particulate and soluble antigen preparations extracted with 3 M KCl or papain from target cells (leukemias) of different haplotype origin (H-2^b, H-2^d) were assayed for their ability to inhibit the destruction of intact ^{51}Cr-labeled target cells by lymphocytes (lymphocyte-mediated cytolysis). The effect of solubilized tumor cell antigens on the binding of killer cell lymphocytes to tumor cell monolayers was also evaluated. In contrast to their serological activity in inhibiting complement-mediated cytotoxicity of these same ^{51}Cr-labeled targets, these preparations, both particulate and soluble, failed to inhibit LMC or to bind to killer lymphocytes (Todd *et al.*, 1975). These findings were supported by previous results of Berke and Amos (1973), Plata and Levy (1974), and Sendo *et al.* (1974), but were contrary to the findings of other investigators (Bonavido, 1974; Wekerle and Feldman, 1974; Wagner and Boyle, 1972) who found inhibition of LMC.

It is clear that more definitive characterization is necessary of the soluble H-2 antigens being tested in the various *in vitro* assays; inhibition of the cytotoxicity of polyspecific antisera is not adequate. Precise specificity controls should always be included in inhibition studies of this nature in which it is widely recognized that sensitivity to target cell lysis is easily influenced.

VI. BIOCHEMICAL PROPERTIES OF SOLUBLE H-2 ANTIGENS

Over the past years, the biochemical analysis of H-2 histocompatibility antigens has been the subject of intensive investigation (Nathenson and Cullen, 1974). We do not intend to review here all the data reported, but we will describe results particularly from our laboratory and others which relate to novel structural features of the H-2 system. H-2 antigen activity has been released by limited proteolysis with papain or solubilized by the nonionic detergent NP-40. This activity has been assayed both by the inhibition of cytotoxicity and by the antibody-binding assay. Purification to a degree of 80–90% has been achieved by a combination of gel filtration, affinity chromatography, and discontinuous polyacrylamide gel electrophoresis (Shimada and Nathenson, 1969; Hess and Davies, 1974; Appella *et al.*, 1975; Peterson *et al.*, 1975). We are now in the process of defining such an H-2^a preparation in terms of its broad biological activities. This material, when subjected to molecular weight analysis, yielded fragments of about 50,000 for the papain-solubilized antigens and about

380,000–130,000 for the NP-40-solubilized material. In dissociating conditions, the papain-solubilized antigens contained two components of approximately 37,000 and 11,000 held together by noncovalent linkage. In the same conditions, the NP-40 material, in addition to the β_2-microglobulin, contained about 60–70% of a material with an apparent molecular weight of 90,000–100,000, whereas the remainder showed a weight of about 50,000. The high molecular weight material was further shown to be composed of 50,000 dalton components upon reduction with β-mercaptoethanol. These results point out that about 40% of the detergent-solubilized H-2 antigens apparently have the form of disulfide-linked dimers. The relevance of these findings to any model proposing an immunoglobulinlike structure for H-2 antigens remains at the moment uncertain since any aggregation through disulfide interchanges has not been ruled out. The difference in molecular weight between the H-2 fragments solubilized by papain and the antigen molecules solubilized by NP-40 appears to be 10,000. This fragment is antigenically silent and represents the hydrophobic region necessary for insertion in the lipid bilayer of the membrane, as has been shown for glycophorin and cytochrome b_5 (Segrest et al., 1971; Spatz and Strittmatter, 1971).

Reports from several laboratories, including our own, have shown that the two-component structures which were first revealed for the human HL-A antigen molecules were also found in the mouse (Silver and Hood, 1974; Rask et al., 1974; Appella et al., 1975). The smaller-component β_2-microglobulin has the molecular weight of 11,000 and appears to be noncovalently bound to the larger component; it dissociates easily under mild conditions such as exposure to a glycine-HCl buffer at pH 2.4. This small component has also been observed in detergent-solubilized H-2 preparations. By the use of rabbit antibodies reactive with the 11,000 dalton component of rat Ag-B antigens, an 11,000 dalton substance from 3 M NaSCN extracts of mouse liver cell membranes has been isolated and purified (Natori et al., 1974). The 11,000 dalton component appears to be the mouse homologue of human β_2-microglobulin. It has homology in amino acid composition to constant domains of mouse immunoglobulins (Table VI). It is indistinguishable antigenically from the 11,000 dalton component isolated from the H-2 antigen molecule. It cross-reacts weakly with rabbit antisera against human β_2-microglobulin (Natori et al., 1975a). In addition, this component is present in plasma and urine of normal mice of different strains (Natori et al., 1976a).

Figure 2 reports the partial amino acid sequence of mouse β_2-microglobulin as compared with the human β_2-microglobulin and the rabbit and dog homologues. Of the 39 residues compared, there are only eight differences from the human protein and the dog homologue, and 11 differences from the rabbit homologue. The data support the conclusion that the mouse protein is a homologue of β_2-microglobulin and indicate that all four proteins are closely related.

Table VI. Amino Acid Composition of Mouse β_2-Microglobulin

Amino acid	Mouse β_2-microglobulin[a] (residues/mol)	Human β_2-microglobulin[b] (residues/mol)	Difference
Aspartic acid	10.3 (10)	12	−2
Threonine	7.1 (7)	5	+2
Serine	6.8 (7)	10	−3
Glutamic acid	11.1 (11)	11	0
Proline	8.1 (8)	5	+3
Glycine	4.5 (4)	3	+1
Alanine	4.7 (5)	2	+3
Half-cystine	1.6 (2)	2	0
Valine	5.2 (5)	7	−2
Methionine	3.8 (4)	1	+3
Isoleucine	5.9 (6)	5	+1
Leucine	4.4 (4)	7	−3
Tyrosine	4.1 (4)	6	−2
Phenylalanine	3.7 (4)	5	−1
Lysine	9.1 (9)	8	+1
Histidine	4.3 (4)	4	0
Arginine	3.5 (4)	5	−1
Tryptophan	2.0 (2)	2	0

[a]The figures for all amino acids are average values from analysis of two different preparations, one from spleen and another from liver. The figures in parentheses are the nearest integer values.
[b]Data from Berggård and Bearn

When aligned for maximum homology, the mouse homologue of β_2-microglobulin appears to more closely resemble the $C_H 3$ region of IgG than any of the other homology regions. The extent of homology between the NH_2-terminal portion of mouse β_2-microglobulin and the homology regions of mouse IgG is similar to that found between the corresponding portions of human and rabbit β_2-microglobulins and the homology regions of human and rabbit IgG.

Studies of the binding activity of the larger component have been carried out with different alloantisera on heteroantisera. The results have shown that the isolated large components retain the H-2 allospecificities of the parental molecules. This assay has also demonstrated most directly that the H-2 specificities coded by the K region and the D region of the H-2 locus are carried by different molecules (Table VII). A rabbit antiserum raised against purified mouse β_2-microglobulin did bind the small component isolated from papain-solubilized H-2 molecules, but did not bind the large component. A rabbit antiserum raised against a preparation of papain-solubilized H-2 did bind both components; this strongly suggests that the large and small component have different antigenic determinants (Natori et al., 1976b).

	1	2	3	4	5	6	7	8	9	10
Mouse	Ile	Gln	Lys	Thr	Pro	Gln	Ile	Gln	Val	Tyr
Human	Ile	Gln	Arg	Thr	Pro	Lys	Ile	Gln	Val	Tyr
Dog	Val	Gln	His	Pro	Pro	Lys	Ile	Gln	Val	Tyr
Rabbit	Val	Gln	Arg	Ala	Pro	Asn	Val	Gln	Val	Tyr

	11	12	13	14	15	16	17	18	19	20
Mouse	Ser	Arg	His	Pro	Pro	Glu	Asn	Gly	Lys	Pro
Human	Ser	Arg	His	Pro	Ala	Glu	Asn	Gly	Lys	Ser
Dog	Ser	Arg	His	Pro	Ala	Glu	Asn	Gly	Lys	Pro
Rabbit	Ser	Arg	His	Pro	Ala	Glu	Asn	Gly	Lys	Asp

	21	22	23	24	25	26	27	28	29	30
Mouse	Asn	Ile	Leu	Asn	Cys	Tyr	Val	Thr	Glu	Phe
Human	Asn	Phe	Leu	Asn	Cys	Tyr	Val	Ser	Gly	Phe
Dog	Asn	Phe	Leu	Asn	Cys	Tyr	Val	Ser	Gly	Phe
Rabbit	Asn	Phe	Leu	Asn	Cys	Tyr	Val	Ser	Gly	Phe

	31	32	33	34	35	36	37	38	39	40
Mouse	His	Pro	Pro	?	Ile	Glx	Ile	Asx	Leu	Leu
Human	His	Pro	Ser	Asx	Ile	Glx	Val	Asx	Leu	Leu
Dog	His	Pro	?	Glx	Ile	Glx	Ile	Asx	Leu	Leu
Rabbit	His	Pro	Ser	Asp	Ile					

Figure 2. A comparison of the amino acid sequences of mouse, human, dog, and rabbit β_2-microglobulin. The data for the human protein are from Smithies and Poulik (1972) and from Peterson et al. (1972); for the dog protein, from Smithies and Poulik (1972); for the rabbit protein, from Cunningham and Berggård (1975); for the mouse protein, from Appella et al. (1976).

Large components of H-2K^k and H-2D^d molecules from H-2^a haplotype tissues have also been prepared after radioiodination and immunoprecipitations and analyzed by gel isoelectric focusing. The patterns of the two samples were the same, indicating that a close similarity exists in the ionic charge of the two types of molecules (Natori et al., 1976b).

Highly purified papain-solubilized H-2 antigens have been subjected to further proteolytic cleavage with thermolysin or other enzymes. Two fragments of 11,000 and 20,000 daltons were obtained. These fragments each appeared to contain a single disulfide bridge of 60–70 amino acids (Peterson et al., 1975). Another quite interesting finding is the interaction between the H-2 antigens and *Staphylococcus* protein A (SpA). The SpA has been shown to react exclusively with the Fc portion of IgG and this interaction with H-2 implies that there is some homology between the two types of molecules. In the absence of data

Table VII. Percent Binding of Radioiodinated H-2
Large-Component Preparations with Various
H-2 Alloantisera

H-2 alloantiserum	^{125}I-labeled H-2 large-component from	
	H-2K^k molecule of H-2.23 specificity	H-2D^d molecule of H-2.4 specificity
Anti-H-2^a polyspecific	53	0[a]
Anti-H-2K^k private	58	-3
Anti-H-2K^k public	34	-5
Anti-H-2D^d private	1	51
Anti-H-2D^d public	-1	-2[b]

[a] Anti-H-2^a polyspecific antiserum did not bind with H-2D^d large component. This indicates that the anti-H-2^a antiserum, although polyspecific, does not contain antibodies directed to H-2D^d specificities in an amount sufficient to produce a significant level of binding with the H-2D^d large component.

[b] The lack of reaction with the anti-H-2D^d public antiserum is probably due to conformational changes which are known to occur during the acid splitting of the H-2 molecules.

on the primary structure of the large components, it is premature to speculate. The model put forward, namely, that the transplantation antigens correspond to constant domains of IgG, although provocative, still lacks hard facts required for it to be completely acceptable.

VII. CONCLUDING REMARKS

The limited amount of transplantation antigens on cells has precluded our obtaining amounts of highly purified material, particularly of the papain-solubilized material, to assay adequately for various biological functions. We have nevertheless proceeded to purification to a degree of 80–90% and are now in the process of assaying these antigen preparations in terms of broad biological activities. This purification has been achieved by combinations of gel filtration, affinity chromatography, and discontinuous polyacrylamide gel electrophoresis. Biological activity, for example, in tolerance induction employing our partially purified chromatographed F2 fraction of H-2^a antigen was obtained with a total dose of approximately 12.0 μg protein (0.4 μg daily × 30 injections) in congenic B10.D2 mice. Assuming that full biological activity is maintained in further purified H-2^a antigen at our estimated 500-fold purification step, then nanogram amounts of purified antigen should have biological activity.

H-2 antigens contain a homologue of β_2-microglobulin. This small component is rather easily dissociable from the large component bearing the H-2 determinants. It is important therefore to assess the role of β_2-microglobulin in modulating H-2 function, by assaying *in vitro* for the biological functions of H-2 devoid of β_2-microglobulin and by assaying *in vivo* if this proves possible. It is known, for example, that β_2-microglobulin is not necessary for HL-A antigens to react with HL-A antibody in the blocking test (Poulik *et al.*, 1974). Also, isolation of the large component of HL-A could be obtained by the use of antibodies directed to human β_2-microglobulin; the 33,000 dalton fragments so prepared carried alloantigenic activity comparable to that of the original 48,000 dalton HL-A preparation (Nakamuro *et al.*, 1975).

Since a small hydrophobic piece of approximately 10,000 daltons is lost in papain solubilization but not through the use of detergents, it becomes necessary to assay for broad biological activity of H-2 antigens solubilized by, for example, deoxycholate; although the hydrophobic piece is presumably antigenically silent, it remains important to compare a purified detergent-solubilized material with purified papain-solubilized material over a broad range of biological activities.

We have no immediate answer to our lack of success in inducing complete immunological tolerance, that is, cell-mediated as well as humoral, in newborn B10.D2 congenic mice through the use of our F2 fraction H-2^a antigen.* Genetic disparity may be the important factor rather than modification or loss of some determinants in the solubilized material. In grafting B10.A to B10.D2, as discussed previously, it is difficult to achieve cell-mediated tolerance with intact lymphoid cells; in contrast, complete tolerance is achieved in nearly 80% of the recipients in B10.D2 to B10.A grafting. In this direction, only one (H2.31) or a few specificities are called into play. Induction of complete tolerance, cell-mediated and humoral, was achieved in approximately 15% of B10.A recipients with soluble (crude soluble) H-2^d antigen obtained from B10.D2 spleen cell membranes. The results of Billingham and Silvers (1960) are of interest here. In their studies of host response (female C57BL strain) to a single, relatively weak transplantation antigen, the Y antigen (determined by the H-Y locus) in C57BL males, it was found (1) that as few as 10,000 lymphoid cells will induce cell-mediated tolerance of a long-lasting nature and (2) that tolerance, although at a reduced frequency, could be induced by extracts prepared from male spleen cells.

Tests for *in vitro* H-2 activity have been attempted. Although antigens on particulate and intact cells appear to be active in a variety of assays, solubilized antigens have restricted or no activity (except in PEC migration inhibition

*In preliminary studies in this laboratory (O. Henriksen, E. Appella, and L.W. Law, unpublished results), cell-mediated tolerance could not be achieved in congenic newborn B10.D2 mice using a 500-fold purified H-2^a antigen preparation, employing the same regimen as that for the F2 fraction antigen.

where specific activity has been found with low concentration of antigen). Such studies need to be continued and the relevance of *in vitro* activities to *in vivo* events need to be defined.

The studies of H-2 antigens have provided us with an excellent model for approaching the problems of solubilization, purification, and biological and biochemical characterization of specific membrane-located tumor antigens (see Law and Appella, 1975).

VIII. REFERENCES

Appella, E., Henriksen, O., Natori, T., Tanigaki, N., Law, L.W., and Pressman, D., 1975, *Transplant Proc.* 7:191.

Appella E., Tanigaki, N., Natori, T., and Pressman, D., 1976, *Biochem. Biophys. Res. Commun.* 70:425.

Berggård, I., and Bearn, A. G., 1968, *J. Biol. Chem.* 243:4095.

Berke, G., and Amos, D.B., 1973, *Transplant Rev.* 17:71.

Billingham, R.E., and Silvers, W.K., 1960, *J. Immunol.* 85:14.

Bonavido, B., 1974, *J. Immunol.* 112:926.

Brent, L., Brooks, C., Lubling, N., and Thomas, A.V., 1972, *Transplantation* 14:382.

Cudkowicz, G., 1968, In: *The Proliferation and Spread of Neoplastic Cells*, p. 661, Williams and Wilkins, Baltimore.

Cunningham, B.A., and Berggård, I., 1975, *Science* 187:1079.

Engers, H.D., Thomas, K., Cerottini, J.-C., and Brunner, K.T., 1975, *J. Immunol.* 115:356.

Graff, R.G., and Nathenson, S.G., 1971, *Transplant. Proc.* 3:249.

Graff, R.J., Mann, D.L., and Nathenson, S.G., 1970, *Transplantation* 10:59.

Hess, M., and Davies, A.L., 1974, *Eur. J. Biochem.* 41:1.

Hilgert, I., 1974, *J. Immunogenet.* 1:153.

Howard J.G., 1973, In: *Defence and Recognition Biochemistry Series*, 1, 10 (H.L. Kornberg and D.C. Phillips, eds.), p. 103, Butterworths, London.

Howard, J.G., Michie, D., and Woodruff, M.F.A., 1961, In: *Transplantation* (O.B.E. Wolstenholme and M.P. Cameron, eds.), p. 138, Little, Brown, Boston.

Klein, J., Hanptfield, M., and Hanptfield, V., 1974, *Immunogenetics* 1:45.

Law, L.W., and Appella, E., 1975, In: *Cancer: A Comprehensive Treatise*, Vol IV, (F.F. Becker, ed.), Plenum Press, New York.

Law, L.W., Appella, E., Wright, P.W., and Strober, S., 1971, *Proc. Natl. Acad. Sci. USA* 68: 3078.

Law, L.W., Appella, E., Strober, S., Wright, P.W., and Fischetti, T., 1972, *Proc. Soc. Natl. Acad. Sci. USA* 69:1858.

Law, L.W., Appella, E., Cohen, J.M., and Dean, J.H., 1973, *Nature* (*London*) New Biol. 246:174.

Law, L.W., Appella, E., Strober, S., Wright, P.W., and Fischetti, T., 1974a, *Transplantation* 18:487.

Law, L.W., Appella, E., Cohen, J.M., and Wright, P.W., 1974b, *Transplantation* 18:14.

Likhite, V., and Sehon, A., 1972, *Science* 175:204.

Maehara, K.T., and McIvor, K.L., 1975, *Cell Immunol.* 15:11.

Maurer, B.A., Dean, J.H., McCoy, J.L., Appella, E., and Law, L.W., 1976, *J. Natl. Cancer Inst.* (in press).

McKenzie, I.F.C., and Snell, G.D., 1973, *J. Exp. Med.* **138**:259.

McKenzie, I.F.C., Koene, R.A., Painter, E., Sachs, D., Winn, H.J., and Russell, P.S., 1970, In: *Proceedings of the Symposium on Immunogenetics of the H-2 System*, p. 231, Karger, Basel.

Murphy, D.B., and Shreffler, D.C., 1975, *Transplantation* **20**:38.

Nakamuro, K., Tanagaki, N., and Pressman, D., 1975, *Transplantation* **19**:431.

Nathenson, S.G., and Cullen, S.E., 1974, *Biochim. Biophys. Acta* **344**:1.

Natori, T., Katagiri, M., Tanigaki, N., and Pressman, D., 1974, *Transplantation* **18**:550.

Natori, T., Tanigaki, N., Appella, E., and Pressman, D., 1975, *Biochem. Biophys. Res. Commun.* **65**:611.

Natori, T., Tanigaki, N., and Pressman, D., 1976a *J. Immunogenet.* (in press).

Natori, T., Tanigaki, N., Pressman, D., Henriksen, O., Appella, E., and Law, L.W., 1976b, *J. Immunogenet.* (in press).

Parish, C.R., 1971, *J. Exp. Med.* **134**:1.

Peterson, P.A., Cunningham, B.A., Berggård, I., and Edelman, G.M., 1972, *Proc. Natl. Acad. Sci. USA* **69**:1697.

Peterson, P.A., Rask, L., Sege, K., Klareskog, L., Anundi, H., and Osterg, L., 1975, *Proc. Natl. Acad. Sci. USA* **72**:1612.

Plata, F., and Levy, J.P., 1974, *Nature (London)* **249**:271.

Poulik, M.D., Ferrone, S., Pellegrino, M.A., Sevier, D.E., Oh, S.K., and Reisfeld, R.A., 1974. *Transplant. Rev.* **21**:106.

Ranney, D.F., Gordon, R.O., Pincus, J.H., and Oppenheim, J.J., 1973, *Transplantation* **16**:558.

Rask, L., Ostberg, L., Lindblom, B., Fernstedt, Y., and Peterson, P.A., 1974, *Transplant. Rev.* **21**:85.

Rosenberg, E.B., Mann, D.C., Hill, J.J., and Fahey, J.L., 1971, *Transplantation* **12**:402.

Segrest, J.P., Jackson, R.L., Andrews, E.P., and Marchesi, V.T., 1971, *Biochem. Biophys. Res. Commun.* **44**:390.

Sendo, F., Aoki, T., and Buafo, C.K., 1974, *J. Natl. Cancer Inst.* **52**:7691.

Shimada, H., and Nathenson, S.G., 1969, *Biochemistry* **8**:4048.

Silver, J., and Hood, L., 1974, *Nature (London)* **249**:764.

Smithies, O., and Poulik, M.D., 1972a, *Proc. Natl. Acad. Sci. USA* **69**:2914.

Smithies, O., and Poulik, M.D., 1972b, *Science* **175**:187.

Spatz, L., and Strittmatter, P., 1971, *Proc. Natl. Acad. Sci. USA* **68**:1042.

Strober, S., Appella, E., and Law, L.W., 1970, *Proc. Natl. Acad. Sci. USA* **67**:765.

Todd, R.F., Stulting, R.D., and Amos, D.B., 1975, *Cell. Immunol.* **18**:304.

Wagner, H., and Boyle, W., 1972, *Nature (London)* New Biology **240**:92.

Wekerle, H., and Feldman, M., 1974, *Eur. J. Immunol.* **4**:240.

Wright, P.W., Law, L.W., Appella, E., and Bernstein, I.D., 1974, *Transplantation* **17**:524.

Solubilization of Biologically Active Cell Surface Antigens

Jack H. Pincus

Life Sciences Division
Stanford Research Institute
Menlo Park, California

I. INTRODUCTION

The importance of the plasma membrane in the maintenance and regulation of a cell's physiological state, its interaction with other cells, and its antigenic individuality has been well established. In addition to acting as a protective barrier against toxic substances and regulating the intracellular ion balance, it has several functions of critical importance to cellular metabolism. Among these are the regulation of nutrient transport (Oxender, 1972), the interactions with polypeptide hormones that regulate certain intracellular events (Cuatrecasas, 1974), and a number of unique enzymatic activities (Coleman, 1973). The external surface of the plasma membrane also contains proteins that are responsible for the recognition of cells of the same type (Moscona, 1965).

Several of the components exposed at the external surface of the plasma membranes of both lymphoid and nonlymphoid cells are of particular interest to immunologists. The membranes of B lymphocytes contain immunoglobulin molecules that are believed to be responsible for antigenic recognition (Sell and Gell, 1965; Ada and Byrt, 1969; Raff *et al*; 1970). Such cells also possess receptors for the Fc portion of IgG (Basten *et al*; 1972) and the activated third component of complement (Nussenzweig and Pincus, 1972). The presence of θ antigen on T lymphocytes is unique for these cells (Reif and Allen, 1964). Membrane glycoproteins function as receptors for plant lectins (Greaves and Janossy, 1972), many of which, upon interaction with lymphoid cells, cause the initial events that result in cell division. A number of surface proteins are allelo-

87

morphic and thus responsible for antigenic individuality. Among these are the blood group antigens, the histocompatibility antigens responsible for allograft rejection, the antigenic determinants involved in the mixed leukocyte reaction (Meo et al; 1973; Bach et al; 1972), and the neoantigens that appear on the surface of cells that have undergone a neoplastic transformation (Price and Baldwin, 1974).

The characterization of cell surface proteins can be achieved on one of several levels—intact cells, isolated plasma membranes, and individual membrane components. Through the use of intact cells, a definition of the complete biological response associated with a particular membrane activity can be achieved. The immunological response to any membrane antigen in situ can also be studied. In addition, by using an electron microscope, the distribution of antigens and other proteins exposed to the external surface, for which ligands are available, can be studied. Experiments performed on the isolated membrane can illustrate the complexity of its protein constituents, which of these are glycoproteins, and which ones may be responsible for a particular antigenic activity. The early, membrane-associated events of any biological process can also be studied in detail. A comprehensive biochemical study of any individual membrane-associated biological activity, however, involves the separation of its constituents from other components. In the case of membrane proteins the initial step in such an undertaking involves solubilization with the concomitant retention of biological activity.

The success with which biologically active membrane proteins have been solubilized is quite variable. The methodology is largely empirical, and it is not always clear why a particular reagent successfully solubilizes some activities and not others. Generalizations as to the usefulness of any given procedure therefore cannot be made. In many cases, even though solubilized proteins exhibit biological activity, biochemical differences between these and the same proteins in the membrane have not been established.

The purpose of this chapter is not to review solubilization procedures per se, since most protocols developed may only apply to a particular system. A general discussion of the isolation of membrane proteins and the associated problems of cell sources and membrane preparation will first be presented. In order to illustrate the rationale and problems associated with the development of specific methodology, the solubilization of three membrane-associated proteins of interest to immunologists will be considered in detail.

II. GENERAL PROBLEMS ASSOCIATED WITH THE ISOLATION OF MEMBRANE PROTEINS

A. Cell Sources

The success of any biochemical isolation procedure is, in part, dependent on the availability of cells or tissue containing a relative abundance of the component of interest. This consideration is particularly important with respect to membrane proteins since only 1.5-13.8% of the total cellular protein is in the membrane (Crumpton and Snary, 1974); and membrane isolation procedures often result in low yields. Thus large amounts of a given tissure may be required to obtain very small amounts of purified plasma membranes. It is easily seen how the problem can be further compounded if the protein of interest represents a small fraction of the total cell membrane.

Whole tissue has largely been used as the starting material for the isolation of membrane proteins. Even though this may be the only available source of cells, there are several problems associated with its use. Some tissues, such as kidney and lung, contain a considerable amount of connective tissue, causing difficulties in homogenization and resulting in a reduction in the yields of particulate subcellular fractions. Furthermore, most tissues are composed of a heterogeneous cell population and, even when thoroughly washed, are contaminated with residual blood cells. Thus, if the membrane protein of interest is not present on all cells, an inordinately large tissue mass may be required. This is especially true with tumor tissue since a large portion of a solid tumor may be necrotic, and the number of viable cells that can be obtained from the tumor mass may be very small.

If an allelic membrane antigen or a tumor antigen not common to all tumors of the same type is sought, a further complication in the use of whole tissues is the impossibility of using pooled random samples of organs obtained from outbred individuals. Although inbred animals represent a partial solution to this problem, most of these are small (rodents), and a large number of animals may be required for a single experiment. It is obvious that this approach is not applicable to human tissue. However, the recent development of a cell separator (Aminco Celltrifuge) offers a solution for the collection of large amounts of blood cells from a single donor. It is possible to use the same donor on more than one occasion, thus assuring a continuous supply of cells. This technique has been used to collect peripheral leukocytes (E. Etheridge, personal communication) and platelets (Voigtman et al., 1974) for the extraction of human histocompatibility (HL-A, human leukocyte locus A) antigens.

An alternative to the use of whole tissue is the use of cultured cells. Tissue culture techniques permit the large-scale growth of a relatively homogeneous cell population. This approach is especially advantageous when working with allelic membrane antigens or tumor-specific antigens. Lymphoblastoid cell lines have been grown in suspension culture (Moore et al., 1967) yielding sufficient numbers of cells for biochemical studies and used for the isolation of HL-A antigens (Mann et al., 1968; Reisfeld et al., 1970). An advantage to their use in such studies is that, compared to peripheral lymphocytes obtained from the same individual, the cultured cells have a higher antigenic content (Pellegrino et al., 1972a). A murine lymphoma (L1210) grown in suspension culture has similarly been used for the isolation of mouse histocompatibility (H-2) antigens (Ranney et al.,

1973; Götze and Reisfeld, 1974) and plasma membrane glycoproteins (Hourani et al., 1973). The large-scale growth of adherent cells has been complicated by the large surface area required to achieve this. However, the recent development of a culture flask with a spiral plastic sheet (House et al., 1972) permits the growth of large quantities of such cells in a reasonable volume of culture medium, making it possible to generate sufficient amounts of adherent cells for membrane protein isolation.

The cultured cell counterpart of every normal cell is not always available and thus, in many instances, whole tissue must be used. In addition, several variables attendant to the use of tissue culture lines must be considered. The establishment of a cell in culture may result in the loss of a membrane-associated activity, thus rendering it unsuitable for use, or the phenotype may be altered, resulting in an altered cell surface (Moore and Woods, 1972). In these instances, the membrane proteins isolated may not be representative of those on normal cells. Furthermore, the expression of a number of cell surface proteins may vary with the cell cycle (Buell and Fahey, 1969; Cikes and Friberg, 1971; Götze et al., 1972; Pellegrino et al., 1972b; Hourani et al., 1973). Nevertheless, the control of any or all of these variables is not insurmountable. A few preliminary experiments can determine the cell line on which the surface proteins of interest are representative of normal cells and the appropriate growth conditions that result in maximum expression.

B. Membrane Preparation

The isolation of the plasma membrane, prior to membrane protein solubilization, permits the removal of the bulk of the cellular protein and, at least in theory, facilitates the subsequent protein purification. The subject of membrane purification and criteria of purity has been reviewed (Warren and Glick, 1971; Wallach and Lin, 1973; Crumpton and Snary, 1974) and will be discussed here only in general terms.

The ability to obtain purified plasma membranes in high yields is dependent on the development of conditions for maximum cell breakage and procedures for the efficient separation of the plasma membrane from other cellular and subcellular components. Although the general principles are the same for all cells, many of the published schemes are successful only when used on the specific cell or tissue for which they were designed. Therefore, it is necessary to develop schemes for each individual cell or tissue that yield a maximum of highly purified membranes.

Whole tissue can be disrupted by gentle homogenization in an isotonic buffer with a ground glass homogenizer, resulting in maximum cell rupture with minimum damage to subcellular particles. This procedure is not effective for single-cell suspensions or cultured cells. One approach to the disruption of these types of cells has been nitrogen decompression (Kamat and Wallach, 1965), which fragments the plasma membrane into small vesicles with a minimum of nuclear breakage. A more generally used approach is hypotonic swelling in the presence of membrane-stabilizing agents, such as fluorescein mercuric acetate, zinc chloride, tris ions, or divalent metals, followed by cell rupture using a Dounce homogenizer (Warren *et al.*, 1966). When this procedure is used on nucleated cells, large membrane fragments are usually obtained, one exception being HeLa cells in which large cell ghosts are produced (Boone *et al.*, 1969).

The precise hypotonic buffer, membrane stabilizing agent, swelling time, and the extent of homogenization must be empirically determined for each cell type in order to achieve maximum cell rupture with minimum nuclear breakage. One may encounter difficulties with this technique when cells grown on monolayers are used, even after removal of the cells from the surface, since a large percentage often do not rupture. However, recent experiments with a human colon carcinoma cell line indicate that treating the cells in a calcium-free Tyrode's buffer for 1-2 h prior to hypotonic swelling and Dounce homogenization may overcome these difficulties (J. H. Pincus, unpublished observation).

Once lysis has been achieved, isolation of cell membranes from a lysate generally depends on their difference in density and involves the use of differential centrifugation and/or density gradient centrifugation. These procedures are lengthy and the yields of purified plasma membranes are often not quantitative. Two recent developments that offer alternatives to strict density fractionation, and may prove superior in some cases, are worth mentioning. Based on the fact that different cellular membranes differ in chemical composition (Bosmann *et al.*, 1968), Brunette and Till (1971) have applied the aqueous two-phase polymer systems developed by Albertson (1960), for separating particles on the basis of differences in surface properties, to the isolation of L-cell membranes. The procedure is fast (less than 2 h) and the yields are good. These principles have been applied successfully to the isolation of plasma membranes from a cultured mouse lymphoma (L1210) (Hourani *et al.*, 1973) and rat liver (Lesko *et al.*, 1973). The second method, termed "affinity density perturbation" (Wallach *et al.*, 1972), is based on the specific receptor content of the plasma membrane. A ligand is covalently bound to a high-density particle, which is then allowed to react with a membrane, causing an increase in density and allowing separation. Concanavalin A (Con A) bound to K29 coliphage has thus been used to fractionate pig lymphocyte plasma membranes containing the Con A receptor.

As with conditions for hypotonic lysis, the exact procedure for fractionation of plasma membranes depends on the cell used. Appropriate manipulations, based on the principles outlined above, should result in a highly purified plasma membrane obtained in a suitable yield.

C. Solubilization of Cell Surface Components

1. Theoretical Problems Associated with the Solubilization of Biologically Active Components: Composition and Organization of the Plasma Membrane

In order to develop techniques for the solubilization of biologically active cell surface components, it is first necessary to understand the constitution and organization of the plasma membrane. The plasma membrane is composed of three major components—proteins, lipids, and carbohydrates. Proteins are the predominant component, being present in a weight ratio of 1.5–4 times that of lipids (Korn, 1969). The majority of the carbohydrate is present as oligosaccharide chains linked to asparagine, serine, or threonine in membrane glycoproteins (Jamieson and Greenwalt, 1971). Lipids are present as neutral lipids and phospholipids.

Based on thermodynamic considerations and experimental data, Singer and Nicolson (1972) have proposed a model for the organization of these components in the membrane, referred to as the "fluid mosaic model." In this model, the phospholipids of the membrane are arranged as a bilayer with the hydrophilic heads exposed at the cytoplasmic and external surfaces and the hydrophobic tails sequestered away from the aqueous environment. The membrane proteins can be divided into two classes: (1) peripheral proteins which are not strongly associated with the membrane lipids, and (2) integral proteins, representing the major portion of the protein of most membranes, which are intimately associated with lipids. Proteins of this latter class are probably amphipathic, and their hydrophobic segments are embedded in the interior of the membrane alternating with phospholipids and forming an interrupted bilayer (see Figs. 2 and 3 of Singer and Nicolson, 1972). Such integral proteins may be partially embedded in the phospholipid bilayer or may completely traverse it, as has been shown to be the case for the major human erythrocyte glycoprotein (Bretscher, 1971; Segrest et al., 1973). In addition to their interaction with lipids, the interaction of either class of membrane proteins with each other to form homo- or heteroaggregates is also possible and has not been experimentally ruled out.

Under physiological conditions, membrane lipids are in a fluid state. The "fluid mosaic model" indicates that the integral proteins are free to undergo lateral diffusion within the plane of the membrane. However, recent evidence suggests that at least some proteins that traverse the phospholipid bilayer may interact with a submembranous assembly composed of microtubules and microfilaments that restricts their mobility (Edelman et al., 1973). This could result in a short-range order of certain membrane proteins.

The organization of proteins in a lipid bilayer as illustrated in the "fluid mosaic model" and their interactions with submembranous components result in a supramolecular structure that may be necessary for the maintenance of certain biological activities. In addition, the maintenance of specific lipid–protein inter-actions and a defined microenvironment characteristic of the membrane may also contribute to this. Since solubilization involves the disruption of the supra-molecular structure and, in many instances, the loss of lipid–protein or protein-protein interactions, those agents that solubilize with the minimal alteration of the constraints necessary for maintaining biological activity will be the most successful.

2. Methods for Solubilizing Membrane Proteins

Solubilization of membrane proteins is achieved by compounds that cause their release into aqueous media. The ease with which this is accomplished is a function of whether the protein is peripheral or integral, and, in the latter case, the extent of its association with membrane phospholipids. Peripheral proteins can be readily solubilized, free of lipids, by using mild nondenaturing conditions. Examples of two such proteins found on the inner surface of the erythrocyte membrane are spectrin (Marchesi and Steers, 1968) and glyceraldehyde 3-phosphate dehydrogenase (Kant and Steck, 1973; Shin and Carraway, 1973). On the other hand, the release of integral proteins involves using conditions that dis-rupt the phospholipid bilayer, and often causes protein denaturation (Coleman, 1973). As mentioned above, these conditions may result in the loss of biological activity.

Membrane proteins in aqueous solution are in a different microenvironment than that of the membrane. Thus solubilized proteins may exhibit biological ac-tivity, but their properties in solution may differ from the corresponding membrane-bound activities. This was first observed for mitochondrial ATPase, in which the soluble enzyme was shown to have lost its sensitivity to several inhibi-tors (Racker, 1967). Similarly, membrane-bound adenylate cyclase is activated by hormones, whereas the detergent-solubilized form, although catalytically ac-tive, loses this sensitivity (Pilkins and Johnson, 1974). A careful comparison of the biological properties of membrane-bound and solubilized antigens has not been made. Although such soluble proteins may still combine with antibodies made against their membrane-bound counterparts or remain immunogenic, this only suggests that gross alterations have not occurred. It thus seems necessary to define carefully the biological activity of antigens in the membrane with respect to their avidity for antibodies and doses needed to obtain an immune response in order to determine how truly "native" solubilized antigens are.

Several methods that have been used for the solubilization of membrane pro-teins of interest to immunologists are listed in Table I. When different proce-dures are used to isolate the same protein, the final product may not be the same in all cases. Unfortunately, sufficient data are not available to permit a compari-son of the different products.

The exact conditions for the solubilization of any membrane protein can only be empirically determined and Table I is therefore meant to serve merely as a guide. A general discussion of the merits of each method may, however, aid in developing an approach to the problem.

Controlled proteolytic digestion has been used to solubilize several membrane enzymes (Coleman, 1973) and a number of cell surface antigens (see Table I). This technique is generally most successful for proteins that do not show an obligatory lipid requirement for biological activity. However, optimal conditions for proteolytic solubilization may result in large losses of the activity originally present in the membrane (Shimada and Nathenson, 1969). This is probably due to proteolysis secondary to solubilization. In addition, the solubilized product, although biologically active, may not be representative of the same protein in the membrane. This was shown to be the case for microsomal cytochrome b_5 by Strittmatter and collaborators. Both enzymatic (Strittmatter and Velick, 1957) and detergent (Spatz and Strittmatter, 1971) extraction procedures have been used to solubilize this protein from beef hepatic microsomes. Comparison of amino acid sequence of the respective products demonstrated that the hydrolytic procedures digested a short polypeptide region extensively and left a hydrophobic segment of approximately 40 residues in the membrane (Spatz and Stittmatter, 1971). The reattachment of solubilized cytochrome b_5 to microsomal membranes occurred only with the detergent-extracted protein that contained the hydrophobic segment and this retained the amphipathic characteristics of a "native" membrane protein.

The brief exposure of cellular suspensions to low-frequency sound results in the release of cell surface proteins into aqueous media. This method has been used for the solubilization of histocompatibility antigens from a variety of tissues and cells (Kahan and Reisfeld, 1971) and more recently for tumor-specific antigens (Hollinshead et al., 1972). The mechanism by which this occurs is not entirely understood but may involve the physical disruption of noncovalent interactions. The technique involves the use of expensive equipment and carefully controlled experimental conditions. Under optimal conditions, the release of only 12–15% of the total histocompatibility antigen activity, from a number of tissues, has been achieved (Reisfeld and Kahan, 1970a). Because of the technical problems and low yields, this method is not widely used.

Detergents act by disrupting the lipid matrix and releasing those proteins that interact with membrane lipids. The mechanism of detergent solubilization and the nature of the solubilized product have recently been reviewed in detail (Helenius and Simons, 1975). Nonionic detergents have been the most useful as solubilizing agents that preserve biological activity. Many of these, however, are denaturing and the choice of the appropriate detergent and optimal solubilization conditions is largely empirical. It may be possible to obtain selective solubilization of some proteins with a given detergent by changing the ionic strength (Kyte, 1972; Yu et al., 1973).

A recent approach to the systematic selection of detergents has been devel-

Table I. Methods Used for the Solubilization of Membrane Proteins
of Immunological Interest

Method	Reagent used	Protein solubilized	References
Controlled enzymatic digestion	Papain	H-2 antigens	Shimada and Nathenson (1969)
		HL-A antigens	Mann et al. (1969)
			Miyakawa et al. (1971)
			Cresswell et al. (1973)
		Thymus leukemia antigen	Muramatsu et al. (1973)
		Tumor-specific antigens	Baldwin et al. (1971)
			Drapkin et al. (1974)
			Billing and Terasaki (1974)
	Trypsin	H-2 antigens	Edidin (1967)
	Phospholipase A	H-2 antigens	Kandutsch and Stimpfling (1962)
	β-Glucosidase	Tumor-specific antigens	Baldwin et al. (1974)
Low-frequency sound		H-2 antigens	Kahan (1965)
		HL-A antigens	Kahan and Reisfeld (1967, 1971)
		Tumor-specific antigens	Holmes et al. (1970)
			Hollinshead et al. (1972)
Detergents	Triton X-100	H-2 antigens	Kandutsch (1960)
	Nonidet P-40	H-2 antigens	Schwartz and Nathenson (1971)
		HL-A antigens	Dautigny et al. (1973)
		Cell surface immunoglobulin	Kennel and Lerner (1973)
		θ-Antigen	Letarte-Muirhead et al. (1974)
	Sodium lauryl sarcosinate	HL-A antigens	Reisfeld and Kahan (1970b)
	Sodium decyl-sulfate	H-2 antigens	Manson and Palm (1968)
	Sodium deoxycholate	H-2 antigens	Snary et al. (1974)
Hypertonic salt extraction	3 M KCl	H-2 antigens	Ranney et al. (1973)
			Götze and Reisfeld (1974)
		HL-A antigens	Reisfeld et al. (1971)
			Voigtman et al. (1974)
			Pincus et al. (1975)
		Tumor-specific antigens	Meltzer et al. (1971)
			Gutterman et al. (1972)
			Pellis et al. (1974)
Other noncovalent bond-breaking agents	Lithium diiodosalicylate	Tumor membrane glycoproteins	Hourani et al. (1973)
			Kuo et al. (1973)
		Carcinoembryonic antigen	Rosai et al. (1972)

oped by Umbreit and Strominger (1973). Detergents are selected on the basis of their HLB (hydrophobic lipophilic balance) number (Schick, 1967), which measures the relative hydrophobicity of a detergent. The ability of nonionic detergents to solubilize several membrane enzymes appears to correlate with this property.

At low detergent/protein ratios, particles containing lipid, protein, and detergent are released (Kagawa, 1972). At higher ratios, lipids are released from the complex as mixed detergent–lipid micelles, and lipid-binding sites on the protein are saturated with detergent (Helenius and Simons, 1975). In the latter cases, the complete removal of the detergent, which is acting to stabilize the protein in solution, may cause irreversible aggregation of the protein with a loss of biological activity, as has been observed in the isolation of H-2 antigens with Triton X-100 (Kandutsch, 1960). Therefore, the presence of lipid or its substitution by detergent molecules may, in many cases, be necessary for the demonstration of biological activity.

Finally, two reagents that solubilize some membrane proteins and can be quantitatively removed without affecting solubility or biological activity are 3 M KCl and lithium diiodosalicylate (LIS). These will be discussed at greater length in subsequent sections.

D. Development of Solubilization Schemes

As stated earlier, specific rules for the development of a solubilization scheme are not available. The cell source, method of membrane preparation, and choice of solubilization procedure must all be experimentally determined. To illustrate the logic involved in the development of such schemes and some of the specific problems that may be encountered, the solubilization of three immunologically relevant cell surface activities will be considered in detail.

III. PLASMA MEMBRANE GLYCOPROTEINS

A. Glycoprotein-Associated Activities and Membrane Location

In most cells that have been studied, glycoproteins are oriented in the membrane with their oligosaccharide side chains projecting at the outer surface (Winzler, 1970). Many of these glycoproteins exhibit carbohydrate-associated activities of interest to immunologists: (1) The plant lectins bind to specific sugars on the side chains of glycoproteins (Allan et al., 1971; Nicolson and Singer, 1971; Marchesi et al., 1972), resulting in the agglutination of transformed cells

(Inbar and Sachs, 1969; Lis and Sharon, 1973; Nicolson, 1974) or stimulation of DNA synthesis in resting lymphocytes (Greaves and Janossy, 1972). (2) The major erythrocyte membrane glycoprotein (glycophorin) contains M and N blood group antigens and the receptor for influenza virus (Marchesi and Andrews, 1971). (3) Malignant transformation may result in new or altered glycoproteins appearing on the cell surface (Krupey *et al.*, 1968; Buck *et al.*, 1970; van Beek *et al.*, 1973). Some of these may function as tumor antigens (Shier, 1971; Baldwin *et al.*, 1974).

The most extensively studied membrane glycoprotein has been the glycoprotein from the human erythrocyte (Marchesi and Andrews, 1971; Segrest *et al.*, 1973; Marchesi *et al.*, 1973; Steck, 1974). This is an amphipathic transmembrane protein. Its *N*-terminal region containing the oligosaccharide side chains is exposed at the outer surface. A hydrophobic amino acid sequence (Segrest *et al.*, 1973) is presumably sequestered in the phospholipid bilayer and interacts with membrane lipids. The *C*-terminal region is located at the inner membrane surface. In aqueous solution, the protein forms an aggregate with a molecular weight of approximately 500,000–600,000 (Springer *et al.*, 1966), the monomeric molecular weight being approximately 30,000 (Grefrath and Reynolds, 1974).

There is no direct evidence to indicate that glycoproteins in other cell types are similarly oriented. However, recent experiments on the Con A induced capping of lymphocyte membrane glycoproteins suggest that these interact with cytoplasmic structures (microtubules) at the inner membrane surface (Yahara and Edelman, 1973). Therefore, glycoproteins in other cells may also span the membrane and may be amphipathic in nature. Thus, for the purpose of developing solubilization procedures, it is safe to assume that glycoproteins in all cells are integral membrane proteins.

B. Isolation of Plasma Membrane Glycoproteins

Most of the information available on the nature of glycoproteins has been obtained by studying glycopeptides obtained by proteolytic cleavage of intact cells (Langley and Ambrose, 1964; Buck *et al.*, 1970, 1974; Codington *et al.*, 1970; Glick *et al.*, 1973; Neri *et al.*, 1974). With the exception of the human erythrocyte, as noted above, intact cell surface glycoproteins have not been isolated in sufficient quantities to permit their biochemical characterization. This has been due, in part, to an insufficient number of cells available as starting material and the tedious procedures that have been necessary for the preparation of plasma membranes. Procedures for cell growth, membrane preparation, and protein solubilization were combined in a scheme that permits the isolation of milligram quantities of membrane glycoproteins (Hourani *et al.*, 1973).

1. Choice of Cells and Growth Conditions

Based on the principles outlined in Section II, the initial consideration in developing an isolation procedure was given to the choice of cells. Although most cell membranes contain glycoproteins, the use of a tumor cell that is agglutinated by lectins not only serves as a starting material for glycoprotein isolation but also provides a convenient and simple means, by measuring inhibition of agglutination, for testing a cell-associated activity of the solubilized product. In order to reproducibly obtain large quantities of a relatively homogeneous tumor cell population, cultured tumor cells were chosen.

For these studies, L1210, a DBA/2 murine lymphoma adapted to grow in suspension culture (Hutchison *et al.*, 1966), was selected. These cells have an approximate doubling time of 12 h (J. H. Pincus, unpublished observation) and can be maintained in continuous culture in cytogenerators to routinely yield sufficient numbers of cells for preparative biochemical studies. L1210 cells are also agglutinated by a number of plant lectins, demonstrating that this property has not been lost during prolonged cultivation.

The agglutinability of L1210 cells by Con A as a function of cell density was first tested to determine whether it showed any variation. If so, this property could be used as an index for optimal growth conditions for glycoprotein expression and extraction. As seen in Table II, cells grown to a density of 8.4×10^5/ml are less agglutinable than those grown to 5.4×10^5/ml. Cells grown to very high densities are not agglutinated by any concentration of Con A. In pilot experiments using techniques described below, only those cells grown under conditions in which they are maximally agglutinable by Con A exhibited reproducible membrane glycoprotein patterns when examined by sodium dodecylsulfate-polyacrylamide gel electrophoresis. The yield of glycoproteins

Table II. Agglutination of L1210 Cells, Grown to Different Densities, by Concanavalin A

Cell density (cells/ml)[a]	Lowest Con A concentration (mg/ml) causing maximum agglutination[b]
5.4×10^5	0.032
8.4×10^5	0.500
1.5×10^5	Not agglutinable
2.1×10^6	Not agglutinable

[a] Final density to which cells were grown.
[b] Determined using a final cell concentration of 1×10^6/ml in phosphate-buffered (0.02 M, pH 7.2) saline (0.15 M). Maximum agglutination as determined microscopically is defined as 95% of the cells in large clumps, with only rare single cells visible.

obtained from such cells was also the highest. The agglutinability of L1210 cells by Con A thus appears to be an index for determining optimal growth conditions in order to obtain reproducible glycoprotein expression and maximal yields of the solubilized product. Therefore, based on the data in Table II, cells were always grown to densities of approximately 6×10^5/ml.

2. Cell Lysis and Plasma Membrane Isolation

Many of the published procedures for cell lysis proved to be unsatisfactory for L1210 cells. Two major problems were encountered. In some cases, such as when divalent cations at concentrations greater than 5 mM were used, the cells would swell but could not be ruptured, presumably because of extensive membrane stabilization. Under other conditions, as exemplified by 10 mM tris at slightly alkaline pH (7.4–8.5), cell rupture could be achieved but nuclear breakage was also quite extensive. Conditions for lysis of these cells thus had to be developed *de novo*.

Optimal conditions for lysis of L1210 cells consist of swelling washed cells in 10 vol of a solution containing 2 mM $NaHCO_3$, 0.2 mM $CaCl_2$, and 5 mM $MgCl_2$, the pH of the solution being 6.8. It should be noted that the ions, their concentration, and the pH all are critical for achieving maximum swelling and lysis. Cell rupture can be achieved by slow Dounce homogenization until at least 90% of the cells are broken, as determined by phase contrast microscopy. These lysing conditions result in maximum cell breakage with minimum nuclear damage.

Separation of plasma membranes from the homogenate can be achieved by a modification of the two-phase polyethylene glycol–dextran method of Brunette and Till (1971). This technique requires only 2.5 h for completion, and the resulting yields of plasma membranes are good. Moreover, the polymers used in this procedure may have a protective effect on the membranes and membrane proteins (Albertson, 1970).

The general protocol for the isolation of plasma membranes is diagrammed in Fig. 1. The method involves the collection of the lysed cellular and subcellular particles by centrifugation and purification of the plasma membrane fraction by distribution in the two-phase polymer system. As pointed out by Brunette and Till (1971), the exact procedure for polymer fractionation varies among cell lines. The conditions for L1210 membranes were thus derived experimentally and are directly applicable only to these cells (Hourani *et al.*, 1973).

The purity of the plasma membrane fraction can be established with respect to protein recovered, enzyme markers recovered, and electron microscopic appearance. Table III illustrates these data. The protein recovery is in good agreement with that of Brunette and Till (1971) for an L-cell membrane preparation. The majority of the Na^+, K^+-activated ATPase, a plasma membrane marker enzyme, is recovered with the isolated membrane. There is very little contamina-

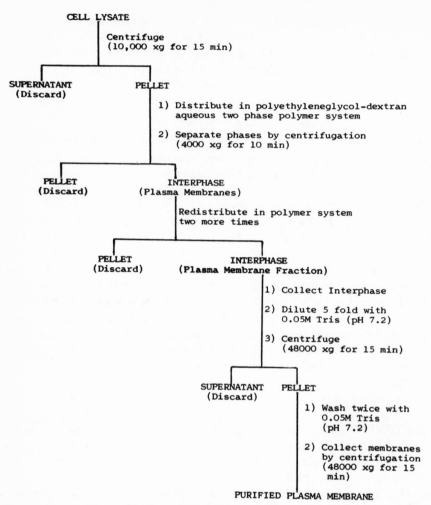

Figure 1. Protocol for purification of L1210 plasma membranes. For more specific details, see Hourani *et al.* (1973).

tion with NADH diaphorase, a marker for smooth endoplasmic reticulum. Electron microscopy of preparations negatively stained with 2% phosphotungstic acid shows sheets of membranes, large fragments rolled into myelin forms, and occasional vesicles. In a number of preparations examined, contamination with nonmembranous material was rarely seen. Thus, on the basis of both biochemical and morphological criteria, the methodology developed results in a highly purified plasma membrane fraction.

By using 5×10^{10} cells (approximately 50 g wet weight), a plasma membrane fraction containing 270 mg of protein can be obtained. The methods for

**Table III. Protein and Enzyme Recoveries in Isolated
Plasma Membranes**

Component	Recovery in membrane fraction (percentage of homogenate)	Marker for
Protein	9.3	–
(Na$^+$, K$^+$)-ATPase	72.9	Plasma membrane
NADH diaphorase	4.2	Smooth endoplasmic reticulum

cell lysis and membrane preparation work on fresh cells as well as those stored frozen in 12.5% dimethylsulfoxide and rapidly thawed before use. The latter fact permits the accumulation of large quantities of cells which can then be processed as a single batch. It is thus possible to isolate plasma membranes in sufficient quantity and purity for the subsequent solubilization of membrane glycoproteins.

3. Solubilization and Purification of Membrane Glycoproteins

Solubilization of L1210 glycoproteins can be effectively achieved by using lithium diiodosalicylate (LIS). This reagent has been used to extract the major human erythrocyte membrane glycoprotein in a water-soluble form (Marchesi and Andrews, 1971). Based on studies of Robinson and Jencks (1965) using model hydrophobic peptides, it appears to be a highly effective dissociating agent. Unlike detergents, LIS can be removed after the extraction without the solubilized protein precipitating. In addition, the extent of removal of the reagent can be followed spectrophotometrically since LIS has a characteristic absorption at 323 nm with a molar extinction coefficient of 4000 (Marchesi and Andrews, 1971).

The procedure used for glycoprotein solubilization and purification is outlined in Fig. 2. Addition of LIS results in a complete clarification of the solution both visually and microscopically. The glycoproteins can be separated from the remainder of the solubilized membrane proteins and lipids by virtue of the fact that they are insoluble in 25% phenol (final concentration). The preparation at this point is contaminated with nucleic acid which can be removed by digestion with staphylococcal nuclease (Cuatrecasas et al., 1967) for 4-6 h. By starting with 270 mg of total membrane protein, it is possible to obtain an average of 6 mg of purified soluble glycoprotein.

4. Properties of the Solubilized Glycoproteins

The sodium dodecylsulfate–polyacrylamide gel electrophoretic analysis of L1210 membranes and the isolated glycoproteins is shown in Fig. 3. When

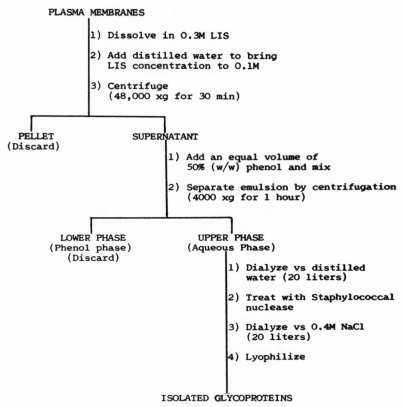

Figure 2. Procedure for the solubilization and fractionation of L1210 plasma
membrane glycoproteins. For more specific details, see Hourani *et al.* (1973).

stained for protein with Coomassie blue, the glycoprotein extract shows only six
of the bands present in the membrane. When gels of the membrane and the extract are stained for carbohydrate, four bands are found (I–IV), in both cases indicating that all of the glycoproteins in the membrane are extracted. The non-
glycoprotein-containing components in the extract represent either acidic
components that are not extracted by phenol or components that remain noncovalently associated with the glycoproteins throughout the extraction procedure. The extract contains all of the sugars characteristic of membrane glycoproteins (Hourani *et al.*, 1973). Only traces of ribose are found, indicating little
contamination with RNA. Of significance is the absence of glucose, indicating
little if any contamination with glycolipid (Kraemer, 1971).

The ability of the extract to inhibit the agglutination of L1210 cells by lec-

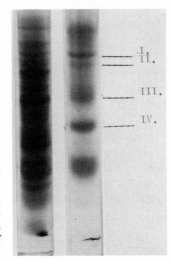

Figure 3. Sodium dodecylsulfate–polyacrylamide gels of L1210 plasma membranes (left) and isolated membrane glycoproteins (right). The gels shown are stained for protein with Coomassie blue. Roman numerals indicate those components which stained for carbohydrate, with periodic acid–Schiff on companion gels.

tins is shown in Table IV. At approximately equal concentrations of lectin and glycoprotein, agglutination is completely inhibited. The solubilized glycoproteins thus retain this carbohydrate-associated lectin receptor activity.

An additional confirmation that these isolated glycoproteins are representative of their plasma membrane counterparts can be obtained by raising antisera to the solubilized materials in rabbits. The antisera are specifically cytotoxic to intact L1210 cells (Hourani *et al.*, 1973), indicating that the components in the extract are membrane components, are accessible at the cell surface, and do not undergo any gross conformational changes during isolation.

Table IV. Inhibition of Lectin Agglutination of L1210 Cells by the Isolated Membrane Glycoprotein Fraction

Lectin	Specificity	Lowest concentration of lectin (mg/ml) causing maximum agglutination	Lowest concentration of glycoprotein (mg/ml) causing inhibition of agglutination
Con A	α-D-Mannose	0.062	0.105
Lens culinaris hemagglutinin	α-D-Mannose	0.20	0.12
Wheat germ agglutinin	*N*-Acetyl-D-glucosamine	0.036	0.043

C. Application to Other Membrane Glycoproteins and Prospects for Further Fractionation

LIS has been successfully used for the solubilization of carcinoembryonic antigen from colon carcinoma (Rosai *et al.*, 1972) and tumor membrane glycoproteins from mammary adenocarcinoma (Kuo *et al.*, 1973). The general approach described here, with appropriate modifications for specific cells, may thus be applicable to the isolation of other membrane glycoproteins.

In this study, further fractionation of individual glycoproteins from the mixture or from the nonglycosylated components was not attempted. Recent experiments on the fractionation of glycoproteins by affinity chromatography on lectin columns (Adair and Kornfeld, 1974) suggest that by using a number of columns with lectins of different specificities the individual components in a mixture might be separated.

IV. EXTRACTION OF HISTOCOMPATIBILITY ANTIGENS

A. A Biochemical Study of a Polymorphic System

Among the allelic cell surface components that function as alloimmunogens are the histocompatibility antigens. These membrane proteins are responsible, at least in part, for the host immune response against transplanted tissue from incompatible donors that ultimately leads to graft rejection.

The genetics and serology of the histocompatibility antigens have been widely studied and have been shown to exhibit extensive polymorphism in outbred populations. In most species that have been studied, a number of genes code for such cell surface proteins, each of which can cause varying degrees of allograft immunity. However, one set of antigenic determinants, termed "major histocompatibility antigens," is strongly immunogenic and responsible for the rapid rejection of transplanted tissue. This has been designated HL-A in man and H-2 in mice. These strong transplantation antigens have received considerable attention within the last several years.

The solubilization and purification of histocompatibility antigens are necessary in order to gain an understanding of the molecular basis for their genetic polymorphism. Solubilized transplantation antigens may also be useful as probes of the immune system to help gain an understanding of the events occurring in allograft immunity and to develop protocols for immune tolerance. Finally, the function of these cell surface proteins as alloimmunogens is probably secondary to their physiological function. Biochemical studies may thus aid in elucidating their primary function.

B. Detection of Histocompatibility Antigens

At present, the only known biological property of histocompatibility antigens is their role as alloimmunogens. Therefore, methods for detection are based on the *in vivo* demonstration of transplantation immunity in an allogeneic host or the *in vitro* reactivity with alloantibodies, as measured by complement-mediated immune cytolysis (cytotoxicity). These techniques involve the use of biological or cellular systems and can be used for the detection of both cell-bound and solubilized histocompatibility antigens.

In vivo methods involve immunization of an allogeneic host with either whole tissue or solubilized antigen. Host immunity can then be demonstrated by accelerated (second-set) rejection of a tissue graft possessing the same histocompatibility antigens as the immunogen. This is probably the most biologically significant assay since it is a true measure of transplantation immunity. Other *in vivo* measurements of immunity include the production of alloantibodies by cell-bound or solubilized antigens and the elicitation of delayed-type hypersensitivity reactions by solubilized materials in hosts that have been preimmunized with whole tissue or intact cells (Kahan and Reisfeld, 1969). It is not certain whether the latter two assays are necessarily measuring the same factors that are responsible for accelerated graft rejection.

Even though *in vivo* assays are the only way of comparing the immunogenic potency of cell-bound antigens to their solubilized counterparts, a quantitative evaluation may require a large number of animals. In addition, the time required for the completion of such assays may range from days to weeks. Therefore, they are not practical for the routine testing of solubilized antigens during the development of methods for solubilization and purification.

The most widely used *in vitro* assay for the detection of histocompatibility antigens has been the microdroplet cytotoxicity test initially developed by Terasaki and McClelland (1964) and modified by Mittal *et al.* (1968). In addition to detecting antigens on surfaces of cells, the method has been adapted for the assay of solubilized human (Pellegrino *et al.*, 1972c) and mouse (Pincus and Gordon, 1971) histocompatibility antigens by measuring their ability to inhibit the cytotoxic effect of alloantibodies. A detailed discussion of the assay and the factors affecting it, such as the sensitivity of the antisera, the choice of target cells, and specificity controls, has been published (Pellegrino *et al.*, 1973a) and will not be dealt with in detail here.

The amount of solubilized protein required to inhibit 50% of the cytotoxicity of a given antiserum at the last dilution where the antiserum is cytotoxic to 95% of the cells is referred to as the ID_{50} and contains 1 unit of antigen. From this value, the specific activity (units/mg) and total antigen activity can readily be obtained. If the amount of antigen on the cells, as determined by quantitative absorption (Pellegrino *et al.*, 1972a), is known, an approximate yield can also be calculated. Inhibition of cytoxicity thus provides a means of quantitating cell-bound and solubilized histocompatibility antigens. In addition, the assay is relatively rapid and many can be performed simultaneously. It is thus more suitable for use in evaluating solubilization and purification methods than *in vivo* assays.

Radioimmunoassays have the advantage that, unlike the abovementioned *in vitro* assays, they do not appear to be affected by the presence of solubilizing reagents that may be toxic. Such assays that are currently used for histocompatibility antigens depend on the prior availability of purified soluble antigens for the preparation of radioactive ligands (Miyakawa *et al.*, 1971). A recently developed radioimmunoassay, however, detects the binding of alloantisera to glutaraldehyde-treated target cells by using ^{125}I-antiFab (Letarte-Muirhead *et al.*, 1974). This assay is based on the presence of cell-bound antigens and has been successfully used to measure solubilized rat histocompatibility antigens in detergents. It would appear that this type of assay is a better index of the differences between the cell-bound and solubilized antigens than the conventional radioimmunoassays.

C. Methods for Solubilizing Histocompatibility Antigens

Histocompatibility antigens from a number of species have been solubilized essentially by four methods: sonication, proteolytic digestion, detergent extraction, and salt extraction. As discussed in Section II, sonication results in low yields and is no longer widely used. The products of proteolytic digestion may not be representative of the membrane-associated counterpart, and the yields of solubilized antigens may be very low. This is exemplified by the fact that when papain was used to solubilize H-2 antigens, 4000 mouse spleens were needed to obtain 1.43 mg of purified antigen (Shimada and Nathenson, 1969). This represents a yield of 2% of the total antigenic activity present in the crude membrane preparation.

Several attempts at using detergents for solubilizing histocompatibility antigens have been made. These include nonionic detergents such as Triton X-100 (Kandutsch, 1960), Nonidet P-40 (Schwartz and Nathenson, 1971), and Triton X-114 (Hilgert *et al.*, 1969), and ionic detergents such as deoxycholate, decyl- and dodecylsulfate (Metzgar *et al.*, 1967), and sodium lauryl sarcosinate (Reisfeld and Kahan, 1970b). Most of these compounds achieve the solubilization of antigenic activity. Removal of the detergent, however, renders the products insoluble in aqueous solutions at neutral pH. Thus, under the experimental conditions that have been used, "truly water-soluble" histocompatibility antigens cannot be obtained.

As mentioned in Section III, LIS has the dissociating properties of a strong detergent but can be quantitatively removed without the resultant insolubility of detergent-solubilized membrane proteins. In fact, Mann (1972a) has used the tris salt of diiodosalicylic acid (TIS) to extract human histocompatibility antigens in yields of 7-12%. Attempts to solubilize active murine histocompatibility antigens from L1210 cells with either LIS or TIS, at concentrations of 0.01-0.3 M, have been unsuccessful (J. H. Pincus, unpublished). It is also noteworthy that the addition of 0.1 M LIS to an active preparation of H-2^d antigen, solubilized from L1210 cells with 3 M KCl (see below), followed by its subsequent removal, results in a total loss of the antigenic activity (J. H. Pincus, unpublished). This suggests that these compounds, which are very useful for solubilizing glycoproteins, either denature antigenic determinants or irreversibly dissociate noncovalent interactions between molecules that are necessary for the detection of antigenic activity. Thus such compounds are not generally useful for the solubilization of histocompatibility antigens.

The abovementioned problems of low yield, ill-defined products, and insolubility occurring upon removal of reagents do not occur when cell surface antigens are extracted with hypertonic salt solutions. This method, although potentially quite useful, is not straightforward. The detailed discussion which follows is thus designed to aid in understanding the mechanism of hypertonic salt extraction so that conditions may be adjusted to extract antigens effectively from different cell sources.

D. Solubilization of Histocompatibility Antigens with 3 M KCl

Several years ago, Reisfeld *et al.* (1971) demonstrated the effectiveness of 3 M KCl as a solubilizing agent for HL-A antigens from cultured human lymphoblasts. Up to 85% of the cell surface antigen activity, as determined by quantitative absorption, could be recovered in soluble form. Fractionation of the crude extract by preparative polyacrylamide gel electrophoresis resulted in the recovery of approximately 50% of the antigenic activity in one fraction that exhibited a single component on reelectrophoresis. The method thus permits high recoveries of histocompatibility antigens that are soluble in aqueous solution, in the absence of the solubilizing agent. This extraction procedure has also been applied to tumor-specific antigens (Meltzer *et al.*, 1971; Gutterman *et al.*, 1972; Pellis *et al.*, 1974), although the crude extracts have not been extensively purified and the quantities of antigen solubilized have not been estimated.

1. Conditions Associated with Optimal Antigen Extraction by 3 M KCl

In order to achieve optimal yields of solubilized antigens by using 3 M KCl, one must consider several facts. Cells should be suspended at a ratio of 10^9 cells per 20 ml of 3 M KCl in phosphate-buffered (0.015 M, pH 7.4) saline (0.15 M); lower molarities of KCl are less effective (Reisfeld *et al.*, 1971). An analysis of the time course of the extraction indicates that at 4°C the maximal extraction requires 16 h, the majority of the antigen being released between 8 and 16 h (Reisfeld *et al.*, 1974). Furthermore, the KCl extraction technique is effective only when used on intact viable cells; significantly lower yields are obtained when largely nonviable cells, frozen and thawed cells, or cell membrane preparations are used (Reisfeld *et al.*, 1971).

Based on these observations, Mann (1972b) demonstrated that the addition of "cell sap" to a crude lymphoid cell membrane preparation resulted in a good yield of KCl-solubilized HL-A antigens. It was then concluded that intracellular proteases contained in the cell sap facilitated the solubilization process. This postulate has been directly tested by using several substrates for proteolytic enzymes and assaying the extract for proteolytic activity (Oh *et al.*, 1974). Under the conditions used for extraction, significant proteolytic activity is not detectable; therefore, the major mechanism of hypertonic salt extraction does not appear to involve proteolysis. However, the requirement for intracellular components may indicate that the metabolic state of the cell at the time of extraction is critical in determining the effectiveness of KCl solubilization.

2. Extraction of Murine Histocompatibility Antigens

Recent interest has centered on the solubilization of murine H-2 antigens since these proteins can be evaluated *in vivo* for immunogenic potency. The 3 M KCl extraction procedure on cultured cell lines appears to be highly suitable for these experiments, since the potential exists for the extraction of large quantities of antigen that remains soluble under physiological conditions in the absence of the solubilizing agent. Although cultured "normal" murine lymphoblasts are not available, lymphoid tumor cell lines, adapted to growth in suspension culture, that possess the H-2 serological specificities can be readily obtained. Since L1210 cells (see Section III) possess the H-2^d antigenic specificities, this line was used for extraction experiments.

The results of solubilizing four antigenic determinants characteristic of the H-2^d gene product by using "standard" conditions for KCl extraction (Reisfeld *et al.*, 1971) are illustrated in Table V. Three of the determinants assayed were obtained in low yields and a fourth could not be detected in the extract. When cultured L1210 cells that have been injected intraperitoneally into DBA/2 mice and propagated as an ascites tumor were extracted, with the exception of determinant 4, even less antigen was solubilized. The extraction of two additional ascites tumors showed further variability. The quantity of antigen extracted from Meth A, with the exception of determinant 4, was similar to that in ascites-propagated L1210. Although the H-2^d antigens could be serologically demonstrated on BALB/RL2 (L. J. Old, personal communication), they were not present in the KCl extract. It should further be stressed that even though determinant 8 could be detected on all four cell lines used, it was never found in any of the extracts. Thus, with these mouse tumors, low and variable yields of solubilized H-2^d anti-

Table V. Activity of 3 M KCl Solubilized Antigens from Murine Tumor Cells Containing H-2^d Antigens

Cell source	Antigen activity $(\times 10^{-3})^a$					Yield^e				
	3	4	8	31	33^b	3	4	8	31	33
L1210, culture	40	20	0	130	0	9	9	0	9	–
L1210, ascites	15	119	0	15	0	–	–	–	–	–
Meth A^c	9	37	0	9	0	–	–	–	–	–
BALB/RL2^d	0	0	0	0	0	–	–	–	–	–

[a] ID_{50} units/10^9 cells, determined by the method of Pincus and Gordon (1971).
[b] Specificity control.
[c] Ascites variant and BALB/c methylcholanthrene-induced fibrosarcoma kindly provided by Dr. Lloyd J. Old.
[d] Ascites variant of BALB/c radiation-induced leukemia kindly provided by Dr. Lloyd J. Old.
[e] Determined by quantitative absorption according to the method of Pellegrino et al. (1972a).

gens were obtained with 3 M KCl. A similar variability between cultured L1210 ascites cells, and DBA/2 mouse spleen cells has been reported (Götze and Reisfeld, 1974).

An analysis of the yields of HL-A antigens solubilized from a number of cultured human lymphoblastoid cell lines has shown that the recoveries depend on the cell line used, are not always good, and are not related to the relative HL-A antigenic density (Pellegrino et al., 1973b). The variable recovery has been suggested to be the result of metabolic differences between the different cell lines (Reisfeld et al., 1974). This explanation may also account for the variability observed above when cultured tumor cells were used.

3. Dependence of 3 M KCl Extraction on Cell Growth

Using synchronized cells, Cikes and Friberg (1971) observed a variation in H-2 antigen expression throughout the cell cycle, the greatest amount being detected during the G_1 phase. With L1210 cells, Götze et al. (1972) observed an increased sensitivity to specific H-2 antibody-mediated cytolysis during the G_1 phase of the cell cycle and when the majority of the cells divided and entered G_1. Götze et al. (1972) then examined the yield of H-2 antigen solubilized from L1210 cells with 3 M KCl as a function of cell growth. Significantly higher antigenic activities were solubilized from cells in mid log phase than those in late log phase or stationary phase. Similar experiments on the extraction of HL-A antigens (Ferrone et al., 1974) from cultured human lymphoblasts demonstrated that the immunological potency of soluble preparations obtained from cells grown to late log phase or early resting phase was greatest even though the expression of HL-A antigen expression did not vary during the cell cycle. These results indicate that antigen expression *per se* does not account for the variability observed during KCl extraction; rather, it appears to be a function of the growth state of the cell.

Since the extractions illustrated in Table V were performed on cultured L1210 cells in late log phase, the experiments were repeated on cells grown to mid log phase. The yield of antigen improved, but the increase was only two- to threefold (J. H. Pincus, unpublished). Thus, even under optimal conditions, the yields of KCl-solubilized H-2 antigen from murine lymphoid tumors do not approach those of HL-A antigens extracted from human lymphoblastoid cell lines. Although the reason for this is not clear, it may reflect a fundamental metabolic difference between human and mouse cultured lymphoblastoid cells. However, from the above considerations, it does appear that 3 M KCl solubilization of membrane components is not simply a salt extraction but also definitely depends on cell-related factors.

E. Extraction of HL-A Antigens from Human Platelets

An understanding of the cellular events that facilitate the KCl extraction technique would be a major step toward standardizing extraction conditions and maximizing antigen yields. It would be desirable to conduct such studies on a cell that has a relatively simple membrane so that a determination of the components extracted under the different conditions can be made. Peripheral blood platelets fulfill this criterion. In addition: (1) they possess the same HL-A antigenic determinants as leukocytes (Colombani *et al.*, 1970); (2) they can be isolated from peripheral blood under conditions that alter the metabolism of several intracellular components, and these changes can be correlated with antigen extractability; (3) their membranes have been well characterized and the protein components exposed at the cell surface identified (Phillips, 1972), thus facilitating the identification of those surface components extracted. Therefore, Pincus *et al.* (1975) extracted human platelets isolated under different conditions with 3 M KCl in an attempt to elucidate those metabolic factors that facilitate HL-A antigen solubilization.

Platelets isolated from whole blood of individual donors, by differential centrifugation, were extracted for 16 h at 4°C with 3 M KCl (15 ml of 3 M KCl/10^9 platelets). The subsequent processing of the extract is outlined in Fig. 4. Three fractions were tested for antigenic activity: (1) the fraction extracted with 3 M KCl (KCl extract); (2) a fraction obtained by extraction of the residue insoluble in 3 M KCl with isotonic saline (saline extract), and (3) the residue that was insoluble in either solvent (residue). Although the saline-extracted antigen could represent material that simply adhered to the pellet, there was suggestive evidence (see below) that it represented a different form of the antigen than that present in the KCl extract.

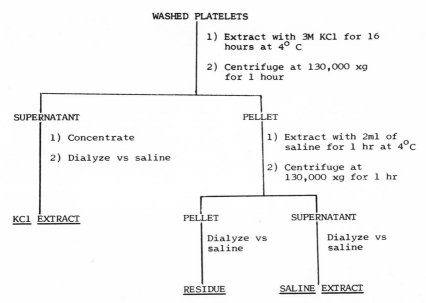

Figure 4. Procedure for the solubilization of HL-A antigens from human platelets. Platelets were prepared from freshly drawn heparinized blood by centrifuging at 2200g for 30 min and washing twice in a Tyrode's buffer (pH 7.4) without calcium but containing either 0.01 M EDTA, 0.01 M caffeine, 0.01 M theophylline, or 10^{-6} M PGE_1 plus 10^{-3} M theophylline. Erythrocytes and leukocytes were separated from the platelets by centrifugation at 250g for 20 min. Residual erythrocyte contamination was then reduced by repeated centrifugation at 1000g for 1 min and the platelets were sedimented at 1000g for 30 min.

The effect of platelet preparative methods on the extractability of HL-A 2 by 3 M KCl as measured by specific inhibition of cytotoxicity is shown in Table VI. These data represent results obtained from 120 preparations. Extraction of platelets that have been isolated in 0.01 M EDTA does not result in antigen solubilization. This result is not due to inactivation of the antigenic determinants since activity is recovered in the residue. These data are consistent with experiments of Oh et al., (1974), who have demonstrated that extraction of cultured lymphoblastoid cells with 3 M KCl in the presence of 0.01 M EDTA results in a 90% reduction of the HL-A antigen solubilized. Although antigen could be solubilized from platelets prepared in 0.001 M EDTA, in agreement with Voigtman et al. (1974), only a small percentage of the recovered activity was found in either soluble extract.

Extraction of platelets prepared in 0.01 M caffeine, 0.01 M theophylline, or prostaglandin E_1 (PGE_1, 10^{-6} M) plus theophylline (10^{-3} M) results in the successful solubilization of HL-A antigens. In some theophylline preparations, all of the activity is solubilized (3B) and none is detected in the residue. The distribution of antigen activity in the two soluble extracts obtained from caffeine-

**Table VI. Effect of Platelet Preparative Method on the Extractability
of HL-A 2 by 3 M KCl**

Expt.[b]	Method of platelet preparation[c]	Recovered HL-A 2 activity $(\times 10^{-3})^a$			Distribution $(\%)^d$		
		KCl extract	Saline extract	Residue	KCl extract	Saline extract	Residue
1A	0.01 M EDTA	0	0	203.3	0	0	100
1B	0.001 M EDTA	15.5	6.7	203.8	7	4	90
2A	0.01 M caffeine	90.0	27.2	99.8	42	12	46
2B	0.01 M caffeine	16.8	110.0	95.8	8	49	43
2C	0.01 M caffeine	0	87.0	132.0	0	39	61
3A	0.01 M theophylline	55.0	38.0	125.7	25	16	57
3B	0.01 M theophylline	43.7	152.0	0	22	78	0
4	10^{-6} M $PGE_1{}^e + 10^{-3}$ M theophylline	82.6	16.2	176.0	30	6	63

[a] Total ID_{50} units recovered in each fraction. At the highest concentration tested (1 mg/ml); none of the fractions inhibited antisera against determinants not present on or cross-reactive with the platelets used for extraction.
[b] Each experiment represents platelets prepared from a single donor.
[c] Platelets prepared in Tyrode's buffer without calcium but containing the compounds indicated.
[d] Distribution of the activity recovered in all three fractions.
[e] Prostaglandin E_1.

prepared platelets is variable (2A and 2B) and dependent on the platelet donor. In some cases, activity can only be found in the saline extract (2C), suggesting that saline extraction of the residue remaining after KCl extraction may not simply be removing adherent antigenic activity but may represent a different form of the antigen. With the exception of several theophylline-prepared platelets, as noted above, significant HL-A activity is always recovered in the residue. Although it has been reported that all of the antigen on platelets detectable by quantitative absorption can be solubilized with 3 M KCl (Pellegrino *et al.*, 1974), this may be due to the fact that absorption techniques underestimate the total platelet HL-A content.

The conditions used for the preparation of platelets that yield active soluble antigen involve the use of reagents that elevate platelet cyclic AMP (cAMP) levels (Salzman *et al.*, 1972). It is known that high concentrations of EDTA inhibit adenylate cyclase. The cAMP levels in platelets isolated under different conditions were determined and are listed in Table VII. Caffeine-prepared platelets can be divided into two groups, those in which cAMP levels do not differ from

Table VII. cAMP Levels in Platelets Prepared under Different Conditions

Expt.	Method of preparation[a]	cAMP levels[b] (pmol/10^9 platelets)	Increase[c]	p[d]
1	0.01 M EDTA	4.76 ± 1.35	–	
2A	0.01 M caffeine	3.98 ± 1.97	0.88	>0.05
2B	0.01 M caffeine	13.21 ± 4.59	2.78	<0.01
3	0.01 M theophylline	17.02 ± 5.53	3.58	<0.001
4	10^{-6} M PGE_1 + 10^{-3} M theophylline	61.73 ± 11.36	12.97	<0.005

[a] Platelets prepared in Tyrode's buffer without calcium but containing the compounds indicated.
[b] Determined according to the method of Gilman (1970).
[c] Increase relative to EDTA-prepared platelets.
[d] Based on the t test of two means.

those in EDTA-prepared platelets and those in which significantly higher values are observed. This is consistent with the variability observed in the solubilization studies and may reflect variable donor responses to this agent. Platelets prepared in theophylline or PGE_1 plus theophylline consistently exhibit significantly higher cAMP values than EDTA-prepared platelets. These results suggest that cAMP levels, prior to KCl extraction, may influence the yield of solubilized HL-A antigens. In this regard, Pellegrino et al. (1974) have successfully extracted HL-A antigens with 3 M KCl from platelets prepared in 0.03 M adenosine. It is noteworthy that this compound is also capable of increasing platelet cAMP levels (Haslam, 1973).

The apparent increase in solubilized antigen under conditions that result in elevated cAMP could be from an altered antigenicity or from a true increase in protein solubilized. Since the number of platelets resulting in 50% inhibition of cytotoxicity, within experimental error, is the same regardless of the method of platelet preparation (Pincus et al, 1975), the increased solubilization cannot result from altered antigenicity. Therefore, the increase in soluble antigen activity must be due to an increased amount of membrane protein solubilized. That this is the case can be seen in Table VIII. Extraction of ^{125}I-labeled platelets indicates that a greater percentage of protein-bound iodine is recovered in both of the soluble extracts when platelets are prepared in theophylline. It should be noted that even after a 16-h extraction, a significant portion of the radiolabel is recovered in the residue. Furthermore, an analysis of the protein-bound radioactivity profiles of each of the fractions and the intact platelets from both of the platelet preparations by sodium dodecylsulfate–polyacrylamide gel electrophoresis (Fairbanks et al., 1971) does not show any qualitative differences between EDTA- or theophylline-prepared platelets (Pincus et al., 1975). The increase in

Table VIII. Distribution of Radioiodinated Protein after
3 M KCl Extraction of ^{125}I-Labeled Platelets[a]

Method of platelet preparation[b]	Distribution of protein-bound radiolabel (%)		
	KCl extract	Saline extract	Residue
0.01 M EDTA	5	4	91
0.01 M theophylline	13	7	80

[a]Platelets labeled using the lactoperoxidase-catalyzed iodination procedure as described by Phillips (1972).
[b]Platelets prepared in Tyrode's buffer without calcium but containing the compounds indicated.

the quantity of radiolabeled protein solubilized by 3 M KCl extraction from platelets prepared under conditions resulting in increased cAMP thus appears to be generalized.

F. Mechanism of cAMP Potentiation of KCl Extraction

As stated earlier, KCl extraction is dependent on the state of the cell and appears to be facilitated by an intracellular metabolic event(s). The successful solubilization of HL-A antigens from human platelets is, at least in part, contingent upon their preparation under conditions resulting in increased cAMP levels. Generally, total solubilization of all the antigenic activity or the total iodinatable cell surface protein cannot be achieved. While the reason for this is not apparent at this time, it may be caused by the degradation of cAMP by platelet phosphodiesterase during the course of the extraction.

Increased platelet cAMP results in the activation of membrane-bound protein kinases which cause the phosphorylation of specific membrane proteins at the inner membrane (Booyse et al., 1973). While there is no direct evidence for the necessity of such protein phosphorylation to occur prior to or during the KCl extraction, such an alteration in membrane proteins could result in subtle changes in protein–protein or lipid–protein interactions. The extent to which this occurs may then determine the degree to which the antigen is soluble in 3 M KCl or is extractable only into isotonic saline, as is the case with caffeine-treated platelets from certain donors. Further experimentation is necessary to test these hypotheses.

Whether cAMP also plays a role in the KCl solubilization of cell surface antigens from other cells remains to be established. However, extraction of HL-A antigens from cultured lymphoblasts is most effective when cells in late log phase or early resting phase are used (Ferrone et al., 1974). This is the point in cell growth at which cAMP levels would be expected to be the highest. Thus cAMP may also play a role in the KCl solubilization of other cell types.

Unlike the glycoprotein extraction described in the previous section, KCl solubilization is more intricate and involves intracellular metabolic factors, one of which appears to be cAMP. By considering these events, it appears possible to improve the yields of antigens solubilized from whole cells. It may also be possible, by controlling such metabolic variables and using the appropriate additives, to manipulate extraction conditions and obtain good yields of KCl-solubilized antigen from isolated membranes. This would reduce the complexity of the initial extract and facilitate the subsequent purification of antigenic activities.

G. Biological Activities of 3 M KCl Solubilized Murine H-2 Antigens

A true test of the biological activity of a solubilized extract involves an analysis of its ability to induce *in vivo* transplantation immunity. Crude KCl extracts of L1210 cells, containing H-2^d serological specificities, can immunize allogeneic hosts and cause accelerated skin graft rejection and antibody production (Ranney *et al.*, 1973; Götze and Reisfeld, 1974), indicating that they are biologically active. However, the possibility that this *in vivo* immunization is aided by other nonantigenic components of the extract cannot be ruled out. A critical evaluation of the biological activity of KCl-solubilized antigen must therefore await the availability of sufficient amounts of purified materials to perform such *in vivo* biological testing.

V. MIXED LEUKOCYTE REACTION (MLR) DETERMINANTS

A. Definition

When unsensitized peripheral blood leukocytes from two unrelated individuals are mixed and cultured for several days, a cell–cell interaction occurs that results in a significantly higher number of blast cells than found in corresponding unmixed cultures (Bain *et al.*, 1964). When untreated cells are used, this response is bidirectional, with each cell being capable of acting as both stimulator and responder. However, by treating one of the cell populations with X-irradiation or antimitotic drugs such as mitomycin C, a unidirectional response can be obtained. Although the MLR was initially assessed morphologically, by the appearance of blast cells, it is now generally evaluated by measuring the enhanced incorporation of tritiated thymidine into DNA in mixed cultures.

The MLR appears to be a general phenomenon associated with lymphoid tissues from many species (Sørensen, 1972). Although it does not require the use of sensitized cells, it appears to be immunospecific (Ling and Kay, 1975) and related to a genetic disparity between the donor leukocytes. It was originally believed to be the result of histocompatibility differences between the cells tested (Bain and Lowenstein, 1964; Bach and Bach, 1971). However, recent evidence indicates that both human (Kissmeyer-Nielsen *et al.*, 1970; Dupont *et al.*, 1971) and mouse (Bach *et al.*, 1972; Meo *et al.*, 1973) mixed leukocyte reactivities are the result of another gene product, coded for by a chromosomal locus closely linked to the histocompatibility locus.

B. Potential for *in Vitro* Studies on the Biological Activities of Solubilized Membrane Antigens

The MLR represents a biological reaction that is defined *in vitro* and permits the ability of solubilized antigenic determinants to stimulate responder cells to be readily evaluated and compared to the unidirectional cellular reaction. In addition, it is possible to study the specific interaction of these antigenic determinants with their receptors and to elucidate the membrane-associated metabolic events in the responder cell that result from this.

C. Factors Other Than Antigenic Recognition Affecting the MLR

1. Requirement for Whole Viable Cells for Stimulation

Results from several laboratories have demonstrated that only intact viable cells, or cells in which only DNA synthesis has been arrested, can participate as stimulators in the MLR. Leukocytes disrupted by freezing and thawing are inactive as stimulators (Hardy and Ling, 1969; Schellekens and Eijsvoogel, 1970). Similarly, heat treatment abolishes a cell's ability to produce an MLR without qualitatively affecting its histocompatibility antigens (Gordon and Maclean 1965; Schellekens and Eijsvoogel, 1970). Furthermore, leukocytes treated with ultraviolet light (Lindahl-Kiessling and Safwenberg, 1971), iodoacetic acid (Schellekens and Eijsvoogel, 1970), or glutaraldehyde (Hardy *et al.*, 1970; Bubbers and Henney, 1975) are ineffective as stimulators. The stimulator cell thus appears to play a greater role in the MLR than merely presenting antigenic determinants to the responder cell.

2. Other Stimulator Cell Requirements

A further investigation of the stimulator cell's properties that are necessary for an MLR has been carried out by using human allogeneic peripheral blood leukocytes (Ranney and Pincus, 1975). In agreement with the results of Bubbers and Henney (1975) for mouse cells, a very brief treatment of stimulator cells with glutaraldehyde (0.015% for 10 s) is sufficient to abolish their ability to induce a unidirectional MLR. A similar loss of stimulating capacity results from fixation with lanthanum chloride (10^{-3} M). These treatments do not drastically alter the cell surface since fixed cells can serve as targets for HL-A antibody-mediated cytolysis and cell-mediated lympholysis. In addition, their ability to bind Con A is not significantly altered.

Pretreatment of the stimulator cells with colchicine, a drug which binds to tubulin and prevents microtubule assembly (Olmstead and Borissy, 1973), abolishes the unidirectional MLR. As seen in Table IX, a concentration dependence is observed, with the maximum effect at 10^{-4} M. This may reflect the fact that colchicine binding is reversible (Olmstead and Borissy, 1973), and upon washing of the stimulator cells, the effect of the higher concentrations on microtubules is longer lasting. Similar results can be obtained with vincristine, another microtubule-disrupting agent at similar concentrations. Lumicolchicine, a photo-

Table IX. Effect of Colchicine and Lumicolchicine Pretreatment of Stimulator Cells on the Unidirectional MLR

Pretreatment[a]	Concentration	Cells[b]	Tritiated thymidine incorporated (counts/min)[c]	Ratio[d]
Untreated control	–	A + Am	683 ± 102	–
		A + Bm	55,805 ± 1278	81.7 ± 1.9
Colchicine	10^{-4} M	A + Am	823 ± 20	–
		A + Bm	5,456 ± 415	6.6 ± 0.5
	10^{-5} M	A + Am	1,161 ± 91	–
		A + Bm	43,558 ± 1694	37.5 ± 1.4
	10^{-6} M	A + Am	1,181 ± 104	–
		A + Bm	60,001 ± 535	50.8 ± 0.4
Lumicolchicine	10^{-4} M	A + Am	672 ± 86	–
		A + Bm	46,565 ± 3389	69.3 ± 5.0
	10^{-5} M	A + Am	714 ± 103	–
		A + Bm	51,203 ± 2384	71.7 ± 3.3
	10^{-6} M	A + Am	804 ± 63	–
		A + Bm	54,678 ± 1127	68.0 ± 1.4

[a] Mitomycin C treated stimulator cells treated for 1 h with colchicine or lumicolchicine and washed before mixing with responder cells.
[b] All experiments were carried out using Ficoll-Hypaque purified peripheral blood leukocytes. The letters A and B denote cells obtained from nonidentical leukocyte donors. Controls consist of mixing untreated and mitomycin-treated cells from the same donor (A + Am).
[c] Obtained after a 5-day incubation period and overnight pulse with tritiated thymidine. Data are expressed as counts/min ± standard deviation from the mean.
[d] Ratio of tritiated thymidine incorporation into experimental vs. control cultures ± standard deviation from the mean.

inactivated derivative of colchicine that does not bind to tubulin, is ineffective, indicating that colchicine specifically affects microtubules. The effects with the microtubule-disrupting agents are not the result of a carryover of these drugs to the responding cell since the addition of drug-treated cells to untreated cells from the same individual does not affect the stimulation of the untreated cells by mitogens (Ranney and Pincus, 1975).

An antiserum against the MLR determinants on the stimulator cell was not available when these studies were performed, and a direct test as to whether any of these treatments affect the antigenic determinants could not be performed. However, as observed with fixed cells, no alteration in anti HL-A antibody-mediated cytolysis, cell-mediated lympholysis, or binding of Con A could be detected in cells treated with the microtubule-disrupting alkaloids colchicine and vincristine (Ranney and Pincus, 1975). Therefore, all of the treatments listed above appear to affect factors other than antigenic determinants.

D. Prospects for Solubilizing Biologically Active MLR Determinants

The collective results just presented indicate that the ability of the stimulator cell to initiate a one-way MLR requires more than recognition of antigenic determinants by the responder cell. It appears that, at least in part, active cellular metabolism and an intact microtubular system are mandatory. One possible explanation for these observations is that a motile cell with a specific superstructural arrangement of membrane proteins may be necessary to activate the responder cell. Thus one aspect of fixation, similar to that of ultraviolet irradiation (Lindahl-Kiessling and Safwenberg, 1971), is to abolish motility. In addition, microtubules may restrict the mobility of certain membrane components (Edelman et al., 1973; Berlin et al., 1974; Nicolson, 1974) and participate in maintaining a specific membrane supermolecular structure.

It has been possible to demonstrate murine I-region determinants, which are responsible for the MLR (Bach et al., 1972), in detergent-solubilized (Nonidet P-40) extracts of spleen cells (Cullen et al., 1974). However, attempts at using crude cell extracts, solubilized by any of several methods, to stimulate allogeneic lymphocytes have resulted either in a lower level of stimulation than observed in the unidirectional MLR or in a failure to obtain a blastogenic response (see Oppenheim, 1972; Ranney et al., 1973; Ling and Kay, 1975). It is not possible to determine which components of those extracts that did induce blastogenesis are responsible for stimulation. Furthermore, the experiments were done at a time when it was believed that only histocompatibility antigenic differences were responsible for the MLR, and it cannot be determined whether the solubilized products tested contained the MLR antigenic determinants. Since the available evidence as cited above indicates that more is required of the stimulator cell than presentation of antigenic determinants to the responding cell, it follows that solubilized MLR determinants, even though serologically detectable, should not be able to induce blastogenesis.

VI. CONCLUSION

At the present time, protocols for the effective solubilization of biologically active cell surface components must be empirically developed every time a new activity, or new cell, is studied. As a guide to achieving this, some general considerations concerning the choice of cell or tissue as starting material, methods for preparation of plasma membranes, and reagents for solubilization have been described, and the merits and disadvantages of each have been evaluated. Specific methodology for three cell surface biological activities of interest to immunologists has been dealt with at length to illustrate some of the difficulties that may be encountered, and, if possible, how these can be resolved. While it is relatively simple to solubilize glycoprotein-associated activities from isolated plasma membranes, the same techniques appear largely unsuitable for solubilizing histocompatibility antigens. The use of 3 M KCl to extract these proteins is apparently facilitated by cellular metabolic events, at least one of which appears to be cAMP levels. At this time, this procedure cannot effectively be used on isolated membranes. Still other antigenic determinants such as those involved in the mixed leukocyte reaction are not biologically active when solubilized. Perhaps the only generalization that can be made is that any given protocol is not universally suitable or optimally effective for solubilizing every membrane-associated activity from every cell type. It is only by a systematic approach that the appropriate conditions for obtaining optimum quantities of solubilized, biologically active membrane proteins can be achieved.

Although an increasing effort is being devoted to the solubilization of immunogenic cell surface components for biological testing, generally this has been carried out with crude extracts. The extent to which the activity of the antigens in these extracts is influenced by other components acting as carriers cannot be determined. This evaluation will only be possible when at least partially purified extracts with few protein components, in addition to the antigen, are used.

With the exception of the Rh antigen, whose activity in solution shows a phospholipid requirement (Green, 1972), the requirement for membrane lipids to maintain or enhance solubilized cell surface antigenic activities has not been investigated. Since the cell surface antigens that have been investigated so far are not solubilized by mild treatments such as low ionic strength or chelating agents, they are probably integral proteins. Such molecules in solution, if representative of their membrane counterparts, should be capable of inserting into liposomes or artificial phospholipid membranes. Although such reconstitution experiments have been done successfully with a number of membrane enzymes (Coleman, 1973) and are necessary to restore the activity of some solubilized bacterial enzymes (Kundig, 1974), they have not been attempted with membrane antigens. Therefore, a detailed biochemical analysis of soluble membrane antigens should include studies on the partial or total requirements for membrane lipids and a comparison of the biological properties of soluble, reconstituted, and membrane-associated proteins. However, in order to achieve a reconstituted state representative of that in the native membrane, it is necessary to use a well-defined soluble preparation since a complex mixture of soluble membrane proteins does not properly reconstitute (Razin, 1974). Thus, the answer to many of these questions must await the availability of more highly purified membrane antigens.

With the development of better methodology for solubilization, purification, and study of cell surface antigens, it will be possible to undertake more detailed biochemical and biological studies than are currently possible. The future holds exciting prospects for understanding of the cell surface and the functional nature of its antigenic components.

ACKNOWLEDGMENTS

This work was supported in part by Veterans Administration Research Funds (Project No. 4819, MRIS No. 7084) and a contract from the National Heart and Lung Institute (No. 1-HB-3-2958). I wish to thank Mrs. Vienna L. Bennett and Mr. Floyd C. Wiseman for their technical assistance and Miss Dorothy Shelangoski for typing the manuscript.

VII. REFERENCES

Ada, G.L., and Byrt, P., 1969, *Nature (London)* **222**:1291.
Adair, W.L., and Kornfeld, S., 1974, *J. Biol. Chem.* **249**:4699.
Albertson, P.A., 1960, *Partition of Cell Particles and Macromolecules*, Wiley, New York.
Albertson, P.A., 1970, *Adv. Protein Chem.* **24**:309.
Allan, D., Auger, J., and Crumpton, M., 1971, *Exp. Cell Res.* **66**:362.
Bach, F.H., and Bach, M.L., 1971, *Transplant. Proc.* **3**:942.
Bach, F.H., Widmer, M.B., Bach, M.L., and Klein, J., 1972, *J. Exp. Med.* **136**:1430.
Bain, B., and Lowenstein, L., 1964, *Science* **145**:315.
Bain, B., Vas, M.R., and Lowenstein, L., 1964, *Blood* **23**:108.
Baldwin, R.W., Bowen, J.G., and Price, M.R., 1974, *Biochim. Biophys. Acta* **367**:47.
Baldwin, R.W., Glaves, D., Harris, J.R., and Price, M.R., 1971, *Transplant. Proc.* **3**:1189.
Basten, A., Miller, J.F.A.P., Sprent, J., and Pye, J., 1972, *J. Exp. Med.* **135**:610.
Berlin, R.D., Oliver, J.M., Ukena, T.E., and Yin, H.H., 1974, *Nature (London) New Biol.* **247**:45.

Billing, R., and Terasaki, P.I., 1974, *J. Natl. Cancer Inst.* **53**:1635.
Boone, C.W., Ford, L.G., Bond, H., Stuart, D.C., and Lorenz, D., 1969, *J. Cell Biol.* **41**:378.
Booyse, F.M., Guiliani, D., Marr, J.J., and Rafelson, M.E., Jr., 1973, *Ser. Haematol.* **6**:351.
Bosmann, H.B., Hagopian, A., and Eylar, E.H., 1968, *Arch. Biochem. Biophys.* **128**:51.
Bretscher, M.S., 1971, *Nature (London) New Biol.* **231**:229.
Brunette, D.M., and Till, J.E., 1971, *J. Membr. Biol.* **5**:2.
Bubbers, J.E., and Henney, C.S., 1975, *J. Immunol.* **114**:1126.
Buck, C.A., Glick, M.C., and Warren, L., 1970, *Biochemistry* **9**:4567.
Buck, C.A., Fuhrer, P.J., Soslau, G., and Warren, L., 1974, *J. Biol. Chem.* **249**:1541.
Buell, D.N., and Fahey, J.L., 1969, *Science* **164**:1524.
Cikes, M., and Friberg, S., 1971, *Proc. Natl. Acad. Sci. USA.* **68**:566.
Codington, J.F., Sanford, B.H., and Jeanloz, R.W., 1970, *J. Natl. Cancer Inst.* **456**:637.
Coleman, R., 1973, *Biochim. Biophys. Acta* **300**:1.
Colombani, J., Colombani, M., and Dausset, J., 1970, in: *Histocompatibility Testing–1970*, (P.I. Terasaki, ed.), p. 79, Munksgaard, Copenhagen.
Cresswell, P., Turner, M.J., and Strominger, J., 1973, *Proc. Natl. Acad. Sci. USA.* **70**:1603.
Crumpton, M.J., and Snary, D., 1974, in: *Contemporary Topics in Molecular Immunology*, Vol. 3 (G.L. Ada, ed.), p. 27, Plenum Press, New York.
Cuatrecasas, P., 1974, *Annu. Rev. Biochem.* **43**:169.
Cuatrecasas, P., Fuchs, S., and Anfinsen, C.B., 1967, *J. Biol. Chem.* **242**:1541.
Cullen, S.E., David, C.S., Shreffler, D.C., and Nathenson, S.G., 1974, *Proc. Nat. Acad. Sci. USA.* **71**:648.
Dautigny, A., Bernier, I., Colombani, J., and Jollès, P., 1973, *Biochim. Biophys. Acta* **298**:783.
Drapkin, M.S., Appella, E., and Law, L.W., 1974, *J. Natl. Cancer Inst.* **52**:254.
Dupont, B., Nielsen, L.S., and Svejgaard, A., 1971, *Lancet* **2**:1336.
Edelman, G.M., Yahara, I., and Wang, J.L., 1973, *Proc. Natl. Acad. Sci. USA.* **70**:1442.
Edidin, M., 1967, *Proc. Natl. Acad. Sci. USA.* **57**:1226.
Fairbanks, G., Steck, T.L., and Wallach, D.F.H., 1971, *Biochemistry* **10**:2606.
Ferrone, S., Pellegrino, M.A., Dierich, M.P., and Reisfeld, R.A., 1974, *Curr. Top. Microbiol. Immunol.* **66**:1.
Gilman, A.G., 1970, *Proc. Natl. Acad. Sci. USA.* **67**:305.
Glick, M.C., Kimhi, Y., and Littauer, U.Z., 1973, *Proc. Natl. Acad. Sci. USA.* **70**:1682.
Gordon, J., and Maclean, I.D., 1965, *Nature (London)* **208**:795.
Götze, D., and Reisfeld, R.A., 1974, *J. Immunol.* **112**:1643.
Götze, D., Pellegrino, M.A., Ferrone, S., and Reisfeld, R.A., 1972, *Immunol. Comm.* **1**:533.
Greaves, M., and Janossy, G., 1972, *Transplant. Rev.* **11**:87.
Green, F., 1972, *J. Biol. Chem.* **247**:881.
Grefrath, S.P., and Reynolds, J.A., 1974, *Proc. Natl. Acad. Sci. USA.* **71**:3913.
Gutterman, J.U., Mavligit, G., McCredie, K.B., Bodey, G.P., Freireich, E.J., and Hersh, E.M., 1972, *Science* **177**:1114.
Hardy, D.A., and Ling, N.R., 1969, *Nature (London)* **221**:545.
Hardy, D.A., Knight, S., and Ling, N.R., 1970, *Immunology* **19**:329.
Haslam, R.J., 1973, *Ser. Haematol.* **6**:333.
Helenius, A., and Simons, K., 1975, *Biochim. Biophys. Acta* **415**:29.
Hilgert, I., Kandutsch, A.A., Cherry, M., and Snell, G.D., 1969, *Transplantation* **8**:451.
Hollinshead, A.C., McWright, C., Alford, T.C., Glew, D., and Gold, P., 1972, *Science* **177**:887.
Holmes, E.C., Kahan, B.D., and Morton, D.L., 1970, *Cancer* **25**:373.
Hourani, B.T., Chace, N.M., and Pincus, J.H., 1973, *Biochim. Biophys. Acta* **328**:520.
House, W., Shearer, M., and Maroudas, N.G., 1972, *Exp. Cell Res.* **71**:293.

Hutchison, P., Ihenson, O.H., and Bjerngood, M.R., 1966, *Exp. Cell Res.* **42**:157.
Inbar, M., and Sachs, L., 1969, *Proc. Natl. Acad. Sci. USA*. **63**:1418.
Jamieson, G.A., and Greenwalt, T.J., ed., 1971, *Glycoproteins of Blood Cells and Plasma*, Lippincott, Philadelphia.
Kagawa, Y., 1972, *Biochim. Biophys. Acta* **265**:297.
Kahan, B.D., 1965, *Proc. Natl. Acad. Sci. USA*. **53**:153.
Kahan, B.D., and Reisfeld, R.A., 1967, *Proc. Natl. Acad. Sci. USA*. **58**:1430.
Kahan, B.D., and Reisfeld, R.A., 1969, *Science* **164**:514.
Kahan, B.D., and Reisfeld, R.A., 1971, *Bacteriol. Rev.* **35**:59.
Kamat, V.B., and Wallach, D.F.H., 1965, *Science* **148**:1343.
Kandutsch, A.A., 1960, *Cancer Res.* **20**:262.
Kandutsch, A.A., and Stimpfling, J.H., 1962, *Transplant. Ciba Found. Symp.*, p. 72.
Kant, J.A., and Steck, T.L., 1973, *J. Biol. Chem.* **248**:8457.
Kennel, S.J., and Lerner, R.A., 1973, *J. Mol. Biol.* **76**:485.
Kissmeyer-Nielsen, F., Svejgaard, A., Sorensen, S.G., Nielsen, L.S., and Thorsby, E., 1970, *Nature (London)* **228**:63.
Korn, E.D., 1969, *Annu. Rev. Biochem.* **38**:263.
Kraemer, P.M., 1971, in: *Biomembranes*, Vol. I (L.A. Manson, ed.), p. 62, Plenum Press, New York.
Krupey, J., Gold, P., and Freedman, S.O., 1968, *J. Exp. Med.* **128**:387.
Kundig, W., 1974, *J. Supramol. Struct.* **2**:695.
Kuo, T., Rosai, J., and Tillack, T.W., 1973, *Int. J. Cancer* **12**:532.
Kyte, J., 1972, *J. Biol. Chem.* **247**:7642.
Langley, O.K., and Ambrose, E.J., 1964, *Nature (London)* **204**:53.
Lesko, L., Donlon, M., Marinetti, G., and Hare, J.D., 1973, *Biochim. Biophys. Acta* **311**:173.
Letarte-Muirhead, M., Acton, R., and Williams, A.F., 1974, *Biochem. J.* **143**:51.
Lindahl-Kiessling, K., and Safwenberg, J., 1971, *Int. Arch. Allergy* **41**:670.
Ling, N.R., and Kay, J.E., 1975, *Lymphocyte Stimulation*, p. 123, North-Holland, Amsterdam.
Lis, H., and Sharon, N., 1973, *Annu. Rev. Biochem.* **43**:451.
Mann, D.L., 1972a, in: *Transplantation Antigens* (B.D. Kahan and R.A. Reisfeld, eds.), p. 287, Academic Press, New York.
Mann, D.L., 1972b, *Transplantation* **14**:398.
Mann, D.L., Rogentine, G.N., Fahey, J.L., and Nathenson, S.G., 1968, *Nature (London)* **217**:1180.
Mann, D.L., Rogentine, G.N., Fahey, J.L., and Nathenson, S.G., 1969, *J. Immunol.* **103**:282.
Manson, L.A., and Palm, J., 1968, in: *Advances in Transplantation* (J. Dausset, J. Hamburger, and G. Mathe, eds.), p. 301, Munksgaard, Copenhagen.
Marchesi, V.T., and Andrews, E.P., 1971, *Science* **174**:1247.
Marchesi, V.T., and Steers, E., Jr., 1968, *Science* **159**:203.
Marchesi, V.T., Jackson, R.L., Segrest, J.P., and Kahane, I., 1973, *Fed. Proc.* **32**:1833.
Marchesi, V.T., Tillack, T.W., Jackson, R.L., Segrest, J.P., and Scott, R.E., 1972, *Proc. Natl. Acad. Sci. USA* **69**:1445.
Meltzer, M.S., Leonard, E.J., Rapp, H.J., and Borsos, T., 1971, *J. Natl. Cancer Inst.* **47**:703.
Meo, T., Vives, J., Miggiano, V., and Shreffler, D.C., 1973, *Transplant. Proc.* **5**:377.
Metzgar, R.S., Flanagan, J.F., and Mendes, N.F., 1967, in: *Histocompatibility Testing–1967*, (E.S. Curtoni, P.L. Mattiuz, and R.M. Tosi, eds.), p. 307, Munksgaard, Copenhagen.
Mittal, K.K., Mickey, M.R., Singal, D.P., and Terasaki, P.I., 1968, *Transplantation* **6**:913.
Miyakawa, Y., Tanigaki, N., Yagi, Y., and Pressman, D., 1971, *J. Immunol.* **107**:395.
Moore, G.E., and Woods, L., 1972, *Transplantation* **13**:155.
Moore, G.E., Gerner, R.F., and Franklin, H.A., 1967, *J. Am. Med. Assoc.* **199**:519.

Moscona, A.A., 1965, in: *Cells and Tissue Culture*, Vol. I (E.N. Wilmer, ed.), p. 197, Academic Press, New York.

Muramatsu, T., Nathenson, S.G., Boyse, E.A., and Old, L.J., 1973, *J. Exp. Med.* **137**:1256.

Neri, G., Smith, D.F., Gilliam, E.B., and Walborg, E.F., Jr., 1974, *Arch. Biochem. Biophys.* **165**:323.

Nicolson, G.L., 1974, *Int. Rev. Cytol.* **39**:89.

Nicolson, G.L., and Singer, S.J., 1971, *Proc. Natl. Acad. Sci. USA* **68**:942

Nussenzweig, V., and Pincus, C.S., 1972, in: *Contemporary Topics in Immunobiology*, Vol. 1 (M.G. Hanna, ed.), p. 69, Plenum Press, New York.

Oh, S.K., Pellegrino, M.A., and Reisfeld, R.A., 1974, *Proc. Soc. Exp. Biol. Med.* **145**:1272.

Olmstead, J.B., and Borissy, G.G., 1973, *Annu. Rev. Biochem.* **43**:507.

Oppenheim, J.J., 1972, in: *Transplantation Antigens*, (B.D. Kahan and R.A. Reisfeld, eds.), p. 357, Academic Press, New York.

Oxender, D.L., 1972, *Annu. Rev. Biochem.* **41**:777.

Pellegrino, M.A., Ferrone, S., and Pellegrino, A., 1972a, *Proc. Soc. Exp. Biol. Med.* **139**:484.

Pellegrino, M.A., Ferrone, S., Natali, P.G., Pellegrino, A., and Reisfeld, R.A., 1972b, *J. Immunol.* **108**:573.

Pellegrino, M.A., Ferrone, S., and Pellegrino, A., 1972c, in: *Transplantation Antigens*, (B.D. Kahan and R.A. Reisfeld, eds.), p. 433, Academic Press, New York.

Pellegrino, M.A., Ferrone, S., Pellegrino, A., and Reisfeld, R.A., 1973a, in: *Proceedings of the International Symposium on Standardization of HL-A Reagents, Copenhagen*, Vol. 18, p. 209, Karger, New York.

Pellegrino, M.A., Ferrone, S., Pellegrino, A., and Reisfeld, R.A., 1973b, *Clin. Immunol. Immunopathol.* **1**:817.

Pellegrino, M.A., Ferrone, S., Pellegrino, A., Oh, S.K., and Reisfeld, R.A., 1974, *Eur. J. Immunol.* **4**:250.

Pellis, N.R., Tom, B.H., and Kahan, B.D., 1974, *J. Immunol.* **113**:708.

Phillips, D.R., 1972, *Biochemistry* **11**:4582.

Pilkins, S.J., and Johnson, R.A., 1974, *Biochim. Biophys. Acta* **341**:388.

Pincus, J.H., and Gordon, R.O., 1971, *Transplantation* **12**:509.

Pincus, J.H., Kahan, B.D., and Mittal, K.K., 1976, *Immunochemistry* (in press).

Price, M.R., and Baldwin, R.W., 1974, *Br. J. Cancer* **30**:382.

Racker, E., 1967, *Fed. Proc.* **26**:1335.

Raff, M.C., Sternberg, M., and Taylor, R.B., 1970, *Nature (London)* **225**:553.

Ranney, D.F., Gordon, R.O., Pincus, J.H., and Oppenheim, J., 1973, *Transplantation* **16**:558.

Ranney, D.F., and Pincus, J.H., 1975, *Fed. Proc.* **34**:1011.

Razin, S., 1974, *J. Supramol. Struct.* **2**:670.

Reif, A.E., and Allen, J.M.V., 1964, *J. Exp. Med.* **120**:413.

Reisfeld, R.A., and Kahan, B.D., 1970a, *Adv. Immunol.* **12**:117.

Reisfeld, R.A., and Kahan, B.D., 1970b, *Fed. Proc.* **29**:2034.

Reisfeld, R.A., Pellegrino, M., Papermaster, B.W., and Kahan, B.D., 1970, *J. Immunol.* **104**:560.

Reisfeld, R.A., Pellegrino, M.A., and Kahan, B.D., 1971, *Science* **172**:1134.

Reisfeld, R.A., Ferrone, S., and Pellegrino, M.A., 1974, in: *Methods in Membrane Biology*, Vol. 1 (E.D. Korn, ed.), p. 143, Plenum Press, New York.

Robinson, D.R., and Jencks, W.P., 1965, *J. Am. Chem. Soc.* **87**:2470.

Rosai, J., Tillack, T.W., and Marchesi, V.T., 1972, *Int. J. Cancer* **10**:357.

Salzman, E.A., Kensler, P.C., and Levine, L., 1972, *Ann. N.Y. Acad. Sci.* **201**:61.

Schellekens, P.T.A., and Eijsvoogel, V.P., 1970, *Clin. Exp. Immunol.* **7**:229.

Schick, M.J., ed., 1967, *Nonionic Surfactants*, Dekker, New York.

Schwartz, B.D., and Nathenson, S.G., 1971, *J. Immunol.* **107**:1363.

Segrest, J.P., Kahane, I., Jackson, R.L., and Marchesi, V.T., 1973, *Arch. Biochem. Biophys.* **155**:167.

Sell, S., and Gell, P.G.H., 1965, *J. Exp. Med.* **122**:423.

Shier, W.T., 1971, *Proc. Natl. Acad. Sci. USA* **68**:2078.

Shimada, A., and Nathenson, S.J., 1969, *Biochemistry* **8**:4048.

Shin, B.C. and Carraway, K.L., 1973, *J. Biol. Chem.* **248**:1436.

Singer, S.J., and Nicolson, G.L., 1972, *Science* **175**:720.

Snary, D., Goodfellow, P., Haymen, M.J., Bodmer, W.F., and Crumpton, M.J., 1974, *Nature (London)* **247**:457.

Sørensen, S.F., 1972, *Acta Pathol. Microbiol. Scand.*, Sect. B., Suppl. 230.

Spatz, L., and Strittmatter, P., 1971, *Proc. Natl. Acad. Sci. USA* **68**:1042.

Springer, G.F., Nagai, Y., and Tegtmeyer, H., 1966, *Biochemistry* **5**:3254.

Steck, T.L., 1974, *J. Cell Biol.* **62**:1.

Strittmatter, P., and Velick, S.F., 1957, *J. Biol. Chem.* **228**:785.

Terasaki, P., and McClelland, J., 1964, *Nature (London)* **204**:998.

Umbreit, J.N., and Strominger, J.L., 1973, *Proc. Natl. Acad. Sci. USA* **70**:2997.

van Beek, W.P., Smets, L.A., and Emmelot, P., 1973, *Cancer Res.* **33**:2913.

Voigtman, R., Uhlenbeck, G., Pardoe, G.I., and Rogers, K., 1974, *Eur. J. Immunol.* **4**:674.

Wallach, D.F.H., and Lin, P.S., 1973, *Biochim. Biophys. Acta* **300**:211.

Wallach, D.F.H., Kranz, B., Ferber, E., and Fischer, H., 1972, *FEBS Lett.* **21**:29.

Warren, L., and Glick, M.C., 1971, in: *Biomembranes*, Vol. 1 (L. Manson, ed.), p. 257, Plenum Press, New York.

Warren, L., Glick, M.C., and Nass, M.K., 1966, *J. Cell. Physiol.* **68**:269.

Winzler, R.J., 1970, *Int. Rev. Cytol.* **29**:77.

Yahara, I., and Edelman, G., 1973, *Exp. Cell Res.* **81**:142.

Yu, J., Fishman, D.A., and Steck, T.L., 1973, J. *Supramol. Struct.* **1**:233.

Surface Immunoglobulins of B and T Lymphocytes: Molecular Properties, Association with the Cell Membrane, and a Unified Model of Antigen Recognition

John J. Marchalonis

Molecular Immunology Laboratory
The Walter and Eliza Hall Institute of Medical Research
Royal Melbourne Hospital, Victoria, Australia

I. INTRODUCTION*

Surface immunoglobulins of lymphocytes probably function in the recognition of antigens by these cells. Considerable evidence suggests that surface immunoglobulin molecules contain the same set of V-region combining sites for antigen as do circulating antibodies to that antigen (Binz and Wigzell, 1975; Cosenza and Köhler, 1972; Eichmann and Rajewsky, 1975; McKearn, 1974; McKearn *et al.*, 1974) but that the constant region of the receptor immunoglobulin heavy chain might differ from the constant region of circulating antibody in its capacity to become associated with the plasma membrane and to function in the initiation of lymphocyte differentiation. Therefore, knowledge

*Abbreviations: B_2M, β_2-microglobulin; DNP, 2, 4-dinitrophenyl hapten; H antigens, histocompatibility antigens; H-2, histocompatibility antigens encoded by murine major histocompatibility locus; Fv, immunoglobulin fragment consisting of the variable region of light chain in association with the variable region of the heavy chain; HRBC. horse erythrocytes; MRBC, mouse erythrocytes; SRBC, sheep erythrocytes; (T,G)-A--L, synthetic polypeptide consisting of tyrosyl, glutamyl, alanyl, and lysyl residues; Ig, immunoglobulin; Ia antigens, proteins specified by genes in the I (immune-response) region of the locus encoding H-2 antigens.

of the structure of lymphocyte surface immunoglobulin is crucial to an understanding of the molecular mechanisms of antigen-specific lymphocyte activation.

A number of recent extensive reviews (Bach, 1973; Greaves *et al.*, 1973; Ladoulis *et al.*, 1975; Marchalonis, 1974a, 1975; Roelants, 1972; Warner, 1974) analyze studies involving the binding of anti-immunoglobulins to lymphocytes and the resulting inhibition of function of T and B lymphocytes. The general conclusions are as follows: (1) surface immunoglobulin, primarily of the IgM class, is readily detectable on B cells of various species, and (2) surface immunoglobulin of T cells requires rigorous conditions for detection, but it also resembles IgM antigenically. This chapter will consider chiefly recent developments in the analysis of physicochemical properties of isolated surface immunoglobulins and the roles of these molecules in antigen recognition. A model will be presented that surface immunoglobulin serves as the recognition unit of a receptor complex which is involved in the initiation of specific immune differentiation of lymphocytes.

II. ISOLATION OF LYMPHOCYTE SURFACE IMMUNOGLOBULIN

Various experimental approaches have proved useful in the isolation and analysis of lymphocyte surface immunoglobulins. These include (1) radioiodination of tyrosines in exposed membrane proteins by means of lactoperoxidase (Baur *et al.*, 1971; Marchalonis *et al.*, 1971; Phillips and Morrison, 1971) coupled with solubilization and use of specific serological precipitation systems (Baur *et al.*, 1971; Marchalonis *et al.*, 1972a), (2) preparation of lymphocyte plasma membranes followed by serological analysis (Chavin, 1974; Demus, 1973; Haustein *et al.*, 1974; Smith *et al.*, 1975), and (3) isolation of surface immunoglobulin complexed to specific antisera which had been bound to the intact cell (Rieber and Riethmüller, 1974a,b; Wilson *et al.*, 1972). All three approaches have been successfully applied to B cells and T cells of various species, as shown in Table I, although use of lacteroxidase-catalyzed radioiodination has been used most extensively. The experimental sequence usually used for murine or human B cells consists of labeling of exposed tyrosines under conditions where only membrane proteins become labeled, then disrupting the cells in a nonionic detergent such as Nonidet P-40 followed by serological precipitation which might be of a direct type (carrier mouse Ig plus rabbit anti-mouse Ig) or a "sandwich" type (rabbit anti-mouse Ig plus goat anti-rabbit IgG). When these conditions are used, 1–3% of soluble macromolecular radioactivity in B-cell membrane proteins is precipitated specifically (Vitetta *et al.*, 1972; Cone and Marchalonis, 1974). Application of the same methodology to thymus lymphocytes results in identification of 0.1% or less of the macromolecular

Table I. Isolation of Lymphocyte Surface Immunoglobulin[a]

Species	Methods used	
	B cells	T cells
Chicken	Surface radioiodination (1)	Surface radioiodination (1)
Mouse	Surface radioiodination (2–7); complexes with anti-immunoglobulin (8)	Surface radioiodination (3,9–12); plasma membrane isolation (13); complexes with anti-immunoglobulin (8,14)
Rat	Surface radioiodination (15); plasma membrane isolation (15)	Surface radioiodination (15); plasma membrane isolation (15)
Pig	Plasma membrane isolation (16)	Plasma membrane isolation (16)
Sheep	Complexes with anti-immunoglobulin (17)	Not tested
Man	Surface radioiodination (18–20); plasma membrane isolation (21); freeze-thaw lysis (22)	Surface radioiodination (3,23,24)
Rabbit	Surface radioiodination (25,26)	Not tested
Goldfish	Surface radioiodination (27)	Surface radioiodination (27)

[a]Sources: 1, Szenberg et al. (1974); 2, Vitetta et al. (1972); 3, Marchalonis et al. (1972a); 4, Abney and Parkhouse (1974); 5, Melchers and Cone (1975); 6, Lisowska-Bernstein et al. (1973); 7, Grey et al. (1972); 8, Wilson et al. (1972); 9, Moroz and Lahat (1974); 10, Boylston and Mowbray (1974); 11, Haustein and Goding (1975); 12, Haustein et al. (1975); 13, Haustein et al. (1974); 14, Rieber and Riethmüller (1974a,b); 15, Smith et al. (1975); 16, Chavin (1974); 17, Ey (1973); 18, Marchalonis et al. (1974b); 19, Kennel and Lerner (1973); 20, Sherr et al. (1972); 21, Demus (1973); 22, Eskeland et al. (1971); 23, Marchalonis et al. (1972b); 24, Moroz and Hahn (1973); 25, P. Smith, and J. J. Marchalonis (unpublished observations); 26, Craig and Cebra (1975); 27, Warr, DeLuca, and Marchalonis (1976).

radioactivity as immunoglobulin (Cone and Marchalonis, 1974). This sort of observation has been taken as evidence that T cells lack surface immunoglobulin (Vitetta et al., 1972); however, the use of other solvent systems has allowed isolation of radioiodinated surface immunoglobulins of T cells (Cone and Marchalonis, 1974; Haustein, 1975) in percentages not greatly different from the range of values obtained for B cells (see below). In particular, surface immunoglobulin of thumus cells (Boylston and Mowbray, 1973; Marchalonis et al., 1972a; Cone and Marchalonis, 1974; Smith et al., 1975; Haustein and Goding, 1975), peripheral T cells (Marchalonis and Cone, 1973; Marchalonis et al., 1974a, 1975), and monoclonal, continuously cultured T lymphoma cells (Marchalonis et al., 1972a; Boylston and Mowbray, 1974; Haustein, 1975; Haustein et al., 1975) has been isolated either by solubilization of radioiodinated cells in acid-urea or by metabolic release when the cells are held under short-term cell culture conditions. The studies involving T lymphoma cells are particularly incisive because many cultured monoclonal cell lines which maintain a strict T-cell phenotype, including a lack of detectable surface Ig by immunofluorescence, synthesize immunoglobulin which can be detected on the surface by proper application of surface labeling and extraction methods (Harris *et al.*, 1973; Haustein *et al.*, 1975; Boylston and Mowbray, 1974).

Similar results have been obtained when plasma membranes of thymus lymphocytes of pigs (Chavin, 1974) and rats (Ladoulis *et al.*, 1975; Smith *et al.*, 1975) are prepared and then assayed for immunoglobulin. Chavin (1974) reported that solubilized porcine thymus membranes contained amounts of IgG comparable to those observed for spleen membranes (0.2%) even though intact thymus cells were negative for immunoglobulin by immunofluorescence while the intact spleen lymphocytes were strongly positive. Smith *et al.*, (1975) obtained similar results with rat thymus and spleen lymphocytes, but more immunoglobulin (2% of total membrane protein), consisting of IgM and IgG molecules, was found. These results parallel the observation of Molnar *et al.*, (1973) that plasma membranes of cells of the murine mammary adenocarcinoma lines TA3/St and TA3/Ha contain comparable amounts of H-2 antigen, although intact TA3/St binds fluorescent anti-H-2 strongly and TA3/Ha cells do not give a detectable reaction.

The initial conviction of many cellular immunologists that T cells lack immunoglobulin stems from an inability to detect immunoglobulin on these cells by binding of fluorescent antibodies (Rabellino *et al.*, 1971). The parallel results for the display of immunoglobulin or histocompatibility antigens on certain cells illustrate the insufficiency of direct binding approaches and emphasizes the importance of isolation of plasma membranes and plasma membrane components.

III. ISOLATED SURFACE IMMUNOGLOBULIN OF B CELLS

It is now well established that the major surface immunoglobulin which is isolated from B cells of various species is a unit comprised of two light chains and two heavy chains which resemble μ-chain in mass and antigenic properties (Marchalonis and Cone, 1973; Vitetta and Uhr, 1973). Human B cells, in addition to this 7 S IgM unit, can possess surface molecules of the IgD class (Fu *et al.*, 1974; Rowe *et al.*, 1973). The IgD class is particularly prominent in fetal life where individual B lymphocytes can possess either surface IgM alone or IgM plus IgD. Very few, if any, normal cells exist which display only IgD; however, chronic lymphocytic leukemia cells bearing only IgD have been observed (Ferrarini *et al.*, 1975). When IgM and IgD coexist on chronic lymphocytic leukemia cells, they share V-region idiotypic determinants (Fu *et al.*, 1975). Figure 1 shows the polyacrylamide electrophoretic pattern of intact (top panel)

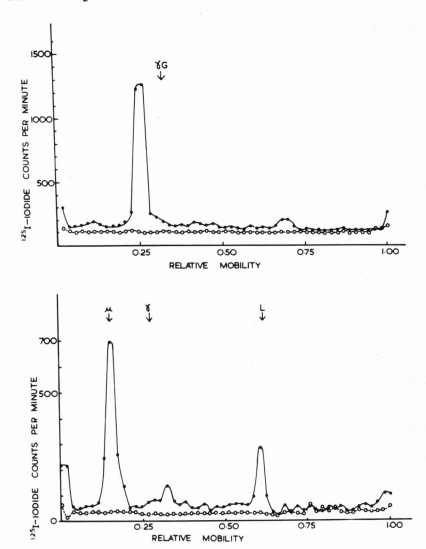

Figure 1. Analysis by polyacrylamide gel electrophoresis in SDS-containing buffers of
^{125}I-labeled surface immunoglobulin of human chronic lymphocytic leukemia cells
(monoclonal B cells). Upper panel: Unreduced samples resolved on 5% gel. Symbols: ●,
specifically precipitated immunoglobulin (rabbit antiserum to human κ-, λ-, and μ-chains
plus IgM carrier); ○, counts associated with control precipitate (chicken IgG plus rabbit
antiserum to chicken IgG). γG↓, location of human IgG marker (molecular weight 150,000).
Lower panel: Samples reduced with 2-mercaptoethanol to cleave interchain disulfide bonds
and analyzed on 10% gel under conditions which resolve light chains and heavy chains.
Symbols: ●, specifically precipitated immunoglobulin; ○, counts associated with control
precipitates. μ, γ, and L indicate positions at which μ-chain, γ-chain, and light chain migrated under these conditions. From Marchalonis *et al*. (1974b).

and reduced (bottom panel) ^{125}I-labeled immunoglobulin isolated from the surface of a human chronic lymphocytic leukemia cell population. The intact molecule possessed a mobility retarded with reference to human IgG (molecular weight 150,000) and was characterized by gel infiltration on Sepharose 6B by an apparent mass of 200,000 daltons. Upon reduction, the molecule was resolved into light chains and heavy chains resembling μ-chains in mobility. Marchalonis *et al.* (1974b) investigated ten such cell populations, finding that all cells which possessed immunoglobulin extractable in Nonidet P-40 possessed 7 S IgM. One of these cell populations yielded both IgM and IgG from its surface, but synthesized only IgM. Studies have not yet been reported using antisera to δ-chain, which should allow specific isolation of surface IgD. Pernis (1975) has stated that the mobilities of δ- and μ-chains are very similar. The likelihood exists that these two polypeptides might not be resolved by polyacrylamide gel electrophoresis in sodium dodecylsulfate-containing buffers in all gel systems presently in use.

Surface immunoglobulin of rabbit peripheral blood lymphocytes gives a pattern identical to that shown for human CLL cells (Smith and Marchalonis, unpublished). It has not yet been possible to obtain definite estimations of the mass of intact chicken B-cell surface IgM because of the pronounced tendency of this molecule to aggregate. The reduced immunoglobulin possessed light chains and μ heavy chains and an additional component of estimated mass 40,000–50,000 which might constitute either the ν heavy chain or a component which binds to antigen–antibody complexes (Haustein *et al.*, 1975; Stevens, 1974). Ivanyi (1975) observed that this type of electrophoretic pattern was typical of secreted 7 S IgM of the chicken, whereas 19 S IgM lacked the component which migrated in an intermediate position. Surface Ig of goldfish splenocytes contained light chains and μ-type heavy chains and existed as disulfide-bonded 7 S molecules (Warr *et al.*, 1976).

Radioiodinated surface immunoglobulin of murine B lymphocytes possesses an intact mass of approximately 200,000 daltons (Marchalonis and Cone, 1973; Vitetta and Uhr, 1973). However, upon cleavage of disulfide bonds, two heavy chains which clearly differ in mobility on polyacrylamide gel electrophoresis are produced (Melcher *et al.*, 1974; Abney and Parkhouse, 1974; Hunt and Marchalonis, 1974; Lisowska-Bernstein *et al.*, 1973). Two surface immunoglobulin chains were also isolated from rat spleen lymphocytes. Antigenically, one of these was IgM and the other IgG, although the mobility of the second heavy chain in SDS-polyacrylamide resembled that of putative mouse δ (Smith *et al.*, 1975). Figure 2 shows the polypeptide chains resolved from reduced ^{125}I-labeled surface immunoglobulin of spleen lymphocytes of congenitally thymic aplastic "nude" (*nu/nu*) mice. A heavy chain identical in gel penetration to μ-chain is present and antigenic evidence confirms the identification as μ-chain. The second heavy chain (peak fractions 18 and 19) is the subject of considerable interest because some investigators argue that it is the murine

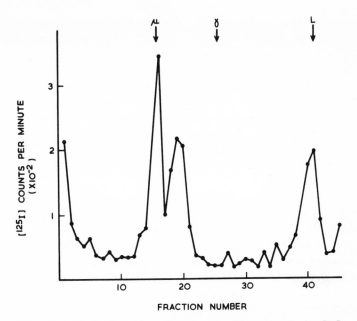

Figure 2. Analysis by polyacrylamide gel electrophoresis in SDS-containing buffers of ^{125}I-labeled polypeptide chains of reduced surface immunoglobulin of murine B cells (from spleens of *nu/nu* mice). μ, γ, and L indicate the positions at which μ-chains, γ-chains, and light chains migrated. Immunoglobulin was isolated using an immunoadsorbent specific for murine κ-chains.

counterpart of the human δ-chain (Vitetta and Uhr, 1975; Abney and Parkhouse, 1974) whereas others report that it possesses μ-chain antigenic determinants (Lisowska-Bernstein *et al.*, 1973). The issue of the identification of the second murine B-cell heavy chain as the homologue of human δ remains unresolved for the following reasons: (1) attempts using anti-δ serum to find cross-reacting molecules in mouse sera have been negative (Neoh *et al.*, 1973), (2) human δ migrates very close to μ-chain on SDS-polyacrylamide gels (Pernis, 1975; Warr and Marchalonis, 1976; Finkelman *et al.*, 1976) whereas the mobility of the putative mouse δ is quite distinct from that of μ, (3) no chemical comparisons between human δ and putative murine δ have been performed, and (4) putative murine δ predominates on cells of older mice in contrast to the prevalence of δ on fetal human B cells (Rowe *et al.*, 1973). In support of the similarity of the murine immunoglobulin to human IgD, Vitetta and Uhr (1975) report that both molecules are particularly susceptible to proteolytic degradations and maintain that addition of inhibitors of proteolysis is required to allow isolation of murine IgD from radioiodinated cell lysates (Vitetta and Uhr, 1975). Others have not encountered this problem in the isolation of murine IgD (Hunt and Marchalonis, 1974; Haustein and Goding, 1975; Goding et al., 1976) even when lysates were allowed to stand at 4°C in the presence of antisera for 3 days prior to centrifugation of precipitates (Marchalonis, unpublished observation). Although the exact nature of the murine second B-cell heavy chain remains to be determined, it is clear that its amount differs in various lymphoid cell populations (Vitetta and Uhr, 1975). B cells of bone marrow origin express mainly surface IgM, whereas the putative IgD-like molecule is predominantly isolated from radiodinated lymph node or Peyer's patch B cells. In analogy to the situation on human B cells, both immunoglobulins may coexist on a subpopulation of B cells, where each might mediate a different response following contact with antigen (Vitetta and Uhr, 1975).

The present conclusion regarding surface immunoglobulins of a number of species is that the predominant immunoglobulin is very similar to the 7 S sub-unit of IgM. In some species, two antigenically distinct surface immunoglobulins exist, and in one species, the mouse, the heavy chains of the B-cell surface im-munoglobulins are clearly distinct in mobility on polyacrylamide gels. Previous studies stating that IgG was the major B-cell surface immunoglobulin were based on binding of fluorescent (Rabellino et al., 1971) or radioiodinated (Jones et al., 1971) anti-immunoglobulins and most likely reflect adherence of IgG molecules to Fc receptors on the cell surface. It is possible, however, that a small per-centage of B cells might synthesize and express IgG molecules on their surface.

IV. ISOLATED SURFACE IMMUNOGLOBULIN OF T CELLS

Surface immunoglobulins of thymus lymphocytes and various T-cell popula-tions of man, mouse, rat, pig, and chicken have been isolated and partially characterized (Table I). Most work has been carried out using various murine T-cell populations because a number of antigenic markers including Thy-1 (θ), Ly-1, 2, 3, and TL are useful surface markers defining T cells (Warner and McKenzie, 1976). Murine T-cell immunoglobulin has been isolated by means of lactoperoxidase-catalyzed surface radioiodination coupled with cell solubiliza-tion by acid–urea (Marchalonis et al., 1972a, 1974a; Cone and Marchalonis, 1974; Boylston and Mowbray, 1973, 1974), acid–urea plus nonionic detergent (Cone, 1976a,b), metabolic release (Marchalonis et al., 1972a; Haustein et al., 1975; Haustein and Goding, 1975), mixtures of urea and nonionic detergent at neutral pH (Haustein, 1975; Haustein et al., 1975), and nonionic detergent plus inhibitors of proteases (Moroz and Lahat, 1974). It has also proved feasible to isolate T-cell immunoglobulin as released complexes with anti-immunoglobulin (Rieber and Riethmüller, 1974a, b; Rieber et al., 1973; Wilson et al., 1972; Rolley and Marchalonis, 1972) and by isolation of plasma membrane followed by solubilization in urea–Nonidet P-40, labeling of solubilized membrane, and serological precipitation (Haustein et al., 1974). Surface immunoglobulin of T cells differs from that of B cells inasmuch as solubilization of radioiodinated cells with nonionic detergents allows isolation of B-cell surface Ig but is ineffective for T cells (Cone and Marchalonis, 1974; Cone, 1976a,b; Haustein, 1975; Smith et al., 1975). This property probably reflects differences in the heavy chains of the molecules and, moreover, might relate to the manner in which the immunoglobulins are associated with membrane components such as lipids. This problem will be considered below.

Figure 3 shows a comparison between reduced surface immunoglobulins of spleen lymphocytes and thymus lymphocytes of CBA mice which was carried out by Haustein and Goding (1975). The former cell population was taken as a B-cell source; the latter constitutes a T-cell source. Two heavy chains were isolated from radioiodinated B cells whether the cells were extracted by 1% Nonidet P-40 (top panel) or by metabolic release (middle panel). In contrast, only one heavy chain was observed in the radioiodinated surface immunoglobulin obtained from thymus lymphocytes by metabolic release (bottom panel). In accordance with other reports, immunoglobulin was not detected in T-cell extracts obtained by detergent lysis (not shown). Haustein and Goding (1975) furthermore emphasize that the mobility of the T-cell heavy chain is slightly faster than that of the classical μ-chain standard. This observation represents a physiochemical difference between surface immunoglobulins of T and B cells which parallels previously reported functional differences (Feldmann and Nossal, 1972; Rieber and Riethmüller, 1974a; Cone et al., 1974; Stocker et al., 1974; Taniguchi and Tada, 1974; Feldmann et al., 1975). It suggests also that such immunoglobulin isolated from T-cell preparations is not the result of contamination of the cell preparations by B cells or plasma cells or by absorption from serum.

In addition to immunoglobulin polypeptide chains, all patterns in Fig. 3 contain a component of R_F 0.55–0.65 (estimated mass 40,000–50,000 daltons) which is present both in the specific antiimmunoglobulin precipitates and in the controls. The component therefore is associated with antigen–antibody complexes. A similar component has been observed elsewhere (Haustein et al., 1975; Stevens, 1974) and might represent the Fc receptor described by Basten et al., (1972). It is interesting that this component has an estimated mass comparable to that of histocompatibility antigens (Snary et al., 1974).

Although thymus lymphocytes have been reported to synthesize too much Ig to be quantitatively accounted for by contamination with other cell types (Moroz and Hahn, 1973), and the Ig synthesis can be blocked using anti-Thy-1 serum plus complement (Moroz and Lahat, 1974), the question of whether or not T cells can synthesize immunoglobulin has remained difficult to resolve satisfactorily. Most T-cell populations contain a small percentage of B cells or plasma cells, and studies demonstrating immunoglobulin biosynthesis have been challenged on this ground (Vitetta et al., 1973). A more direct approach to this problem became feasible when it was shown that some monoclonal murine T

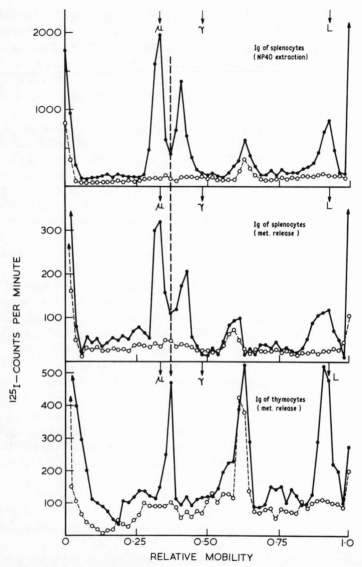

Figure 3. Analysis by polyacrylamide gel electrophoresis in SDS-containing buffers of
^{125}I-labeled surface immunoglobulins of CBA spleen lymphocytes (top and middle panels)
and CBA thymus lymphocytes (bottom panels). Symbols: ●, counts in specifically precipitated
immunoglobulin (mouse IgM plus rabbit antiserum reacting with mouse κ- and μ-chains);
O, counts associated with control precipitate (chicken IgG plus rabbit antiserum to chicken
IgG). Top panel: Spleen lymphocytes were extracted with 1% Nonidet P-40. Middle panel:
Surface protein of spleen lymphocytes was obtained by metabolic release. Bottom panel:
Surface proteins of thymus lymphocytes were obtained by metabolic release. μ, γ, and L
indicate positions at which μ-chains, γ-chains, and light chains migrated. From Haustein and
Goding (1975) with permission of the authors.

lymphoma cells could incorporate radioactive amino acids into detectable immunoglobulin (Harris *et al.*, 1973). Further studies (Haustein *et al.*, 1974, 1975; Boylston and Mowbray, 1974; Feldmann *et al.*, 1975) have confirmed and extended this observation. Evidence that T cells can synthesize surface receptor Ig also comes from studies involving capping and reappearance (Roelants *et al.*, 1973, 1974) of specific receptors for (T,G)-A--L. Since the binding of this synthetic polypeptide is eliminated by antisera to κ- and μ-chains, these authors conclude that specific IgM is removed with antigen and reappears in a metabolic process. It is now clear that a number of monoclonal continuously cultured T lymphoma cells which maintain a strict T-cell phenotype synthesize immunoglobulin, some of which is expressed on their surface. Each monoclonal tumor expresses a characteristic number of surface Ig molecules. Figure 4 presents a comparison between murine T lymphomas and human chronic lymphocytic

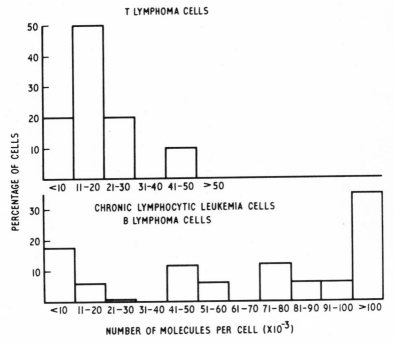

Figure 4. Frequency distributions of estimated numbers of molecules of surface immunoglobulin on T lymphoma cells and monoclonal B cells (chronic lymphocytic leukemia cells and B lymphoma cells). These distributions among monoclonal cells are assumed to reflect distribution of Ig molecules in normal lymphocyte populations. Estimated numbers of molecules per cell were taken from literature values for T lymphomas of mice (Boylston, 1973; Haustein *et al.*, 1975) and B lymphomas and leukemias of man (Lerner, 1972; Eskeland *et al.*, 1971; Marchalonis *et al.*, 1974b; Sherr *et al.*, 1972). The values pooled for construction of the frequency diagrams were obtained by techniques involving binding of antisera of Igs to cell surfaces as well as direct isolation of surface Ig.

leukemia cells (homogeneous B cells) in terms of frequency of cells bearing a certain number of Ig molecules (ordinate) vs. the number of molecules (abscissa). These constructed distributions are presumed to reflect the distributions occurring within normal T and B-cell populations. The estimated number of surface Ig molecules per B cell ranges from fewer than 10^4 to approximately 5×10^5, with a mean of about 8×10^4. This value agrees well with other estimates in the literature (Warner, 1974). The range of surface Ig molecules per cell for T lymphoma cells is between 10^4 and 4×10^4, with an average of 1.7×10^4. Thus B cells "on the average" possess more Ig molecules than do T cells, but there is overlap at the lower end of the B-cell range. I would emphasize that the T lymphoma values were obtained using isolation conditions which gave the "best estimates" of the number of molecules per cell (Haustein *et al.*, 1975); i.e., computations were not made from data obtained using solvents which either apparently enriched (acid–urea) or depleted (NP-40) for Ig. The approximate nature of these calculations is stressed (Marchalonis, 1974b; Marchalonis *et al.*, 1974b), although it should be emphasized that (1) the calculations for B cells are in excellent agreement with values computed by various techniques, and (2) at present no assumption-free method exists for absolute quantitation of membrane Igs.

Haustein *et al.*, (1975) reported that six of six T lymphoma lines possess surface Ig and concluded that this is a general property of T-type cells. Expression of surface Ig was not found to correlate with the presence of an Fc receptor, as was previously suggested by Grey *et al.*, (1972). Figure 5 shows an analysis of intact and reduced radioiodinated surface immunoglobulin of the BALB/c T lymphoma cell WEHI-22 by polyacrylamide gel electrophoresis in SDS-containing buffers. The intact molecule is retarded relative to the IgG standard. This finding is consistent with other reports that T-cell surface immunoglobulin has a molecular weight of approximately 200,000. Upon reduction, the molecule is cleaved into light chains and heavy chains. Only one type of heavy chain is present and that resembles the μ-like chain observed on thymus lymphocytes (see Fig. 3). Antigenic data suggest that the T lymphoma heavy chain is related to the μ-chain of normal IgM but that it is not identical to the serum molecule. In addition to immunoglobulin polypeptide chains, WEHI-22, which possesses an Fc receptor (Harris *et al.*, 1973), has a polypeptide of estimated mass 45,000 daltons which occurs in both the experimental and control precipitates. Other T lymphoma cells, such as WEHI-7, which lack Fc receptors lack this component.

The evidence described here indicates that murine T cells express a surface immunoglobulin of approximate mass 200,000 daltons which consists of light chains and heavy chains similar to μ-chain in gel penetration and in antigenic properties. Similar conclusions obtain for surface immunoglobulin isolated from radioiodinated T cells of rats (Smith *et al.*, 1975) and man (Marchalonis *et al.*, 1972b; Moroz and Hahn, 1973). Moroz and her co-workers have reported that

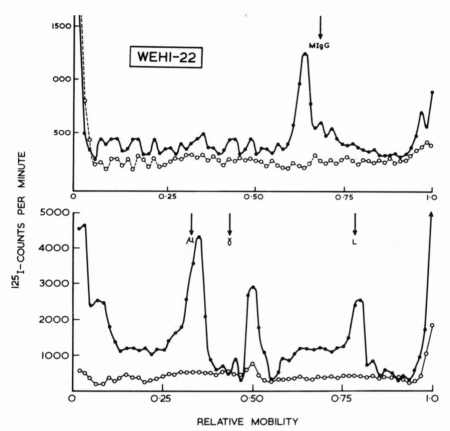

Figure 5. Analysis by polyacrylamide gel electrophoresis in SDS-containing buffers of intact (upper panel) and reduced (lower panel) ^{125}I-labeled surface Ig of WEHI-22 T lymphoma cells. Symbols: ●, counts in specifically precipitated Ig; ○, counts in control precipitate (chicken IgG plus rabbit antiserum to chicken IgG). From Haustein et al. (1975).

the light chains and μ-chains of human thymus Ig (Moroz and Hahn, 1973) and C57Bl mouse thymus Ig (Moroz and Lahat, 1974; Lahat and Moroz, 1975) are not linked covalently via disulfide bonds. The reasons for this discrepancy remain to be determined, but the procedure of Moroz and Hahn (1973) differs from that of other groups because the cells are treated with an alkylating agent prior to radioiodination of membrane proteins. Moreover, Moroz and Lahat (1974) found that BALB/c thymus lymphocytes expressed and synthesized Ig containing α-chains rather than μ-chains. The finding by Chavin (1974) of large amounts of buried IgG in pig thymus membranes warrants comment because this probably reflects a species difference. Kim et al., (1966) have previously shown that the major Ig produced in fetal pigs is 19 S IgG, so an analogy exists between this molecule and IgM in other species in terms of their early appearance in ontogeny.

Presently available data (reviewed above) indicate that B cells of man, mouse, and rat can express two classes of 7 S immunoglobulin. In man, these have been identified as IgM and IgD, both of which can exist on the same cell. When IgM and IgD occur on the same cell, they share variable-region idiotypes. The argument has been made that some mouse B cells possess both IgM and a homologue of IgD, but the conclusive identification of the second class of mouse B cell Ig as IgD requires further analysis. T cells, in contrast, possess only one class of surface immunoglobulin. This molecule contains light chains (either κ or λ) and heavy chains which migrate on SDS-polyacrylamide gels with a mobility clearly distinct from that of murine γ- and putative δ-chains. The mobility of the T-cell Ig heavy chain is slightly faster than that of serum μ-chain. Antigenic studies suggest that this chain is related to serum μ but it is not identical to the serum molecule. This distinction is emphasized by the observation that antisera to μ-chains of mouse myeloma proteins usually do not react with T-cell immunoglobulin (Burckhardt et al., 1974; Boylston and Mowbray, 1974). The 7 S IgM (T) has been shown to differ functionally from surface IgM and IgD of murine B cells in cytophilic properties for macrophages (Cone et al., 1974; Rieber and Riethmüller, 1974b) and by its capacity to act as a collaborative factor in T/B cooperation (Feldmann and Nossal, 1972; Feldmann et al., 1973; Rieber and Riethmüller, 1974a; Taniguchi and Tada, 1974; Dennert, 1973). Further investigation is necessary to establish whether differences between μ (T) and the heavy chains of B-cell origin arise from differences in amino acid sequences in the Fc region or from the presence or absence of carbohydrate moieties.

V. PROBLEMS IN THE ISOLATION OF MEMBRANE PROTEINS WITH REFERENCE TO SURFACE IMMUNOGLOBULIN

Approaches to the solubilization and isolation of membrane proteins are largely empirical, and a number of problems remain to be solved (Helenius and Simons, 1975; Steck and Fox, 1972; Wallach and Winzler, 1974). Proper discussion of these problems is beyond the scope of this chapter and the reader is referred to the above reviews. I would, however, point out some of the difficulties involved in analysis of membranes which have resulted in divergent findings regarding membrane immunoglobulins of B and T lymphocytes.

Membrane proteins, particularly those of an integral nature (Singer, 1974), exist in association with lipid. Solubilization of the protein requires that the membrane lipid, bound to hydrophobic proteins of the protein, be replaced by the hydrophobic portion of a detergent. The "soluble" membrane protein, then, is a complex of protein and detergent, with the hydrophilic portion of the detergent contributing to increased solubility in aqueous solution. Recent studies have clearly shown for various cell membranes that different membrane proteins are differentially solubilized by different detergents (Helenius and Simons, 1975; Liljas *et al.*, 1974; Letarte-Muirhead *et al.*, 1974). In some cases, nonionic detergent alone is not sufficient and urea must be added to the detergent solution to ensure effective release of proteins strongly associated with membrane lipid (Garewal and Wasserman, 1974). These comments are especially relevant to studies using nonionic detergents such as Nonidet P-40 and Triton X-100 which have been used extensively in lymphocyte work because the solubilized complexes tend to retain their antigenicity. In addition to simple complexes of one protein and detergent, detergent micelles, which can be of considerable size (Yedgar *et al.*, 1974), form above certain critical concentration of detergent (Helenius and Simons, 1975). These may trap a variety of membrane proteins and glycoproteins, some of which might be accessible for isolation by serological precipitation and others not (Hart, 1975). It is well established that 0.5% or 1% Nonidet P-40 allows excellent recovery of B-cell surface Ig (Vitetta *et al.*, 1972; Cone and Marchalonis, 1974), but is inadequate for isolation of T-cell surface Ig (Cone and Marchalonis, 1974). Cone (1976a,b) has observed that T-cell Ig appears to associate strongly with detergent micelles in a manner resembling that expected of hydrophobic integral proteins, whereas B-cell surface Ig resembles peripheral proteins more closely and is readily released from the micelle.

Lysis of cells by detergent is an effective means of releasing proteases (Steck and Fox, 1972; Tökés and Chambers, 1975). Moroz and Hahn (1973) found that T-cell Ig could be detected in Nonidet P-40 lysates of T cells if inhibitors of proteolysis were included. This difficulty applies not only to Ig of T cells but also to the IgD-like surface Ig of murine B cells (Vitetta and Uhr, 1975). These authors claim that the B-cell IgD-like molecule was not detected in their early studies (e.g., Baur *et al.*, 1971; Vitetta *et al.*, 1972) because the protein was readily degraded and rendered nonantigenic unless precautions were taken to inhibit proteolytic enzymes.

A crucial difficulty in immunological studies has been the specificity of the antisera used. This issue has also arisen in isolation of histocompatibility antigens and the Thy-1 alloantigen and will continue as an increasing number of surface markers are analyzed. Presently available data for the three types of lymphocyte surface Ig considered here indicated that (1) murine B-cell surface IgM is precipitated specifically by antisera to κ-chains and μ-chains (Marchalonis and Cone, 1973; Vitetta and Uhr, 1973), (2) a murine B-cell surface IgD-like molecule is precipitated specifically by antisera to κ-chains (Abney and Parkhouse, 1974; Vitetta and Uhr, 1975) but only by some antisera to μ-chains (Lisowska-Bernstein *et al.*, 1973), and (3) murine T-cell surface Ig reacts specifically with antisera to κ-chains (Marchalonis and Cone 1973; Boylston and Mowbray, 1973, 1974; Rieber and Riethmüller, 1974a,b; Feldmann *et al.*, 1975) but reacts only with some antisera to μ-chain, notably those produced to serum IgM of normal animals (Burckhardt *et al.*, 1974; Haustein *et al.*, 1975). Thus murine Ig (T) and putative IgD parallel one another in antigenic properties, although poly-acrylamide gel electrophoretic data (Haustein and Goding, 1975) and functional studies (Cone *et al.*, 1974) indicate that the heavy chains of the two molecules must differ structurally.

When studies involving lactoperoxidase-catalyzed radioiodination of surface proteins are used, care must be taken to ensure that the conditions used are suitable for the particular cell type and for the particular proteins under consideration (Haustein, 1975; Haustein *et al.*, 1975; Tsai *et al.*, 1973; Hynes, 1975). As an illustration, labeling conditions suitable for normal T and B lymphocytes are not necessarily adequate for investigation of surface proteins of T lymphoma cells (Haustein, 1975; Haustein *et al.*, 1975).

In principle, no absolutely definitive set of conditions exists for the isolation of particular membrane components, and a variety of strategies of extraction and analysis must be considered. It has been found possible to isolate three types of lymphocyte surface Igs. Surface IgM of B cells is readily isolated using a variety of extraction procedures. Surface IgD of mouse B cells can be extracted using a variety of conditions, but more care must be taken to ensure that it is not lost because of proteolysis. Isolation of IgM (T) from mouse T cells requires the most careful attention to detail because it is not readily isolated by detergent lysis of cells and might be subject to proteolytic degradation.

VI. CAPACITY OF SURFACE IMMUNOGLOBULIN TO BIND ANTIGEN

By definition, a receptor must bind the ligand in question. Since we are considering a surface receptor, it is also necessary to establish that the binding molecule was obtained from the cell surface. Four types of approaches indicate that surface Ig possesses the capacity to combine with antigen. These are as follows: (1) "co-capping" analysis which determines whether antigen and immuno-globulin are associated in the plane of the membrane, (2) isolation of antigen and Ig as complexes from the cell surface, (3) demonstration that radio-iodinated, extracted surface Ig binds antigen, and (4) the isolation of radio-iodinated surface Ig which bears the iodiotype characteristic of a particular anti-body. At the present time, all four approaches have been used for B cells and the first three for T cells.

The first method can be applied to individual antigen-binding lymphocytes which combine with fluorescent antigens. Initially the antigen is uniformly distributed over the surface of the cell, but, if the cells are maintained at 37°C, it forms aggregates or "patches" and eventually accumulates in a large cap at one pole of the cell. This "capped" antigen, presumably complexed with its receptor, is then shed or taken into the cell. An analogous process occurs on the surfaces of B lymphocytes when fluorescent antibody (divalent) to Ig is added. If Ig is the lymphocyte receptor for antigen, antigen and Ig should cap together. This result has been observed for protein and erythrocyte antigens binding to B lymphocytes. It is more difficult to perform this sort of experiment directly with T lymphocytes because these usually do not bind detectable levels of antiglobulins. However, Ashman and Raff (1973) have found that erythrocyte antigens binding to T cells form caps just as they do on B cells. Roelants *et al.* (1973, 1974) have made a strong case that IgM molecules on T cells which bind protein antigens are capped along with the antigen. These data provide evidence consistent with immunoglobulin functioning as the antigen receptor on B and T cells. It is not conclusive proof, however. The same results would be obtained if the true receptor for antigen were not Ig but some molecule which was contiguous with Ig on the same protein island in the fluid lipid of the membrane.

Rolley and Marchalonis (1972) described experiments designed to isolate complexes of dinitrophenylated mouse hemoglobin and cell surface immunoglobulin obtained from spleen lymphocytes of congenitally athymic *nu/nu* mice. This was feasible since B cells of unimmunized mice possesses a high level of lymphocytes (0.1–1.0%) capable of reacting with saturating concentrations (50–100 μg) of ^{125}I-labeled DNP hemoglobin. Similar high numbers of binding cells specific for the DNP hapten were found by other workers (Lawrence *et al.*, 1973; Rutishauser and Edelman, 1972). Cytophilic antibodies apparently did not play a major role in the DNP binding by B cells because the number of antigen-binding cells was not increased by incubation with antisera to DNP (Rolley and Marchalonis, 1972). Complexes of DNP hemoglobin and cell surface Ig were detected by specific coprecipitation using systems specific for DNP and for mouse Ig. Such complexes were isolated from the cell surface by metabolic release at 37°C and by limited proteolysis with trypsin. Moreover, the population of radioiodinated cell surface immunoglobulin was found to mimic the heterogeneous population of antibodies normally found in sera inasmuch as removal of cell surface Ig specifically reactive to DNP by affinity chromatography did not remove the capacity of the Ig pool to combine with other antigens, e.g., horseshoe crab hemocyanin. Further studies involving B-cell populations highly enriched in cells of a given specificity are required to completely establish the structural properties of B-cell receptor immunoglobulin. This study, however, provided direct evidence in support of the hypothesis that B-cell Ig functions as antigen receptor.

A third approach to test the capacity of lymphocyte surface immunoglobulin to bind antigen is to isolate radioiodinated membrane immunoglobulin and determine whether it combines with suitable chosen antigens. This strategy has recently been used to show that a detectable fraction of ^{125}I-labeled surface Ig of normal B cells (spleen cells of *nu/nu* mice) bound to solid-phase DNP-immunoadsorbents. The design of experiments recently performed in this laboratory is depicted in Fig. 6. Since it is now possible to obtain as many as 10^6 cpm in specifically isolated surface Ig of 10^8 B cells, the attempt to ascertain whether about 1% of this amount binds to DNP is feasible. If surface Ig is the only molecule which binds DNP under these conditions, the DNP eluate of the Ig-depleted fraction should contain little detectable protein. If other surface proteins which can be radioiodinated bind DNP, these would be observed in the DNP-eluate of the Ig-depleted fraction. Figure 7 shows that the radioiodinated protein which was specifically eluted from DNP-Sepharose contained μ-chains, light chains, and some putative δ-chains. It was characteristic of eluted DNP-binding surface Ig that the bulk of the ^{125}I counts were associated with the μ-chain. No detectable ^{125}I-labeled protein was specifically eluted from the Ig-depleted fraction of cell surface protein. Further studies using DNP coupled to glutaraldehyde-fixed sheep red blood cells and autoradiographic analysis of eluted ^{125}I-labeled binding proteins (J. J. Marchalonis and E. White, unpublished observations) clearly showed that the putative δ-chain, as well as the μ-chain, was present in surface Ig which binds this hapten. These results are

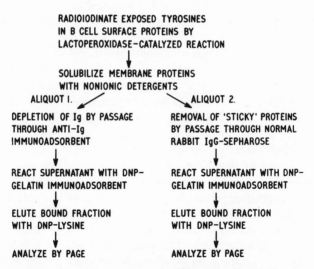

Figure 6. Scheme for isolation of ^{125}I-labeled surface Ig of B cells (from spleens of *nu/nu* mice) which binds to DNP. The DNP-gelatin was coupled to Sepharose-4B by the CNBr method. Elution was performed using 5×10^{-4} M DNP-lysine. The anti-Ig immunoadsorbent was specific for mouse κ and γ chains.

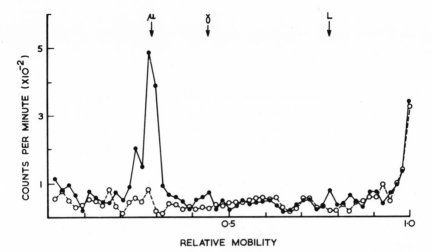

Figure 7. ^{125}I-labeled proteins obtained from the DNP-immunoadsorbent with DNP-lysine (see Fig. 6) Symbols: ●, counts in eluate of cell surface protein mixture which had been passed through normal rabbit IgG-Sepharose (i.e., mouse ^{125}I-surface Ig was present, but "sticky" proteins had been removed); ○, counts in eluate of cell surface protein mixture which had been passed through anti-Ig-Sepharose (i.e., removed mouse Ig and "sticky" proteins).

consistent with the finding that human IgM and IgD can share idiotypes (Fu et al., 1975) and provide direct support for an antigen-binding role of B-cell surface Ig.

Since techniques now exist which allow the biological enrichment of T lymphocytes to a variety of antigens, it is possible to carry out investigations of the binding specificity of ^{125}I-labeled surface immunoglobulins of activated T cells. At this time, studies have been carried out using murine T lymphocytes activated specifically to syngeneic tumor-associated transplantation antigens (Röllinghoff et al., 1973), histocompatibility antigens (Cone et al., 1972), foreign erythrocytes (Cone and Marchalonis, 1973), and foreign proteins (Feldmann et al., 1973). In all cases, detectable amounts of surface immunoglobulin showing specific binding to the activating antigen were observed. As an illustration (Cone and Marchalonis, 1973), helper T cells activated to sheep erythrocytes (SRBC) were obtained by reconstituting lethally irradiated (850 r) CBA mice with syngeneic thymus lymphocytes plus SRBC plus a synthetic polynucleotide adjuvant consisting of a complex of polyadenylic acid and polyuridylic acid. This complex stimulates T cells (Cone and Johnson, 1972), and helper cells appear rapidly, preceding the appearance of antibody-secreting cells. Two days after injection of this mixture, spleens were removed and used as a source of helper T cells to SRBC in an *in vitro* assay consisting of spleens of congenitally athymic (*nu/nu*) mice and added test T-cell populations. The properties of these helper T cells are listed in Table II. It should be stressed that T/B cooperation to SRBC and to protein antigens (keyhole limpit hemocyanin and chicken IgG) does not show a requirement for histocompatible T and B cells. Specifically activated helper T cells to SRBC produced a hemolytic plaque-forming cell response >10 times larger than that supported by normal CBA thymus lymphocytes or by CBA T cells activated (as above) to chicken γ-globin. ^{125}I-labeled surface proteins of the activated T cells were obtained by metabolic release and divided into two aliquots. Ig was removed from one aliquot by specific precipitation; the other was treated with an indifferent immunological precipitation system. The latter aliquot thus contained ^{125}I-labeled surface Ig, but proteins which might adhere to antigen-antibody complexes had been removed. When tested for the presence of radioiodinated proteins binding to SRBC or control erythrocytes, the immunoglobulin-containing sample had high numbers of counts binding to SRBC but very few binding to mouse or horse RBC (Table III). The immunoglobulin-depleted fraction showed no binding to any of the RBCs tested, as would be expected if immunoglobulin were the only specific binding agent. The specific precipitate (anti-mouse immunoglobulin) was analyzed and found to contain IgM-like 7 S immunoglobulin. Further experiments showed that the ^{125}I-labeled surface Ig came from helper T lymphocytes because treatment with antiserum to the θ-alloantigen in the presence of complement blocked helper activity and completely eliminated detection of immunoglobulin. These results were consistent with the low percentage of B cells in these activated populations (<2%) and the virtual absence

Table II. Properties of Helper T Cells to SRBC[a]

Specific
    Did not increase PFC to DRBC
    Helpers to FγG did not increase response to SRBC
    Antigen-specific suicide by soluble ^{125}I fragments
      of SRBC
Contained too few Ig+ cells to account for the amount of Ig
    isolated
Function and isolation of Ig completely eliminated
    by anti-θ + C'
Cooperation does not require identity of H-linked genes

[a]PFC, plaque-forming cells; DRBC, donkey red cells; FγG, chicken IgG; SRBC, sheep red blood cells. Based on data of Cone and Marchalonis (1973) and Stocker and Marchalonis (unpublished observations).

**Table III. Antigen Binding by ^{125}I-Labeled Surface Immunoglobulins
of T Cells (CBA) Activated to Sheep Erythrocytes[a]**

Treatment of ^{125}I-labeled cell surface proteins of specifically activated T cells	^{125}I-radioactivity (cpm $\times$ 10^{-3}) bound to		
	SRBC	HRBC	MRBC
Coprecipitated with chicken IgG and rabbit antiserum to chicken IgG	5.5 ± 0.1	0.2 ± 0.1	0.6 ± 0.3
Coprecipitated with mouse IgG and rabbit antiserum to mouse IgG	0.3 ± 0.1	0.2 ± 0.0	0.5 ± 0.1

[a]SRBC, sheep erythrocytes; HRBC, horse erythrocytes; MRBC, mouse erythrocytes. Cell surface proteins were obtained by metabolic release. The rabbit antiserum to mouse IgG reacted with κ-chains and γ-chains. Data of Cone and Marchalonis (1973).

of cells forming antibodies to SRBC (< 5 PFC/10^6 cells). I would stress that these results were obtained with activated T-cell populations, but the above results of Roelants et al., (1973, 1974) using lymph node T lymphocytes from nonimmunized mice suggest that the receptor on resting T lymphocytes is likewise IgM-like immunoglobulin. The direct isolation results cited here for B and T lymphocyte surface immunoglobulin demonstrate that membrane immunoglobulin can bind foreign antigens and certain tumor antigens and strong alloantigens. Other recognition systems might occur in weak allogeneic interactions such as MLR and GVHR (Marchalonis, 1975). Moreover, the possibility remains that surface immunoglobulin acts in concert with other membrane proteins in the early events of lymphocyte differentiation.

Strayer et al., (1975) have used an analogous procedure demonstrating that approximately 10% of radioiodinated extracted surface Ig of B cells of BALB/c mice hyperimmunized to phosphorylcholine possessed the idiotype characteristic of the phosphorylcholine-binding myeloma protein TEPC-15. Cosenza and Köhler (1972) had previously shown that use of this anti-idiotype serum would suppress antibody formation to phosphorylcholine. The isolation data emphasize the identity between V_H-V_L antigen-combining sites of surface receptors and secreted antibody of different isotype. Several recent studies establish the antigenic similarity of idiotypes of serum antibodies and T-cell receptors for strong histocompatibility antigens (McKearn, 1974; Binz and Wigzell, 1975) and streptococcal antigens (Eichmann, 1975; Eichmann and Rajewsky, 1975). The idiotype-containing molecules have not yet been isolated from the T-cell surface. When idiotype-bearing molecules are eventually isolated from the surface of T cells, such experiments should be carried out using extraction conditions suitable for T-cell immunoglobulin (see above).

VII. ATTACHMENT OF SURFACE IMMUNOGLOBULIN TO THE PLASMA MEMBRANE

Knowledge of the manner in which surface Ig is associated with the plasma membrane is essential to an understanding of the role of this molecule in the specific immune activation of lymphocytes. As was discussed above, surface immunoglobulin possesses the capacity to combine with antigen; however, the mechanism by which the signal generated by binding of antigen is transmitted to the cell's genome is not clear at this time. The most simple hypothesis is to envision that surface Ig is located in the plasma membrane such that its variable-region combining sites for antigen are exposed to the external surroundings and the Fc region is associated with enzymes, e.g., adenyl cyclase, or contractile structures (Yahara and Edelman, 1972), e.g., microtubules, which might function in the initiation of cell differentiation. Since both adenyl cyclase (Robison et al., 1971) and microtubules (Roth et al., 1970) are associated with the inner surface of the plasma membrane, this model would predict that surface immunoglobulin might be a transmembrane protein which actually spans the lipid bilayer. The Fc region of immunoglobulin is of sufficient size (Fc of γ, 45 Å; Poljak, 1973) to cross the lipid bilayer of the membrane ($\sim$ 30 Å wide); however, a number of difficulties challenge this simple hypothesis. If the amino acid sequence of the human μ-chain Ou (Putnam et al., 1973) is representative of membrane-bound μ-chain, the first problem is that the Fc portion does not contain a stretch of residues comparable in hydrophobicity to the residues of glycophorin (Segrest and Feldmann, 1974) which are thought to span the erythrocyte membrane (Steck, 1974). Moreover, surface IgM of B cells has been shown to possess mannose-containing carbohydrate moieties (Hunt and Marchalonis, 1974). If the distribution of glycosyl moieties on surface μ-chain is similar to that on μ (Ou), the fifth glycopeptide (one rich in mannose; Baenziger and Kornfeld, 1974) occurs 14 residues from the C-terminus of the chain (Putnam et al., 1973), so only 13 residues might be available for interaction with membrane lipid. A sequence of 13 amino acids would have a maximum length, when fully extended, of about 45 Å, which is comparable to the width of the lipid bilayer, but the C-terminal 14 residues are not of a pronounced hydrophobic character and such an extended structure is unlikely. If the residues were arranged in an α-helix, the length would be approximately 20 Å. This arrangement would not span the membrane. Fu and Kunkel (1974) have found that certain Fc region antigenic determinants of human μ- and δ-chains are not accessible to fluorescein-labeled antisera and suggest that the C-terminal portion of these chains is "buried." This result supports the above hypothesis, as does work of D. Snary and M. J. Crumpton (cited by Haustein et al., 1974) showing that surface IgM of the human lymphoblastoid line BR18 is firmly bound to the plasma membrane. Similar conclusions can be made for surface Igs of rat (Smith et al.,

1975) and pig (Chavin, 1974) B cells. Studies involving lactoperoxidase-catalyzed radioiodination of murine B cells suggest that the major portion of surface μ-chain is exposed (Marchalonis et al., 1972a; Vitetta et al., 1972). The available data on IgM structure and properties of B-cell IgM would thus suggest that most of the 7 S unit is exposed; however, a small portion of the C-terminal region of the heavy chain is associated directly either with plasma membrane lipid or with another membrane protein which is an integral or transmembrane structure (adaptor). If the latter alternative is correct, the association of μ- or δ-chains with the adaptor molecule need not necessarily occur via strong hydrophobic interactions analogous to the interaction of glycophorin with membrane lipid. Since membrane Ig of mouse B cells contains mannose-rich glycopeptides (Hunt (and Marchalonis, 1974), the binding to the adaptor might result from the binding of glycosyl moieties to a lectinlike protein. Precedent exists for the presence of lectinlike proteins on the surface of mammalian cells (Balsamo and Lilien, 1975; Hudgin and Ashwell, 1974).

It might be argued that Ig surface receptors, since they exist in fairly stable association with the plasma membrane (Melchers and Cone, 1975), must be quite different from serum Igs. However, in the case of surface IgM at least, the heavy chain appears antigenically identical to the μ-chain of serum IgM and possesses an identical mobility when analyzed by polyacrylamide gel electrophoresis under various solvent conditions. Therefore, it is unreasonable to propose that surface μ-chain differs markedly from serum μ-chain. These two chains might differ in carbohydrate content rather than in amino acid sequence. If surface IgM is essentially identical to serum IgM except for state of polymerization, the 7 S IgM is probably associated with the plasma membrane through strong noncovalent association with another protein (the adaptor), rather than via direct hydrophobic interaction with membrane lipid.

Evidence from various approaches also suggests that IgM (T) is tightly associated with the lymphocyte plasma membrane. These observations can be listed as follows: (1) constant-region μ-chain determinants are "buried" on antigen-binding T cells (Hogg and Greaves, 1972), (2) surface Ig of the T lymphoma cell WEHI-22 is sufficiently strongly bound to the plasma membrane to resist vigorous washing (Haustein et al., 1974), (3) IgM (T) becomes associated with micelles formed by nonionic detergents (Cone, 1976a,b), and (4) lactoperoxidase-catalyzed radioiodination of T-cell Ig on the cell surface might only label the Fd portion of the heavy chain, i.e., the ratio of label in light chain to label in heavy chain is approximately 1 : 1 (Marchalonis et al., 1972a). The possibility has been raised that the heavy chain of T-cell Ig is distinct from μ or δ in solubility properties and resembles an integral membrane protein, whereas the latter two chains are extremely similar to those found on the corresponding serum Igs (Cone, 1976a,b). IgM (T), like the B-cell surface molecules, might be associated either with membrane lipid or with an adaptor molecule.

Although direct data supporting this view are not yet available, it is attractive to propose an antigen-recognition complex on the lymphocyte surface (Fig. 8). This complex, by analogy with receptors for certain polypeptide hormones (Birnbaumer *et al.*, 1970; Perkins, 1973), would contain (1) a recognition element (Ig), (2) a regulatory element (the adaptor), and (3) an effector element on the inner face of the membrane, e.g., a nucleotide cyclase or microtubules. Rabbit lymphocytes probably possess a complete complex, because binding of anti-immunoglobulins will initiate cell activation (Sell and Gell, 1965). Mouse B lymphocytes, in contrast, are not stimulated by these reagents (Greaves and Janossy, 1972), so functional receptor complexes might not exist prior to contact with antigen. Activation would require not only binding of antigen but also interaction with the adaptor–effector complex. This event could be considered a mitogenic signal and conceivably might be mediated via contacts between histocompatibility antigens or Ia antigens. Studies are in progress to determine whether the components of apparent mass 40,000–50,000 on SDS-polyacrylamide gel (similar to H-2 antigens) which precipitated with antigen–antibody complexes (see Figs. 3 and 5) might be associated with Ig on the cell surface. This model parallels the case in which antigen binding to IgE, which is cytophilically bound to the surface of a mast cell via interaction of its Fc fragment and cell receptor, elicits production and release of pharmocologically active mediators (Austen *et al.*, 1975; Lichtenstein and Henney, 1975).

A possible qualification to the proposed analogy between hormone-recognition complexes and antigen-recognition complexes is that the density of surface

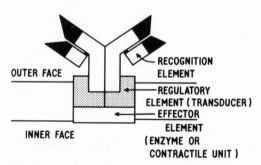

Figure 8. Hypothetical model for lymphocyte surface antigen recognition complex. Recognition element, surface immunoglobulin. V_H–V_L combining sites for antigen are exposed to the solvent. Regulatory elements are associated with the Fc portions of the surface Ig. These regulatory components penetrate the membrane lipid and might span the membrane. Distinct regulatory elements are possible and might be involved in triggering distinct antigen-specific functions of T and B cells. The effector element is associated with the inner surface of the plasma membrane and might be an enzyme or a contractile unit. The possibility exists that different effector elements might be involved in distinct activation processes.

Ig on B cells is much greater than that of receptors for insulin (Cuatrecasas, 1973) or catecholamines (Cuatrecasas *et al.*, 1974) on other cell types. A normal fat cell, for example, contains approximately 10^3 insulin receptors per cell (Cuatrecasas, 1973), which gives a density of 10 or fewer receptors per square micrometer of surface; a B cell, in contrast, possesses 8×10^4 Ig molecules per cell on the average and this computes to a density in the range of $400/\mu m^2$. Therefore, B cells express considerably more Ig than they would require for physiological receptor function. Possibly only a small subset ($< 5\%$) of B-cell surface Ig is directly involved in physiological activation. These molecules would exist in association with the regulatory and effector elements of the complex. The bulk of B-cell Ig, like the functional receptor Ig, would combine with antigen, but this might serve as a means of trapping of antigen, possibly for presentation to other cells such as T cells or macrophages. A distinction between activation for immunity or tolerance might follow from the relative distribution of antigen between Ig in receptor complexes and Ig existing free in the membrane. Alternatively, similar control could be obtained if Ig in both cases is associated with the regulatory element, but different effector units are involved in tolerance and immunity. Possible alternatives are the pair adenylate cyclase and guanylate cyclase (Watson, 1975) or one of these enzymes with the other signal coming from a membrane contractile element. The latter possibility is suggested by the differences in susceptibility of mouse (Sell and Gell, 1965) and rabbit (Greaves *et al.*, 1974) B cells to blastogenic stimulation by binding of anti-immunoglobulins. Murine B-cell surface Igs are extremely mobile within the plane of the membrane and form polar caps readily (Taylor *et al.*, 1971). Surface Ig of rabbit B and possibly T cells (Linthicum and Sell, 1974a, b), in contrast, forms small patches after binding bivalent antibodies but does not show the pronounced tendency to cap which is characteristic of mouse B-cell surface Ig. Moreover, anti-Ig patches are rapidly endocytosed in the rabbit, whereas this process follows cap formation in the mouse. Since interaction of ligands with surface Ig by itself is not sufficient to initiate lymphocyte differentiation in murine B cells (Möller, 1975), it is necessary to propose that specific physiological activation requires at least two components: a recognition unit (Ig) and an effector unit. By analogy with hormone receptor complexes, I have also introduced a regulatory or transducing unit which connects the recognition molecule on the outer face of the membrane with the effector unit on the inner surface. Since Ig is differentiated into recognition (V-region) and effector (C-region) domains (Edelman and Gall, 1969), the obvious candidate for the regulatory unit is the Fc region of the membrane immunoglobulin. In this model, binding of antigen to the V_H-V_L antigen-combining site would induce a conformational change in the Fc region which might be transmitted to the effector molecule. Evidence now exists supporting the concept of a conformational change in serum IgM (Haustein, 1971) and IgG (Schlessinger *et al.*, 1975) antibodies following binding of antigen. The function of the Fc region in signal transduction is further suggested by the existence of two types of surface Igs on some human and murine B cells (see above). These molecules, when present on the same cell, share V-region idiotypes but possess distinct heavy-chain constant regions. Vitetta and Uhr (1975) have argued eloquently that discrimination between the signal for tolerance and that for immunity might result from binding of antigen to surface IgD (immunity) or to surface IgM (tolerance). Experimental evidence militating against this type of model exists, however, because murine bone marrow B cells which have been said to express only IgM (Vitetta and Uhr, 1975) can be made either tolerant or immune (Stocker and Nossal, 1975). A similar situation appears to obtain for lower species such as carp, which apparently possess only IgM in the serum (Marchalonis, 1971) and on lymphocytes (Warr et al., 1976), but which can be rendered immune or tolerant depending on the conditions of antigen presentation (Avtalion et al., 1976). Furthermore, T cells express only one type of surface Ig, yet can be activated specifically or rendered tolerant (Chiller et al., 1970). Clearly the structural differences in the Fc regions of μ-, δ-, and μ(T)-chains have important physiological consequences. Pernis (1975) has shown that surface-associated IgD molecules exert a profound regulatory influence on formation of IgG antibodies in monkeys, and released complexes of IgM(T) and antigen act as collaborative factors in T/B cooperation (Feldmann and Nossal, 1972; Rieber and Riethmüller, 1974b; Taniguchi and Tada, 1974). The above considerations, however, support the requirement for a regulatory unit which is distinct from the Ig recognition unit. The existence of distinct types of regulatory and effector elements would allow precise control of a variety of reactions specifically initiated by the binding of antigen Ig to V_H-V_L combining sites.

VIII. TOWARD A UNIFIED RECEPTOR HYPOTHESIS

General criteria defining a surface receptor can be stated as follows:

1. The molecule must be present on the cell surface.
2. The molecule must bind the ligand in question.
3. Binding of the ligand must initiate the physiological process in question.

All three criteria must be satisfied in order to establish that a putative receptor actually functions in physiological recognition. The first criterion is obvious, but it immediately questions the source of putative recognition factors isolated from the culture fluid of moribund or dead cells. The second condition is a necessary requirement of receptor definition but it is not sufficient. Murine B cells, for example, bind more than 10^6 concavalin A molecules per cell (Stobo et al.,

1972) but are not stimulated by this interaction (Greaves and Janossy, 1972). T cells bind comparable amounts of this lectin and become stimulated to undergo mitogenic transformation. It would thus be proper to conclude that B cells possess surface molecules characterized as concanavalin A binding moieties, but they do not possess receptors (*sensu strictu*) for this mitogen. Another example is the binding of [^{3}H] norepinephrine to intact fat cells (Cuatrecasas *et al.*, 1974). Approximately 5×10^6 molecules bind per cell, which is an extremely high value compared to the binding of another hormone, insulin. The number of norepinephrine molecules bound is at least 500 times greater than the binding capacity for insulin. However, Cuatrecasas *et al.* (1974) determined that the binding of labeled norepinephrine to intact cells seems not to measure catecholamine receptor interactions but rather a membrane catechol-binding protein which might be related to enzyme catechol-O-methyltransferase. These workers suggest that the true receptors are probably quite scarce and might not be detected by the binding approach used.

Surface Ig of both B and T cells apparently meets the first two criteria for the definition of a recognition role for certain antigens. However, a number of caveats must be stated: (1) Establishment of the physical presence of Ig on cell surfaces using some relatively insensitive technique like immunofluorescence is useful as a simple preliminary means of identifying cell types, but it does not demonstrate that Ig is an antigen receptor. The converse argument that failure to find Ig by this method disqualifies Ig as a receptor is also untenable. As Cuatrecasas *et al.* (1974) point out, the number of true hormone receptors is usually quite modest (about 10^3 per fat cell) and the receptors might not be detectable by many binding assays. (2) B cells possess a vast excess of surface Ig molecules (about 10^5 molecules per cell) relative to the number of hormone receptors on most cells. Possibly only a small fraction of this Ig actually carries out a true receptor role (see above). T cells, on the average, possess one-tenth to one-fifth the number of Ig molecules found on B cells. This number is still high compared to the number of insulin receptors, for example, but IgM(T) differs from IgM and IgD of B cells structurally and in its association with the plasma membrane. (3) When defining an antigen receptor, care should be taken to specify what function is under consideration. This comment is straightforward when applied to B cells, but leads to complicated situations with T cells. T cells can carry out a number of recognition functions, some of which do not represent a specific immunological function. In particular, the allogeneic mixed lymphocyte reactions might constitute a recognition system which does not involve Ig variable regions (Crone *et al.*, 1972; Marchalonis, 1975). Moreover, the possibility exists that receptors on helper and suppressor T cells specific for foreign antigens might differ. In this case, the minimal hypothesis would be that recognition is mediated via Ig variable regions, but that the cells differentiate into distinct effector cells. The term "receptors for antigen" in this chapter has been restricted to those recognizing foreign antigens such as foreign erythrocytes and proteins (see above), where the capacity to respond is not under the control of genes linked to the major histocompatibility locus. Similar conclusions have been drawn for some synthetic polypeptides, such as (T,G)-A--L, which are under H-linked genetic control where both B and T cells recognize antigen using Ig receptors (Hämmerling and McDevitt, 1974; Roelants *et al.*, 1973, 1974) but lack the capacity to cooperate in antibody formation (Benacerraf and McDevitt, 1972). The deficiency in this system appears to be at the level of cell cooperation rather than at the level of recognition.

The concept of either T- or B-cell Ig *per se* functioning as a physiological receptor for antigen suffers most difficulty when analyzed in terms of criterion (3). Although B-cell surface Ig binds antigen, this event alone does not suffice to induce differentiation (Möller, 1975). Furthermore, binding of anti-immunoglobulin does not induce blast transformation (Greaves *et al.*, 1974). In contrast, rabbit peripheral B and T lymphocytes can be stimulated by binding of antisera to Igs (Sell and Gell, 1965). Möller (1975) has argued that murine B-cell surface Ig is not a physiological or "triggering" receptor. It focuses antigen onto the cell, but the stimulus for differentiation is essentially a nonspecific mitogenic one. In this chapter, the concept was discussed that Ig is part of an antigen-recognition complex where it serves as the recognition unit but must be in proper juxtaposition with regulatory and effector elements in order to generate a signal for differentiation. The other elements in the system are not yet established. Similar arguments apply to the role of T-cell Ig in the activation of antigen-specific T cells into various effector cells; however, released complexes of T-cell surface Ig and antigen can function in the stimulation of specific B cells.

Figure 9 presents a hypothetical scheme which unifies lymphocyte surface antigen receptors and soluble antigen-specific factors. This model proposes that recognition of a particular antigen in all cases is mediated by an Ig-combining site composed of V_L and V_H regions. Although the usual case would be one in which interaction between V_H and V_L is obligatory to create the combining site (Capra and Kehoe, 1975), the possibility exists that V_H alone might in some situations possess a high degree of binding capacity (Utsumi and Karush, 1964). B cells could possess IgM and IgD sharing idiotype but differing in heavy-chain C-region domains. Circulating antibody might be IgM, IgG, IgA, or IgE but would possess the same idiotype. T-cell IgM(T) likewise would share the V_H-V_L idiotype, but have a heavy chain distinct from μ, δ, and the serum Ig heavy chains. In this scheme, the idiotypes are represented as identical on the basis of antigenic data (see above). In actuality, B-cell and T-cell Igs would be predicted to share V regions specified by immunoglobulin V-region genes, but they would not necessarily be identical. For example, if V regions are encoded by multiple germ lines, B- and T-cell V regions could be identical. If, however, somatic diversification generates V-region genes and diversification continues after the divergence

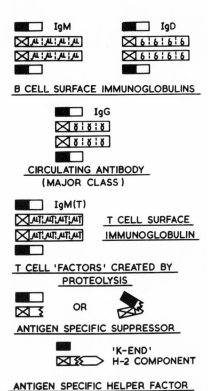

Figure 9. Surface immunoglobulins of B and T cells and their hypothetical relationships to antigen-specific "factors." The "dark" V region of the light chains and "crossed" V region of the heavy chains indicate that receptors of the same specificity share idiotypic determinants, whether they arise from T cells or B cells.

of the stem cells leading to the two cell types, the V-region sequences would be identical in terms of the invariant portions of the sequence specified by germ-line gene prototype, but might differ somewhat in residues altered by the somatic variation mechanism. The genes specifying the C-regions of μ- and δ-chains probably are closely linked within the heavy-chain translocon, whereas the gene encoding the C region of μ(T) might lie outside of the gene cluster (Gally and Edelman, 1972).

This model proposes that antigen-specific helper or suppressor factors also contain immunoglobulin V regions. IgM (T) itself has been shown to act as a specific collaborative factor in T/B cooperation using both *in vivo* (Taniguchi and Tada, 1974) and *in vitro* (Feldmann and Nossal, 1972) systems. Since soluble factors (Munro *et al.*, 1974; Taussig, 1974) are often produced under conditions where cell death and lysis would be expected to occur, proteolytic enzymes might be released to cleave IgM (T) into fragments corresponding to Fab or Fv. Both of these would be specific for antigen because the antigen-combining site would be intact. Such factors would probably act as suppressors because, complexed with antigen, they could give the antigen-specific signal (signal 1 of

Bretscher, 1975), but since they lack the Fc piece they would be unable to deliver the mitogenic signal (signal 2). T. Tada (personal communication) has found that antigen-binding fragments of rat IgM (T) acted as suppressive factors. If only the Fv fragment were involved, this factor would not react with antisera made against Ig light- or heavy-chain C-region determinants and most probably would not react with antisera directed against the Fv fragments of individual myeloma proteins. An antigen-specific helper factor might be generated by the noncovalent association of Fv with H-2 antigen. Since a number of proteins are specified by genes associated with the major histocompatibility locus of the mouse, i.e., H antigens and Ia antigens, the discrimination between "helper" and "suppressor" factors might depend also on which H-associated molecule is complexed to the Fv. A similar explanation has been proposed by Coutinho (1975). This combination is not improbable because H antigens possess the capacity of binding β_2-microglobulin (Poulik et al., 1974; Strominger et al., 1974), which is structurally homologous to an Ig domain (Cunningham et al., 1973). A possible role of H antigens in mitogenesis is feasible because these molecules occur on the surface of most cells and recent evidence suggests that H-2 genotype can be correlated with liver content of cAMP (Meruelo and Edidin, 1975). These authors suggest that H-2 antigens might be involved in the binding of hormones which activate adenylate cyclase. The role of H-2 or H-associated antigens would be implicated, not in antigen recognition, but in determining the capacity of T or B cells to divide or cooperate following contact with antigen (Katz and Benacerraf, 1975; Marchalonis et al., 1974c). The present model postulates that such a hybrid V-region Ig and H-associated antigen molecule complexed with antigen might give both the specific and the mitogenic signals to B cells.

Presently available data allow the conclusion that lymphocyte surface Ig functions as a recognition unit for antigen on the surface of both T and B cells but that interaction with other membrane molecules is necessary for cell differentiation. Although the nature of possible regulatory and effector units of the antigen receptor complex remains to be determined, discrete complexes of at least three proteins have been characterized on erythrocyte membranes (Steck, 1974) and such complexes have been proposed for the recognition and response to certain hormones (Birnbaumer et al., 1970; Perkins, 1973). Characterization and elucidation of the functional interactions among these elements constitute a major problem facing cell biologists.

IX. ADDENDUM

Continuing investigations of surface Igs by a number of laboratories have generated new information which is relevant to the present review.

B Cell Surface Ig. (a) The heavy chain of the putative surface IgD of murine B cells is antigenically distinct from μ chain and contains an allotypic marker which allows the cistron specifying it to be mapped within the heavy chain gene complex. This is a new heavy chain locus and has been designated Ig-5 (Goding *et al.*, 1976).

(b) Comparison of the putative murine δ chain with human δ chain by high resolution disc gel electrophoresis in SDS shows that the two chains possess distinct mobilities with the human δ chain migrating more slowly than the mouse protein (Warr and Marchalonis, 1976; Finkelman *et al.*, 1976).

T Cell Surface Ig. (a) Murine T cells of thymus and T lymphoma cells were found by molecular hybridization techniques to synthesize RNA sequences homologous to kappa chain messenger RNA. On the average thymus cells (99.8% Thy-1 bearing) contained about one half as much K-mRNA as the average spleen B cell, whereas the thymoma cells tested contained about 1/30 of this amount (Storb *et al.*, 1976).

(b) Hämmerling and his associates (Hämmerling *et al.*, 1976a,b) have used chicken antiserum to mouse IgM myeloma proteins to demonstrate by indirect immunofluorescence analysis that T cells express an Ig on their surface which shares some, but not all, antigenic Ig determinants of B cells. The surface Ig of radioiodinated T cells solubilized by Nondidet P-40/6 M urea was precipitated using the chicken antiserum and found to contain light chains of apparent mass 20,000 daltons and heavy chains of mass 71,000 daltons, a value compatible with μ chain. Hämmerling *et al.* (1976b) concluded that their results strongly support the existence of an immunoglobulin molecule on T cells which cross-reacts with IgM.

(c) Murine fetal thymus analagen grown as *in vitro* organ cultures lacked B cells, but possessed surface immunoglobulin comparable to IgM (T) in antigenic and physical properties (Haustein and Mandel, 1976; Haustein *et al.*, 1976).

(d) Thymus lymphocytes of vertebrate species representing lower vertebrate classes such as amphibians (DuPasquier *et al.*, 1972; Charlemagne and Tournefier, 1975), teleosts (Emmrich *et al.*, 1975; Warr *et al.*, 1976), elasmobranchs (Ellis and Parkhouse, 1975) express surface Ig detectable by immunofluorescence analysis using rabbit antisera to serum IgM of these animals. In cases where shedding and reappearance studies were carried out, the data suggest that the thymus Ig is synthesized by the cells themselves. Studies involving surface radio-iodination and isolation of surface Ig show that goldfish thymus cells resemble murine T cells in the solubility properties of their membranes. Moreover the Ig of thymus lymphocytes possessed a heavy chain which migrated slightly faster on SDS polyacrylamide gel electrophoresis than did the surface μ-like chain of spleen lymphocytes (Warr *et al.*, 1976). These differences support the contention that the heavy chain of T cell Ig is distinct from B cell heavy chains and, further-more, the genes encoding the T and B cell heavy chains probably diverged early in vertebrate evolution.

ACKNOWLEDGMENTS

This work was supported by Grants CA20085 and AI-12565 from the United States Public Health Service and by Grant AHA 75-877 from the American Heart Association. I thank Ms. Pat Smith and Ms. Elizabeth White for expert technical assistance. This is publication No. 2165 from the Walter and Eliza Hall Institute of Medical Research.

X. REFERENCES

Abney, E., and Parkhouse, R.M.E., 1974, *Nature (London)* **252**:600.
Ashman, R.F., and Raff, M.C., 1973, *J. Exp. Med.* **137**:69.
Austen, K.F., Lewis, R.A., Stechschutte, D.J., Wasserman, S.I., Leid, R.W., and Goetzl, E.J., 1975, in: *Progress in Immunology II*, Vol. 2 (L. Brent and J. Holborow, eds.), p. 61, North-Holland, Amsterdam.
Avtalion, R.R., Weiss, E., and Mualem, T., 1976, in: *Comparative Immunology* (J.J. Marchalonis, ed.), Blackwell, Oxford, in press.
Bach, J.-F., 1973, *Contemp. Top. Immunobiol.* **2**:189.
Baenziger, J., and Kornfeld, S., 1974, *J. Biol. Chem.* **249**:7270.
Balsamo, J., and Lilien, J., 1975, *Biochemistry* **14**:167.
Basten, A., Miller, J.F.A.P., Sprent, J., and Pye, J., 1972, *J. Exp. Med.* **135**:610.
Baur, S., Vitetta, E.S., Sherr, C.J., Schenkein, I., and Uhr, J.W., 1971, *J. Immunol.* **106**:1133.
Benacerraf, B., and McDevitt, H.O., 1972, *Science* **175**:273.
Binz, H., and Wigzell, H., 1975, *J. Exp. Med.* **142**:197.
Birnbaumer, L., Pohl, S.L., Krans, M.L., and Rodbell, M., 1970, *Adv. Biochem. Psychopharmacol.* **3**:185.
Boylston, A.W., 1973, *Immunology* **24**:851.
Boylston, A.W., and Mowbray, J.F., 1973, cited in *T and B Lymphocytes* (M.F. Greaves, J.J.T. Owen, and M.C. Raff, eds.), p. 116, Excerpta Medica, Amsterdam.
Boylston, A.W., and Mowbray, J.F., 1974, *Immunology* **27**:855.
Bretscher, P.A., 1975, *Transplant. Rev.* **23**:37.
Burckhardt, J.J., Guggesberg, F., and von Fellenberg, R., 1974, *Immunology* **26**:521.
Capra, J.D., and Kehoe, J.M., 1975, *Adv. Immunol.* **20**:1.
Charlemagne, J., and Tournefier, A., 1975, in: *Immunologic Phylogeny* (W.H. Hildemann and A.A. Benedict, eds.), Plenum, New York.
Chavin, S.I., 1974, *Biochem. Biophys. Res. Commun.* **61**:382.
Chiller, J.M., Habicht, G.S., and Weigle, W.O., 1970, *Proc. Natl. Acad. Sci. USA* **65**:551.
Cone, R.E., 1976a, *Progr. Allergy* (in press).
Cone, R.E., 1976b, *J. Immunol.* **116**:847.
Cone, R.E., and Johnson, A.G., 1972, *Cell. Immunol.* **3**:283.
Cone, R.E., and Marchalonis, J.J., 1973, *Aust. J. Exp. Biol. Med. Sci.* **51**:689.
Cone, R.E., and Marchalonis, J.J., 1974, *Biochem. J.* **140**:345.
Cone, R.E., Sprent, J., and Marchalonis, J.J., 1972, *Proc. Natl. Acad. Sci. USA* **69**:2556.
Cone, R.E., Feldmann, M., Marchalonis, J.J., and Nossal, G.J.V., 1974, *Immunology* **26**:49.
Cosenza, H., and Köhler, H., 1972, *Science* **176**:1027.
Coutinho, A., 1975, *Transplant. Rev.* **23**:49.
Craig, S.W., and Cebra, J.J., 1975, *J. Immunol.* **114**:492.
Crone, M., Koch, C., and Simonsen, M., 1972, *Transplant. Rev.* **10**:36.

Cuatrecasas, P., 1973, *Fed. Proc.* **32**:1838.
Cuatrecasas, P., Tell, G.P.E., Sica, V., Parikh, I., and Chang, K.-J., 1974, *Nature (London)* **247**:92.
Cunningham, B.A., Wang, J.L., Berggard, J., and Peterson, P.A., 1973, *Biochemistry* **12**:4811.
Demus, H., 1973, *Biochim. Biophys. Acta* **291**:93.
Dennert, G., 1973, *Proc. Soc. Exp. Biol. Med.* **143**:889.
DuPasquier, L., Weiss, N., and Loor, F., 1972, *Eur. J. Immunol.* **2**:366.
Edelman, G.M., and Gall, W.E., 1969, *Annu. Rev. Biochem.* **38**:415.
Eichmann, K., 1975, *Eur. J. Immunol.* **5**:511.
Eichmann, K., and Rajewsky, K., 1975, *Eur. J. Immunol.* **5**:661.
Ellis, A.E., and Parkhouse, R.M.E., 1975, *Eur. J. Immunol.* **5**:729.
Emmrich, F., Richter, R.F., and Ambroiuns, H., 1975, *Eur. J. Immunol.* **5**:76.
Eskeland, T., Klein, E., Inoue, M., and Johansson, B., 1971, *J. Exp. Med.* **134**:265.
Ey, P., 1973, *Eur. J. Immunol.* **3**:37.
Feldmann, M., and Nossal, G.J.V., 1972, *Transplant. Rev.* **13**:3.
Feldmann, M., Cone, R.E., and Marchalonis, J.J., 1973, *Cell. Immunol.* **9**:1.
Feldmann, M., Boylston, A., and Hogg, N.M., 1975, *Eur. J. Immunol.* **5**:429.
Ferrarini, M., Bargellesi, A., Corte, H., Viale, G., and Pernis, B., 1975, *Ann. N.Y. Acad. Sci.* **254**:243.
Finkelman, F.D., van Boxel, J.A., Asofsky, R., and Paul, W.E., 1976, *J. Immunol.* **116**:1173.
Fu, S.M., and Kunkel, H.G., 1974, *J. Exp. Med.* **140**:895.
Fu, S.M., and Winchester, R.J., and Kunkel, H.G., 1974, *J. Exp. Med.* **139**:451.
Fu, S.M., Winchester, R.J., and Kunkel, H.G., 1975, *J. Immunol.* **114**:250.
Gally, J.A., and Edelman, G.M., 1972, *Annu. Rev. Genet.* **6**:1.
Garewal, H.S., and Wasserman, A.P., 1974, *Biochemistry* **13**:4063.
Goding, J.W., Nossal, G.J.V., Shreffler, D.C., and Marchalonis, J.J., 1975, *J. Immunogenet.* **2**:9.
Goding, J.W., Warr, G.W., and Warner, N.L., 1976, *Proc. Natl. Acad. Sci.* **73**:1305.
Greaves, M.F., and Janossy, G., 1972, *Transplant. Rev.* **11**:87.
Greaves, M.F., Owen, J.J.T., and Raff, M.C., 1973, *T and B Lymphocytes*, Excerpta Medica, Amsterdam.
Greaves, M.F., Janossy, G., Feldmann, M., and Doenhoff, M., 1974, in: *The Immune System, Genes, Receptors, Signals* (E.E. Sercarz, A.R. Williamson, and C.F. Fox, eds.), p. 271, Academic Press, New York.
Grey, H.M., Kubo, R.T., and Cerrottini, J.-C., 1972, *J. Exp. Med.* **136**:1323.
Hämmerling, G., and McDevitt, H.O., 1974, *J. Immunol.* **112**:1726.
Hämmerling, U., Mack, C., and Pickel, G., 1976a, *Immunochemistry*, in press.
Hämmerling, U., Pickel, H.G., Mack, C., and Masters, D., 1976b, *Immunochemistry*, in press.
Harris, A.W., Bankhurst, A.D., Mason, S., and Warner, N.L., 1973, *J. Immunol.* **110**:431.
Hart, D.A., 1975, *J. Immunol.* **115**:871.
Haustein, D., 1971, Untersuchungen zum Mechanismus du Hapten-Antikörper-Reaktion mit Hilfe eines solvatochromen Farbstoffs aus der Reiche der Pyridinium-*N*-(4-hydroxphenyl)-betaine. Doctoral dissertation der Albert-Ludwigs-Universitat Zu Freiberg im Breisgau.
Haustein, D., 1975, *J. Immunol. Meth.* **7**:25.
Haustein, D., and Goding, J.W., 1975, *Biochem. Biophys. Res. Commun.* **65**:483.
Haustein, D., Marchalonis, J.J., and Crumpton, M.J., 1974, *Nature (London)* **252**:602.
Haustein, D., and Mandel, T.E., 1976, submitted.
Haustein, D., Marchalonis, J.J., and Harris, A.W., 1975, *Biochemistry* **14**:1826.
Haustein, P., Marchalonis, J.J., Harris, A.W., and Mandel, T.E., 1976, in: *Leukocyte Membrane Determinants Regulating Immune Reactivity* (V.P. Eijsvoogel, D. Roos, and W.P. Zeijlmaker, eds.), p. 205, Academic Press, New York.

Helenius, A., and Simons, K., 1975, *Biochim. Biophys. Acta* **415**:29.

Hogg, N.M., and Greaves, M.F., 1972, *Immunology* **22**:967.

Hudgin, R.L., and Ashwell, G., 1974, *J. Biol. Chem.* **249**:7369.

Hunt, S.M., and Marchalonis, J.J., 1974, *Biochem. Biophys. Res. Commun.* **61**:1227.

Hynes, R.O., 1975, in: *New Techniques in Biophysics and Cell Biology* (R. Pain and B.J. Smith, eds.), Wiley, New York.

Ivanyi, J., 1975, *Immunology* **28**:1015.

Jones, G., Torrigiani, G., and Roitt, I.M., 1971, *J. Immunol.* **106**:1425.

Katz, P.H., and Benacerraf, B., 1975, *Transplant. Rev.* **22**:175.

Kennel, S.J., and Lerner, R.A., 1973, *J. Mol. Biol.* **76**:485.

Kim, Y.B., Bradley, S.G., and Watson, D.W., 1966, *J. Immunol.* **97**:52.

Kucich, U.N., Bennett, J.C., and Johnson, B.J., 1975, *J. Immunol.* **115**:626.

Ladoulis, C.T., Gill, T.J., III, Chen, S.H., and Misra, D.N., 1975, *Progr. Allergy* **18**:205.

Lahat, N., and Moroz, C., 1975, *Cell. Immunol.* **18**:110.

Lawrence, D.A., Spiegelberg, H.L., and Weigle, W.O., 1973, *J. Exp. Med.* **137**:470.

Lerner, R.A., 1972, *Contemp. Top. Immunochem.* **1**:111.

Letarte-Muirhead, M., Acton, R.T., and Williams, A.F., 1974, *Biochem. J.* **143**:51.

Lichtenstein, L.M., and Henney, C.S., 1975, in: *Progress in Immunology II*, Vol. II (L. Brent and J. Holborow, eds.), p. 73, North-Holland, Amsterdam.

Liljas, L., Lundahl, P., and Hjertén, S., 1974, *Biochim. Biophys. Acta* **352**:327.

Linthicum, D.S., and Sell, S., 1974a, *Cell. Immunol.* **12**:443.

Linthicum, D.S., and Sell, S., 1974b, *Cell. Immunol.* **12**:459.

Lisowska-Bernstein, B., Rinny, A., and Vassalli, P., 1973, *Proc. Natl. Acad. Sci. USA* **70**:2879.

Marchalonis, J.J., 1971, *Immunology* **20**:161.

Marchalonis, J.J., 1974a, *J. Med.* **5**:329.

Marchalonis, J.J., 1974b, *Aust. J. Exp. Biol. Med. Sci.* **52**:535.

Marchalonis, J.J., 1975, *Science* **190**:20.

Marchalonis, J.J., and Cone, R.E., 1973, *Transplant. Rev.* **14**:3.

Marchalonis, J.J., Cone, R.E., and Santer, V., 1971, *Biochem. J.* **124**:921.

Marchalonis, J.J., Cone, R.E., and Atwell, J.L., 1972a, *J. Exp. Med.* **135**:956.

Marchalonis, J.J., Atwell, J.L., and Cone, R.E., 1972b, *Nature (London) New Biol.* **235**:240.

Marchalonis, J.J., Cone, R.E., and von Boehmer, H., 1974a, *Immunochemistry* **11**:271.

Marchalonis, J.J., Atwell, J.L., and Haustein, D., 1974b, *Biochim. Biophys. Acta* **351**:99.

Marchalonis, J.J., Morris, P.J., and Harris, A.W., 1974c, *J. Immunogenet.* **1**:63.

McKearn, T.J., 1974, *Science* **183**:94.

McKearn, T.J., Hamoda, Y., Stuart, F.P., and Fitch, F.W., 1974, *Nature (London)* **251**:648.

Melcher, U., Vitetta, E.S., McWilliams, M., Lamm, M.E., Phillips-Quagliata, J.M., and Uhr, J.W., 1974, *J. Exp. Med.* **140**:1427.

Melchers, F., and Cone, R.E., 1975, *Eur. J. Immunol.* **5**:234.

Meruelo, D., and Edidin, M., 1975, *Proc. Natl. Acad. Sci. USA* **72**:2644.

Möller, G., 1975, *Transplant. Rev.* **23**:126.

Molnar, J., Klein, G., and Friberg, S., Jr., 1973, *J. Transplant.* **16**:93.

Moroz, C., and Hahn, J., 1973, *Proc. Natl. Acad. Sci. USA* **70**:3716.

Moroz, C., and Lahat, N., 1974, *Cell. Immunol.* **13**:397.

Munro, A.L., Taussig, M.J., Campbell, R., Williams, H.W., and Lawson, Y., 1974, *J. Exp. Med.* **140**:1579.

Neoh, S.H., Jahoda, D.M., Rowe, D.S., and Voller, A., 1973, *Immunochemistry* **10**:805.

Perkins, J.P., 1973, *Adv. Cyclic Nucleotide Res.* **3**:1.

Pernis, B., 1975, in: *Membrane Receptors of Lymphocytes* (M. Seligmann, J.L. Preud' homme, and F.M. Kourilsky, eds.), p. 57, North-Holland, Amsterdam.

Phillips, D.R., and Morrison, M., 1971, *Biochemistry* **10**:1766.

Poljak, R., 1973, *Contemp. Topics Mol. Immunol.* 2:1.

Poulik, M.D., Ferrone, S., Pellegrino, M.A., Sevier, D.E., Oh, S.K., and Reisfeld, R.A., 1974, *Transplant. Rev.* 21:106.

Putnam, F.W., Florent, G., Paul, C., Shinoda, T., and Shimizu, A., 1973, *Science* 182:287.

Rabellino, E., Colon, S., Grey, H.M., and Unanue, E.R., 1971, *J. Exp. Med.* 133:156.

Rieber, E.P., and Riethmüller, G., 1974a, *Z. Immun.-Forsch.* 147:262.

Rieber, E.P., and Riethmüller, G., 1974b, *Z. Immun.-Forsch.* 147:276.

Rieber, E.P., Riethmüller, G., and Hadam, M., 1973, in: *Protides of the Biological Fluids* (H. Peeters, ed.), pp. 311–314, Pergamon Press, Oxford.

Robison, G.A., Butcher, R.W., and Sutherland, E.W., 1971, *Cyclic AMP*, Academic Press, New York.

Roelants, G.E., 1972, *Contemp. Top. Microbiol. Immunol.* 59:135.

Roelants, G.E., Forni, L., and Pernis, B., 1973, *J. Exp. Med.* 137:1060.

Roelants, G.E., Rydén, A., Hägg, L.-B., and Loor, F., 1974, *Nature (London)* 247:106.

Rolley, R.T., and Marchalonis, J.J., 1972, *Transplantation* 14:734.

Röllinghoff, M., Wagner, H., Cone, R.E., and Marchalonis, J.J., 1973, *Nature (London) New Biol.* 243:21.

Roth, L.E., Pihlaja, D.J., and Shigenaka, Y., 1970, *J. Ultrastruc. Res.* 30:7.

Rowe, D.S., Hug, K., Forni, L., and Pernis, B., 1973, *J. Exp. Med.* 138:965.

Rutishauser, U., and Edelman, G.M., 1972, *Proc. Natl. Acad. Sci. USA* 69:1596.

Schlessinger, J., Steinberg, I.Z., Givol, D., Hochman, J., and Pecht, I., 1975, *Proc. Natl. Acad. Sci. USA* 72:2775.

Segrest, J.P., and Feldmann, R.J., 1974, *J. Mol. Biol.* 87:853.

Sell, S., and Gell, P.G.H., 1965, *J. Exp. Med.* 122:423.

Sherr, C.J., Baur, S., Grundke, J., Zeligs, J., Zeligs, B., and Uhr, J.W., 1972, *J. Exp. Med.* 135:1392.

Singer, S.J., 1974, *Adv. Immunol.* 19:1.

Smith, W.I., Ladoulis, C.T., Misra, D.N., Gill, T.J., III, and Bazin, H., 1975, *Biochim. Biophys. Acta* 382:506.

Snary, D., Goodfellow, P., Hayman, M.I., Bodmer, W.F., and Crumpton, M.J., 1974, *Nature (London)* 247:457.

Steck, T.L., 1974, *J. Cell Biol.* 62:1.

Steck, T.L., and Fox, C.F., 1972, in: *Membrane Molecule Biology* (C.F. Fox and A Keith, eds.), pp. 27–75, Sinauer Associates, Stamford, Conn.

Stevens, R.H., 1974, in: *Progress in Immunology II*, Vol. 1 (L. Brent and J. Holborow, eds.), p. 137, North-Holland, Amsterdam.

Stobo, J.D., Rosenthal, A.S., and Paul, W.E., 1972, *J. Immunol.* 108:1.

Stocker, J.W., and Nossal, G.J.V., 1975, *Contemp. Topics Immunobiol.* (in press).

Stocker, J.W., Marchalonis, J.J., and Harris, A.W., 1974, *J. Exp. Med.* 139:785.

Storb, U., Hager, L., Putnam, D., Buck, L., Marvin, S., Farin, F., and Clagett, J., 1976, *Proc. Natl. Acad. Sci.*, in press.

Strayer, D.S., Vitetta, E.S., and Köhler, H., 1975, *J. Immunol.* 114:722.

Strominger, J.L., Cresswell, P., Grey, H.M., Humphreys, R.H., Mann, D., McCune, J., Parham, P., Robb, R., Sanderson, A.R., Springer, T.A., Terhorst, C., and Turner, M.J., 1974, *Transplant. Rev.* 21:126.

Szenberg, A., Cone, R.E., and Marchalonis, J.J., 1974, *Nature (London)* 250:418.

Taniguchi, M., and Tada, T., 1974, *J. Immunol.* 113:1757.

Taussig, M.J., 1974, *Nature (London)* 248:235.

Taussig, M.J., Mozes, E., and Isac, R., 1974, *J. Exp. Med.* 140:301.

Taylor, R.B., Duffus, W.P.H., Raff, M.C., and de Petris, S., 1971, *Nature (London)* 233:225.

Tökés, Z.A., and Chambers, S.M., 1975, *Biochim. Biophys. Acta* 389:325.

Tsai, C.M., Huang, C.C., and Canellakis, E.S., *Biochim. Biophys. Acta* **322**:47.

Utsumi, S., and Karush, F., 1964, *Biochemistry* **3**:1329.

Vitetta, E.S., and Uhr, J.W., 1973, *Transplant. Proc.* **14**:50.

Vitetta, E.S., and Uhr, J.W., 1975, *Science* **189**:964.

Vitetta, E.S., Bianco, C., Nussenzweig, V., and Uhr, J.W., 1972, *J. Exp. Med.* **136**:81.

Vitetta, E.S., Uhr, J.W., and Boyse, E.A., 1973, *Proc. Natl. Acad. Sci. USA* **70**:834.

Wallach, D.F.H., and Winzler, K.J., 1974, *Evolving Strategies and Tactics in Membrane Research*, Springer-Verlag, New York.

Warner, N.L., 1974, *Adv. Immunol.* **19**:67.

Warner, N.L., and McKenzie, I.F.C., 1975, in: *The Lymphocyte: Structure and Function* (J.J. Marchalonis, ed.), Dekker, New York.

Warr, G.W., and Marchalonis, J.J., 1976, *J. Immunogenetics*, in press.

Warr, G.W., DeLuca, D., and Marchalonis, J.J., 1976, *Proc. Natl. Acad. Sci.*, in press.

Watson, J., 1975, *Transplant. Rev.* **23**:223.

Wilson, J.D., Nossal, G.J.V., and Lewis, H., 1972, *Eur. J. Immunol.* **2**:225.

Yahara, I., and Edelman, G.M., 1972, *Proc. Natl. Acad. Sci.* **69**:608.

Yedgar, Y., Barenholz, Y., and Cooper, V.G., 1974, *Biochim. Biophys. Acta* **363**:86.

Allotypes of Light Chains of Rat Immunoglobulins and Their Application to the Study of Antibody Biosynthesis

Roald Nezlin and Oscar Rokhlin

Institute of Molecular Biology
USSR Academy of Sciences
Moscow, USSR

I. INTRODUCTION

The study of allotypes of immunoglobulin (Ig) polypeptide chains has thrown considerable light on the structure of antibodies, their biosynthesis, and their genetics. The best-known genetic markers are allotypic determinants of H and L peptide chains from human and rabbit Ig. However, studying genetic regulation of Ig biosynthesis in these species is difficult. Among experimental animals, the most available and genetically thoroughly investigated is the mouse, but Ig genetic markers have been reported only for H chains. The genetics of several dozen highly inbred strains of rats have also been well studied, particularly their Ig, since the recent discovery of their Ig-producing myeloma tumors (Bazin *et al.*, 1973).

Several years ago, allotypic variants of rat L chains were reported (Wistar, 1969; Rokhlin *et al.*, 1970, 1971; Armerding, 1971; Gutman and Weissman, 1971). This was followed by their careful chemical and genetic analysis and successful use for the study of antibody biosynthesis. This chapter is an exhaustive review of the L-chain allotypes of rat Ig.

II. DETECTION OF ALLOTYPES OF RAT Ig

The main approach to distinguishing intraspecies differences in the antigenic structure of animal Ig (allotypes) is by immunization of animals of one inbred strain with Ig isolated from animals of another strain, or, in the case of random-bred animals, by cross-immunization with Ig obtained from an individual animal (Mage et al., 1973). The search for Ig allotypic differences is thereby carried out blindly, is laborious, and does not always lead to positive results.

We have therefore used another approach involving inhibition of radio-immunoadsorption (Rokhlin et al., 1970), which permits the presence of small antigenic differences in various proteins to be readily detected. We have inhibited the reaction between soluble radiolabeled antigen and corresponding pure anti-bodies fixed on diazocellulose (antibody immunoadsorbents) (Rokhlin and Nezlin, 1969).

Three inbred strains of rats were used in the experiment: August, WAG, and MSU. The first experiments were conducted with pure antibodies that were isolated from rabbit antiserum against IgG of WAG rats and fixed on cellulose. The radioactive antigen used was [^{125}I] IgG WAG; the unlabeled antigens used in the inhibition of radioimmunoadsorption were IgG from WAG, August, and MSU rats (Rokhlin et al., 1970, 1971).

It was found that the unlabeled August and WAG IgG completely inhibited WAG [^{125}I] IgG adsorption on anti-WAG IgG adsorbent, whereas that of MSU inhibited the above adsorption by 5–8% less than did the homologous IgG. This effect, which was constantly reproducible, suggested a difference between the antigenic structure of MSU IgG and the structures of August and WAG IgG. This suggestion was verified by repeatedly immunizing August and WAG rats with IgG MSU. The sixth immunization gave rise to antibodies that reacted only with MSU IgG. This fact unambiguously proved the existence of allotypic differences between IgG of the MSU strain and IgG of August and WAG strains. Allotypic markers were thus detected by means of inhibiting radioimmunoadsorption, with the overall population of antibodies to IgG in one of inbred strains being used. Such an approach to identifying allotypic differences avoided carrying out large series of cross-immunizations. It also proved possible to obtain antiallotypic antibodies by immunizing rabbits with rat IgG that was previously cross-adsorbed. The resulting variant of MSU L chains was designated as rat light 1 (RL1), that of WAG and August L chains as RL2.

III. THE MODE OF INHERITANCE OF RL ALLOTYPES AND THEIR DISTRIBUTION IN LABORATORY AND WILD RATS

In order to elucidate the mode of inheritance of RL1 and RL2 allotypic markers, MSU rats were crossed with WAG and August rats, and F1 hybrids

(MWF$_1$ and MAF$_1$, respectively) were crossed with rats of the parent strains. Analysis of backcrosses showed the formation of RL allotypes to be controlled by two allelic genes (Rokhlin *et al.*, 1971). However, we could not exclude the possibility that, not just two, but three or even more allelic variants of rat L chains existed. To clarify this issue, the presence of allotypic markers in different strains was studied with sera obtained from various sources (Table I). As seen in Table I, all the rat strains studied could be classified into two groups: RL1(+) RL2(-) and RL2(+) RL1(-). No strain in which both allotypes were absent was found. It is also seen from Table I that our RL1 allotype was rather similar or identical to allotype SD1 described by Armerding (1971) and to allotype R1-1a described by Gutman and Weissman (1971). Thus it follows that inbred rats have only two allotypic variants of L chains.

Distribution of RL allotypes was also studied in random-bred laboratory albino rats. Of 159 albino rats, 129 (81.2%) had the RL2 allotype only, and 30 rats were heterozygous (Table II). If RL2 rats are homozygous in terms of the

Table I. Distribution of Allelic Variants of L Chains in Different Inbred Strains of Rats

	RL2 (Ik1a; W1; RI-1b)	RL1 (Ik1b; SD1; RI-1a)
Rattus rattus[a]	CAP[b,c]	MSU
Birmingham inbred	LEP[b]	Sprague-Dawley
AA[a]	WP[b]	BD[a]
BB[a]		
Wistar[a,b,c]	AS[b,c]	Fisher
BN[a,b,c,d]	BS[b,c]	DA
BP[a,b]	HS[b]	ACI
AVN[a,b,c]	HW[b]	F344
F45[a]	ACP[c]	ACJ[c]
R[a]	Agus[c]	Albany[c]
RA[a]	Atrichis[c]	COP[c]
L/E[a]	AXC[c]	Copenhagen[c]
Buffalo[a,b,c,d]	BD X/Cub[c]	Gunn[c]
Marshall[a,b,c]	Hypodactyl[c]	OFA[c]
WAG[a,b]	Long-Evans[c]	Okamoto[c]
August[a,b,c]	PVG/e[c]	SH[c]
Lewis[b,c,d]	Selfed[c]	Yoshida[c]
LOU/Ws1[a,c]	Sherman[c]	
E3[b]	Zimmerman[c]	
BDE[b]	W/Fu[d]	
WF[b]		

[a]Data from Rokhlin and Nezlin (1974).
[b]Data from Armerding (1971).
[c]Data from Beckers *et al.* (1974).
[d]Data from Gutman and Weissman (1971).

Table II. Distribution of RL1 and RL2 Allotypes among
Random-Bred Albino Rats and Wild Rats[a]

Rats	Number of rats tested	Number of rats with allotypes			Frequency of RL1 gene
		RL1 RL1	RL2 RL2	RL1 RL2	
Random-bred	159	0	129	30	0.094
Wild from Moscow	36	36	0	0	
Wild from Novosibirsk	124	59	1	64	0.734

[a]From Rokhlin and Nezlin (1974).

RL2 gene, the frequency of this gene amounts to 0.906, that of RL1 gene being 0.094. Thus in inbred and random-bred laboratory rats the RL2 variant is much more prevalent than the RL1.

The results obtained with wild rats caught in Moscow and in Novosibirsk were quite different. It is seen from Table II that Moscow rats had RL1 only and no RL2 whatsoever, either homozygous or in a heterozygous combination. In Novosibirsk rats, the RL1 gene accounted for 0.734 and the RL2 gene for 0.266. As will be shown in Section IV B, the RL1 gene is more active than the RL2 gene in biosynthesis of antibodies, and the obvious frequency of this RL1 gene in wild rats appears to be caused by its higher adaptive value as compared to that of the RL2 gene.

IV. MOLECULAR LOCALIZATION AND ANTIGENICITY OF RL ALLOTYPIC DETERMINANTS

The precise location of allotypic determinants is one of their identifying characteristics. Therefore, it was important to determine on which peptide chain—and, even more precisely, on what region of the chain, the constant (C) or the variable (V) regions—the particular allotypic determinants are localized. When the Ig molecule is split into fragments and chains, the antigenic activity of allotypic determinants can weaken considerably. For example, the antigenic activity of Inv factors of human κ-chains and Gm determinants localized on Fd fragments of human γ-chains is considerably lower than that of the intact Ig molecule. Therefore, it was necessary to account for the possible decrease in antigenic activity of allotypic determinants in isolated chains and fragments.

A. Localization of RL Determinants on κ-Chains

To find which Ig peptide chains contained allotypic determinants, the immunoadsorption procedure was again used. Specifically, the cellulose-fixed H and L peptide chains that retain their antigenic properties on being fixed to an insoluble carrier (Nezlin and Kulpina, 1967; Nezlin and Rokhlin, 1969) were the immunoadsorbent. Antiallotypic antibodies obtained on interstrain immunization were studied for their capacity to be specifically bound to fixed chains. It was shown that these antiallotypic antibodies were absorbed on L chains only. The RL determinants studied were thereby found to be located on L peptide chains, thus enabling one to use this type of determinant as genetic markers to study the formation of any class of Ig (Binz and Lindenmann, 1974; Rokhlin, 1976).

Over 90% of L chains in rats and mice belong to the κ type. It was shown by immunoadsorption that about the same amount of L chains had one or another allotypic determinant, and the RL determinants described were likely to account for allotypic differences in rat κ-chains (Rokhlin et al., 1970, 1971).

B. RL Antigenicity of Isolated L Chains and of Intact IgG Molecules

The effect of quaternary structure of Ig molecules on antigenic activity of RL determinants was also investigated by means of quantitating inhibition of radioimmunoadsorption. Antiallotypic antibodies fixed on cellulose were used as the immunoadsorbent, and $[^{125}I]$IgG of the respective rat strain was applied as the test antigen. The resulting data could be expressed either in terms of the minimum concentration that inhibited antigenic activity or by the percentage of inhibition caused by adding unlabeled L chains or IgG to the reactants. When estimating the antigenic activity, it was, of course, necessary to bear in mind the differences in the molecular weights of IgG and L chains, the latter forming dimers in solution (Vengerova et al., 1972a). The molar ratio of IgG to 2L amounted to 150,000: 40,000 or 3.75. Table III lists the determinations of RL antigenicity at minimum inhibiting concentrations. It will be seen from the data that whereas RL1 antigenicity of isolated L chains was not significantly affected, RL2 determinants were about 4 times less antigenic than intact IgG molecules from the same rat strains.

These differences between the two allotypic determinants were clearly demonstrated in experiments designed to inhibit the activity of isolated L chains and intact IgG molecules as conducted with two types of adsorbents, i.e., fixed antibodies against L chains and antibodies against only allotypic determinants of the same chains. The former adsorbent allowed the changing activity of the sum of determinants to be studied; the latter showed results concerning solely RL

Table III. RL Antigenicity of Isolated L Chains and IgG of MSU (RL1) and
WAG (RL2) Rats as Measured in Inhibition of Immunoadsorption[a]

| | Lowest protein concentration at which the RL antigens were detected (μg/ml) | | | | Molar ratios[b] | |
| | | | | | L MSU [IgG MSU or (1)/(2) × 3.75] | L WAG [IgG WAG or (3)/(4) × 3.75] |
Expt.	L MSU (1)	IgG MSU (2)	L WAG (3)	IgG WAG (4)		
1	0.03	0.08	0.05	0.05	1.39	3.75
2	0.01	0.07	0.05	0.03	0.53	6.37
3	0.09	0.3	0.1	0.07	1.12	5.36
				Mean	1.01	5.16

[a]From Rokhlin et al. (1971).
[b]Molar ratios of 1 indicate no change in antigenicity. Molar ratios greater than 1 indicate a
decrease in antigenicity and ratios less than 1 indicate an increase (Polmar and Steinberg,
1967).

determinants. It is seen from Fig. 1b, d that L chains had a higher inhibiting
activity than IgG when they were added to the adsorbents in equal weight quantities. This was expected since the molecular IgG/L ratio is 3.75. The RL1 antigenic
activity of isolated MSU L behaved similarly, and was also more active than MSU
IgG in equal weight quantities. However, WAG IgG and WAG L added in equal
weight quantities identically inhibited test antigen adsorption to the antiallotypic
adsorbent. This pointed to reduced allotypic antigenic activity of RL2 determinants after L chains were isolated from the Ig molecule. On the other hand,
the overall antigenic activity of WAG L chains was not essentially affected after
isolation as seen from the curve obtained from inhibition on adsorbent with
fixed antibodies against L chains (Fig. 1b). The decreased allotypic activity of
WAG L chains was evidently of a local nature and limited solely to RL2
determinant.

C. Splitting of Rat L Chains into Halves and Their Antigenic Activity

It is generally thought that peptide chains of antibodies are coded by two
different structural genes, variable (V) genes and constant (C) genes for V and C
chain regions, respectively (Nezlin, 1976). When using allotypic determinants as
genetic markers, one should know exactly which marker of these two gene types
is the particular allotypic determinant. Such an exact determination is difficult,
especially when multiple differences between allotypic variants of chains are
found.

To elucidate this point, we studied the possibility of proteolytic splitting of

L chains into halves involving approximately equal C and V regions. Ig peptide chains are known to be constructed of rather compact globular domains connected by a relatively open chain site available to the action of proteases. L chains consist of two domains involving V and C regions. Therefore, it is not surprising that a number of workers have reported the splitting of human L chains with different proteases (Karlsson *et al.,* 1969; Solomon and McLaughlin, 1969). The possibility of such splitting by one or another enzyme is dependent on the sequence of the chain site that connects both domains. It will be shown below that there are Lys and Arg residues in the middle of rat κ-chains which permit trypsin to be used for halving L chains. After incubation in trypsin followed by gel filtration (Fig. 2), the L-chain fragments isolated were equal to their halves (second peak) in a 10–13% yield of the amount of chains used. About 30–40% of the chains were undigested (first peak) and the remaining protein was split

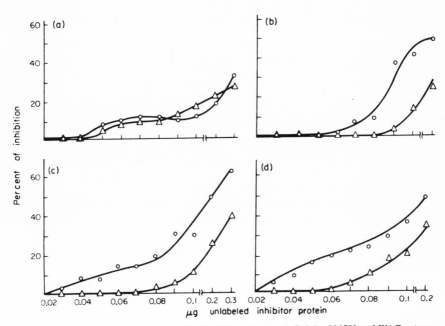

Figure 1. Antigenicity of isolated L chains (O) and intact IgG (Δ) of MSU and WAG rats as measured by inhibition of immunoadsorption. Inhibition of adsorption of [^{125}I]IgG WAG by unlabeled L chains and IgG of WAG rats (a) on anti-RL2 immunoadsorbent and (b) on anti-WAG L-chain immunoadsorbent. Inhibition of adsorption of [^{125}I]IgG MSU by unlabeled L chains and IgG of MSU rats (c) on anti-RL1 immunoadsorbent and (d) on anti-MSU L-chain immunoadsorbent. Immunoadsorption of [^{125}I]IgG in the absence of unlabeled antigens (0% of inhibition) was 2100–2500 cpm. Reprinted by permission of Rokhlin *et al.* (1971).

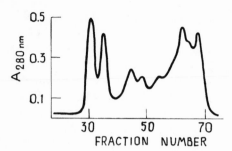

Figure 2. Gel filtration patterns of tryptic hydrolysate of rat L chain (60 mg) on a Sephadex G50 column (2.5 by 100 cm) in 1 N acetic acid. First peak, undigested chains; second peak, halves of L chains. Reprinted by permission of Vengerova *et al.* (1972a).

into more or less large peptides (Vengerova *et al.*, 1972a). Allotypic activity was found in proteins of the first and second peaks only, i.e., in unsplit L chains and their halves.

In order to elucidate the localization of allotypic determinants, it was essential to find whether the configuration of globular domains changed after the halving of L chains. Since the expression of antigen determinants depends on their conformation (Sela, 1969), immunochemical methods were considered suitable to approach this problem (Nezlin and Rokhlin, 1969).

To this end, we used quantitative inhibition of test-antigenic activity by immunoadsorption on cellulose-fixed pure antibodies against intact L chains and RL determinants. These experiments showed that antigenic properties characteristic of intact chains were fully retained after splitting into halves (Vengerova *et al.*, 1972a). This fact held good for allotypic antigenic properties as well. A number of physicochemical data (Björk *et al.*, 1971) also showed that L-chain halves essentially retained the configuration they had in intact chains.

D. Separation of V and C Regions and RL Determinant Localization on the C Region

To separate V and C chain halves, isoelectrofocusing (IEF) was used either in gels or in solutions. Fractionation of normal L chains revealed many bands, essentially at pH 5–6 (Fig. 3a). Almost all rat L chains are of the κ type, and this charge heterogeneity appears to be due to the different structures of their V halves. Therefore, it could be suggested that IEF of L-chain halves would reveal one or two main bands corresponding to C halves and similar in all chains of the particular allotype, as well as many weaker bands corresponding to the spectrum of V halves (Nezlin *et al.*, 1974b). Figure 3b confirms such a separation in gels to produce one strong band (pH 4.6–4.8) and many weaker bands. A similar result was obtained for liquid IEF, which gave a sufficient quantity of V and C halves to be used for further experiments (Nezlin *et al.*, 1975).

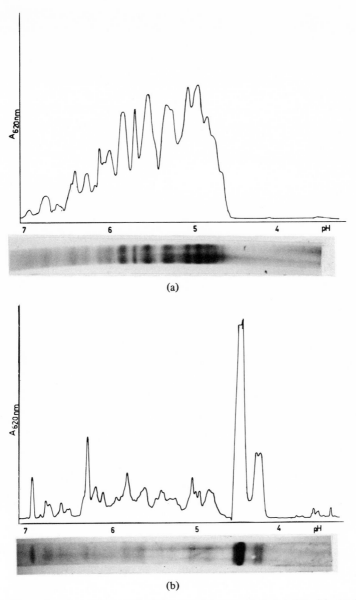

Figure 3. Electrofocusing pattern of L chains of rat Ig (a) and their halves (b). Analytical isoelectrofocusing was performed on columns (0.5 by 10.0 cm) of polyacrylamide gels in 6 M urea (ampholines, pH 3-10). Gels were stained with Coomassie blue. Upper part, densitometric tracing; lower part, photographs of gel columns. Reprinted by permission of Nezlin *et al.* (1974b).

Determination of N-terminal amino acids of the protein in the main IEF peak substantiated the fact that it did indeed account for the C half. In intact L chains from rats, the N-terminal was mainly Asp, whereas the protein of the main peak was Arg together with some Leu and Ala. The presence of three N-terminals indicated that trypsin split L chains at three sites closely spaced in the middle of the chain (see Section VC).

Allotypic antigenic activity of halves extracted from columns of poly-acrylamide gel and of those isolated on preparative columns in liquid was studied by inhibition of immunoadsorption. In all these experiments, only the C half was found to have RL activity. This result was confirmed by comparing the allotypic activity of isolated C halves and intact chains, bearing in mind that if the properties of the allotypic determinant were completely dependent on the C half its allotypic antigenic activity would be no less than twice that of the activity of intact L chains in terms of a unit or protein weight. The experimental results of such a comparison (Fig. 4) produced by inhibition of radioimmunoadsorption substantiated our suggestion that the C half was indeed more active than the intact chain.

It was thus shown that the RL allotypic determinants were localized on the C region and were genetic markers of the structural gene Cκ. The method applied to provide this evidence (IEF of L-chain halves) can also be more generally used to obtain C and V halves for further chemical and other studies. It can also be useful for studying L chains of many animal species, e.g., our recent IEF data on human L-chain halves (Nezlin et al., 1975). Finally, the profile of V halves can serve as a definite characteristic of variability for the particular chain type.

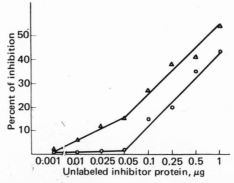

Figure 4. Allotypic antigenic activity of intact L chains (○) and their isolated C halves (△) (both RL2 variant) in inhibition of radioimmunoadsorption. Proteins were mixed with 2 μg of pure antiallotypic antibodies fixed on cellulose, and immediately thereafter the ^{125}I-labeled L chains (specific activity 150,000 cpm/μg) were added. After washing, the amount of ^{125}I bound to the immunoadsorbent was counted. Two micrograms of fixed antibodies was reacted with 3000 cpm of radiolabeled L chains (0 inhibition). From Nezlin et al., 1975.

V. CHEMICAL DIFFERENCES BETWEEN RL ALLELIC VARIANTS

In studying the chemistry of genetic variants in peptide chains from human and rabbit Ig, two types of differences were found: (1) single differences, i.e., differences in one or two amino acids only (Gm and Inv factors in human Ig, d and e rabbit allotypes), and (2) multiple differences, i.e., differences in several amino acid residues (a allotypes of H chains and b allotypes of L chains of rabbit Ig).

The results of investigating both allotypic rat variants that led to the present study of their primary structure are summarized below. The evidence shows that antigenic allotypic differences depend on multiple amino acid substitutions in several sites of the C region.

A. Amino Acid Analysis and Peptide Mapping

One of the previous approaches to examining allotypic differences in peptide chains was amino acid analysis. Thus Reisfeld and Inman (1968) discovered important differences in the multiple amino acids of allelic variants of rabbit κ-chains, which were recently confirmed by data defining their primary structure (Zeeuws and Strosberg, 1975). Our similar analysis of allelic variants of rat L chains also pointed to their multiple differences as substantiated by statistically significant differences in the content of several amino acids. However, it is clear that an analysis of preparations from normal Ig chains, involving a huge number of different V regions, cannot be considered as providing definite and final proof of the point in question. Yet the above data were proved by subsequent experiments. Thus, by studying tryptic peptides by peptide mapping, clear-cut differences between both allelic variants were found in several spots (Vengerova *et al.*, 1972b; Nezlin *et al.*, 1974a). This evidence points to multiple differences between allotypic chain variants, most likely in their C regions.

B. Cyanogen Bromide Splitting

Cyanogen bromide (CNBr) splitting of peptide chains on Met residues is usually used in protein chemistry to obtain large fragments. Amino acid analysis showed that rat L chains contained three or four Met residues, i.e., more than L chains of other species. This suggested the possibility that the positions of these residues are different on the two allelic variants. It is seen from Fig. 5 that fractionation of peptides on RL2 chains treated with CNBr resulted in three peaks. The molecular weight for the third protein peak was about 8000-9000 and that for the second peak about 14,000-15,000 daltons. CNBr action on RL1 chains gave rise to peptides of other dimensions (Fig. 5). The differences in the action

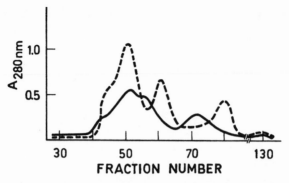

Figure 5. Gel filtration of CNBr cleavage products of rat L chains on a Sephadex G50 (fine) column (2 by 110 cm) equilibrated with 6 M urea and 0.05 M formic acid. RL1 allotype, solid line; RL2 allotype, broken line. Reprinted by permission of Vengerova *et al.* (1972b).

of CNBr on RL1 and RL2 chains may be accounted for by presuming different localizations of Met residues. Indeed, Met 122 was found only in RL1 chains and Met 137 was found only in RL2 chains (Fig. 6). The possibility of amino acid substitution in position 175 is also not excluded. These results were readily reproducible, and such an approach can be used for allocating the particular rat L chain to one or another allelic variant (Vengerova *et al.*, 1972b).

C. Primary Structure

At present, the complete amino acid sequence of one rat Bence-Jones protein S211 (RL2 variant) (Starace and Querinjean, 1975) and the sequence of C regions of pooled L chains isolated from Lew (RL2) and DA (RL1) strains are known (Gutman *et al.*, 1975). The central portion of the L chain has the following sequence:

105   110

–Lys↓–Leu–Gly–Leu–Lys↓–Arg↓–Ala–Asn–Pro–

This sequence explains how chains can be split in half by trypsin (indicated by arrows).

All differences between both allelic variants are located in three places—six substitutions from 122 and 136 residues, two substitutions from 153 to 155, and three substitutions from 184 to 187. According to the model constructed from the results of X-ray studies of human L chains (Poljak *et al.*, 1974; Schiffer *et al.*, 1973), the first group of residues is located inside the C domain but the other two are spaced on the surface close to one another in the region which is also responsible for the human markers Oz, Inv, and Kern (Milstein *et al.*, 1974).

Figure 6. The amino acid sequence of C regions of rat κ Bence-Jones protein S211 and of pooled L chains from Lew and DA rat stains. Reprinted by permission of Gutman *et al.* (1975).

```
       105                 110             115             120             125             130
S211    L  E  L  K  R  A   N  A  A  P  T   V  S  F  P  P   S  T  Z  Z  L   A  T  G  G  A   S  V  V  C
LEW     -  Z  -  -  -  -   -  -  -  -  -   -  -  -  -  -   -  -  -  -  -   T  S  -  -  -   T  -  -  -
DA      -  Z  -  -  -  -   B  -  -  -  -   -  -  -  -  -   M  -  -  -  -   T  S  -  -  -   T  -  -  -

       135                 140             145             150             155             160
S211    L  M  N  K  F  Y   P  R  D  I  S   V  K  W  K  D   G  T  E  R  B   G  V  L  B  S   V  T
LEW     -  -  B  -  -  -   -  -  -  -  -   -  -  -  -  -   -  S  -  [ ] R   -  -  -  -  -   -  -
DA      F  V  B  -  -  -   -  -  -  -  -   -  -  -  -  -   -  S  -   Z  R   -  -  -  -  -   -  -

       165                 170             175             180             185             190
S211    B  Z  B  S  K  D   S  T  Y  S  M   S  S  T  L  S   L  T  K  A  D   Y  Q  S  H  N   L  Y  T  C
LEW     -  -  -  -  -  -   -  -  -  -  -   -  -  -  -  -   -  -  -  V  Z   -  -  S  -  -   -  -  -  -
DA      -  -  -  -  -  -   -  -  -  -  -   -  -  -  -  -   -  -  -  V  Z   -  -  R  -  -   -  -  -  -

       195                 200             205             210
S211    Q  V  V  H  K  T   S  S  S  P  V   V  W  K  N  F   N  R  N  E  C
LEW     -  V  -  -  -  -   -  -  -  -  -   V  -  -  -  S   -  -  -  -  -
DA      -  -  -  -  -  -   -  -  -  -  -   -  -  -  -  S   -  -  -  -  -
```

Probably the same two regions of the chain are the important parts of the RL antigenic determinants. These results are in good agreement with data regarding the antigenicity of other proteins. For example, all antigenic determinants of the myoglobin molecule occupy surface location (Atassi, 1975).

VI. INTERACTION OF RL1 AND RL2 ALLELIC GENES IN Ig BIOSYNTHESIS

A. Molecular Ratio of RL1 and RL2 Allotypes for Normal Ig in F_1 Hybrids and Heterozygous Backcrosses

The predominance of the RL1 allelic variant in wild rats (Section III) suggested that the RL1 allelic gene has a greater adaptive value than the RL2 allelic gene. Hence the RL1 gene should be more active in Ig biosynthesis of heterozygous RL1–RL2 rats than the RL2 gene.

The relative roles of RL1 and RL2 genes in Ig biosynthesis were evaluated by studying the molecules with RL1 and RL2 chains in MAF_1 and MWF_1 hybrids (Rokhlin et al., 1972; Rokhlin and Nezlin, 1973, 1974). The quantitation of RL1 and RL2 molecules in normal Ig of F_1 hybrids from direct and reciprocal crosses indicated that 60% of Ig molecules contained RL1 chains and 40% contained RL2 chains (Rokhlin et al., 1971). The increased activity of RL1 gene was also retained in F_1 × August and F_1 × WAG backcrosses, which suggested that RL1 gene activity was dependent on the properties of the gene rather than on the MSU-strain genotype.

It was shown above that RL determinants were markers of the C region of L chains. However, it was difficult to explain the difference in the activity of RL genes by a different structure of C regions. The higher activity of RL1 gene than of RL2 gene was probably caused by its functional properties, i.e., by V genes that were linked to the C gene of RL1. As a rule, only those V and C genes are expressed that are located on one chromosome, i.e., that are in the cis-position (Kindt et al., 1970). Quite possibly, the increased content of RL1 molecules in the sera of normal F_1 reflected V genes linked to the RL1 C gene being more active in the formation of antibodies than V genes linked to the RL2 C gene. To check this suggestion, we investigated the activity of RL1 and RL2 genes in the formation of antibodies to haptens.

B. The Role of RL Allelic Genes in the Formation of Antibodies to Haptens

In heterozygotes, only one of two alternative allotypic markers is carried on a given peptide chain (Dray and Nisonoff, 1965). Most work on the role of allelic genes of L and H chains in the biosynthesis of antibodies with different specificity has made use of random-bred, thus nonidentical, animals. Therefore, it is difficult to arrive at definite conclusions as to the regularity with which antibody-producing cells differentiate according to allelic genes when utilizing genetically nonidentical animals. Although in some humans, given antibodies belong to the Inv (1,2) allelic variant, in others antibodies of the same specificity belong to the Inv (3) variant (Cooper and Steinberg, 1970). In some b4b5 rabbits, the amount of b4 allotype in the given antibodies is higher, whereas in others b5 allotype predominates (Catty et al., 1969; Zappacosta and Rossi, (1972). However, it is not clear at all whether such variation is from genotypic differences in individuals or whether lymphoid cell differentiation on allelic genes is simply a random process. Therefore, we studied allelic gene interaction under the conditions of genetically identical background, using F_1 hybrids from crossing inbred rats from strains with alternative allelic variants.

The experiments reported below were concerned with the amount of molecules with allelic variants of L chains in preparations of antibodies to two haptens—DNS (1-dimethylaminonaphthalene-5 sulfonyl) and AB (azobenzoate) isolated from antisera of hybrids MAF_1 and MWF_1 (Rokhlin et al., 1972; Rokhlin and Nezlin, 1973). Antibodies were fractionated according to affinity (Kitagawa et al., 1965) by eluting antibodies adsorbed on immunoadsorbents with hapten solutions of various concentration. The amount of RL1 and RL2 molecules was determined in every fraction of antibodies isolated from individual F_1 rats after each immunization, by using anti-RL1 and anti-RL2 antibody-immunoadsorbents.

The amount of RL1 molecules in antibodies to DNS from MAF_1 hybrids is given in Fig. 7. As shown in Fig. 7a, molecules with RL1 chains in antibodies to DNS exceeded by 1.5-2 times those with RL2 chains. Even more important, RL1 molecules exceeded RL2 molecules in practically all individual MAF_1 rats. Quite the opposite was true with MWF_1 (Fig. 7b). It should be noted that individual rats had pronounced differences in the amount of allelic variants, the ratio of RL1 to RL2 molecules ranging from 4 : 1 to 1 : 4. Although MWF_1 rats were of the same genotype, the activity of their RL1 and RL2 genes in the formation of antibodies to DNS was quite different in individual hybrids. The individual differences in the ratio of allelic variants were observed when the average group RL1/RL2 ratio was 1 : 1.

Fractionation by affinity of antibodies to DNS isolated after the third immunization showed that RL1 gene activity was higher than that of RL2 gene only in a particular fraction, i.e., the fraction eluted with 2×10^{-3} M DNS-OH (Fig. 7c). The antibodies of this fraction accounted for almost 50% of the overall amount of antibodies to DNS. Other fractions of antibodies to DNS contained molecules with RL1 and RL2 chains in an approximately equal amount, and there were no differences whatsoever between MAF_1 and MWF_1 hybrids.

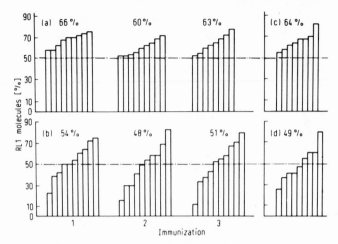

Figure 7. Content of RL1 molecules in anti-DNS antibodies isolated after first, second, and third immunizations. Each column gives the value of RL1 molecules in anti-DNS antibodies of a single rat. Numbers on top show mean percentages of RL1 molecules. The percentage of RL2 molecules is equal to 100% – % RL1. (a) Anti-DNS antibodies from MAF_1. (b) Anti-DNS antibodies from MWF_1. (c,d) Lowest-affinity anti-DNS antibodies eluted by 2×10^{-3} M DNS-OH after third immunization from (c) MAF_1 and (d) MWF_1. Reprinted by permission of Rokhlin and Nezlin (1973).

A similar picture was found in the case of antibodies to AB. During biosynthesis of these antibodies, as with antibodies to DNS, each F_1 type displayed a different expression of its RL1 and RL2 genes. The differences between MAF_1 and MWF_1 were noted after the second immunization and were retained after the third one. As seen from Fig. 8a, for MAF_1 hybrids, the ratio of RL1 and RL2 molecules in the fraction of anti-AB antibodies eluted with 1×10^{-2} M of o-nitrobenzoate was on the average 1 : 1 in the group, but individual rats displayed pronounced differences in the ratio. On the other hand, individual MWF_1 rats had no essential differences in allelic genes. The mean ratio of RL1 to RL2 variants was 70% to 30%, and all MWF_1 rats studies had higher activity of the RL1 gene during biosynthesis of antibodies to AB.

Thus the biosynthesis of antibodies to DNS and to AB reflected the same two regularities in the expression of the allelic genes of L chains. First, if one of the allelic genes was more active in the formation of antibodies of particular specificity than the alternative allele, this unequal activity was a constant feature for all F_1 under study. Second, if the allelic variant ratio in antibodies of the particular specificity was on the average 1 : 1, and it was possible to speak of a "functional" equality of allelic genes, individual rats displayed pronounced differences in the ratio of allelic variants within a genetically identical group of F_1 hybrids. The results obtained can be interpreted as follows.

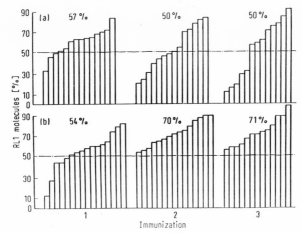

Figure 8. Content of RL1 molecules in anti-AB antibodies eluted by 1×10^{-2} M o-nitrobenzoate after second and third immunizations and by 1×10^{-1} M o-nitrobenzoate after first immunization. (a) MAF_1. (b) MWF_1. For details, see caption of Fig. 7. Reprinted by permission of Rokhlin and Nezlin (1973).

1. Antigen Independence of the Differentiation of Antibody-Producing Cells with Respect to Allelic Genes

V genes are expressed together with the C gene that is located with them on one chromosome. It was therefore possible to determine the contribution of the paternal and maternal V_L genes to the formation of particular antibodies by studying their allotypic composition.

The allelic variant ratio of L chains was on the average 1 : 1 for MWF_1 hybrids in antibodies to DNS as well as in MAF_1 antibodies to AB. In these cases, it was possible to speak of a "functional" equality of allelic V_L genes. These F_1 displayed pronounced differences in the activities of RL1 and RL2 genes in forming antibodies with a particular specificity. The individual differences could not be explained by genotypic differences in individual animals, for only genotypically identical F_1 were studied. The individual differences in the activity of allelic genes could not be accounted for by the selective action of antigen either, for it was difficult to conceive the existence of any reason why in one RL1 RL2 rat the antigen should induce cell differentiation toward the RL1 variant and in another RL1 RL2 rat with similar genotype the same antigen should favor the RL2 variant.

Therefore, the variability in expression of allelic genes which is observed in the case of their "functional equality" is inherent in the very process of differentiation of antibody-producing cells in respect to allelic genes, viz., this process is random. Hence lymphoid cell differentiation according to allelic genes took place before antigen acted on the cells.

Experimental evidence on allotypic suppression and surface Ig in embryos and newborn heterozygous animals also indicated that differentiation according to allelic genes was independent of antigen (Mage, 1974). However, neither embryos nor newborn animals are subject to substantial antigen action, and it remains unclear whether the differentiation under study was also independent of antigen in adult animals or whether it was specific for a particular ontogenetic stage.

The data obtained show that differentiation of lymphoid cells in respect to allelic genes is antigen independent in adult animals.

2. Heterozygosity of V Genes as a Cause of Unequal Activity of Allelic Genes

The unequal ratio of allelic variants in antibodies of DNS in MAF_1 hybrids and antibodies to AB in MWF_1 hybrids pointed to hereditary functional differences in RL1 and RL2 allelic genes. In rabbits it was shown that each allelic variant of the b locus has an amino acid sequence characteristic of the V region. It is thus likely that allelic variants of rabbit κ-chains differ not only in the structure of the C but also in that of the V region (Waterfield *et al.*, 1973). It is also probable that the above-mentioned higher activity of the RL1 gene as compared to that of the RL2 gene in antibody biosynthesis resulted from a structural difference between V genes linked to corresponding RL genes.

Thus heterozygosity according to V genes is common, and the frequency of the allotypic variant depends on the number and diversity of V genes linked to the particular C gene (Mage, 1974). Quite possibly it was heterozygosity according to V genes (i.e., different specificity of allelic V genes) that caused the phenomenon of allelic exclusion; otherwise, the formation of functionally inactive hybrid molecules in cells would have been inevitable. In its turn, V-gene heterozygosity could participate in the selection, thus doubling the amount of coded specificity.

VII. THE GERM-LINE NATURE OF ONE FRACTION OF ANTI-AB RAT ANTIBODIES

Considerable evidence has accumulated recently in favor of the germ-line hypothesis for the origin of antibody variability (Wigzell, 1973; Williamson *et al.*, 1975). One rather useful approach to prove the hypothesis is to study the properties of antibodies in individual animals. The presence of a population of antibodies with similar V regions in different animals of an inbred strain supported the germ-line theory of inheritance of V genes. Yet the most important substantiation of this hypothesis was provided by data on the idiotypic properties of antibodies. It was shown that individual mice of a given strain had antibodies with similar idiotypic determinants whose structure was known to depend on V regions (Eichmann, 1972; Potter and Lieberman, 1970). Furthermore, these idiotypic determinants could be inherited as a simple Mendelian trait (Eichmann *et al.*, 1974).

Another approach is to study allelic allotypic markers in antibodies from heterozygous F_1 animals. We conducted experiments with antibodies against AB obtained from heterozygous rats. In order to achieve the finest separation of antibodies, use was made of the most effective resolving method—IEF—that allowed antihapten antibody fractions to be separated with a very high degree of homogeneity. Two criteria were used to characterize the resulting fraction: (1) the ratio between the two allelic RL variants and (2) the affinity of antibodies (i.e., capacity to undergo elution from AB-adsorbent at a particular hapten concentration).

Figure 9 shows IEF profiles of anti-AB antibodies from two rats with nearly identical spectra to those in six other rats (Rokhlin *et al.*, 1975). Those rat anti-AB antibodies were characterized by considerable homogeneity, and isoelectric points mainly between pH 5.4 and 5.9 in all animals studied. Subsequent analysis

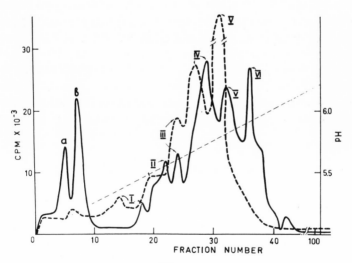

Figure 9. Electrofocusing pattern of pure ^{125}I-labeled anti-AB antibodies isolated from two individual MWF_1 rats. Analytical electrofocusing was performed on columns (0.5 by 10.0 cm) of polyacrylamide gels in 6 M urea (ampholines pH 5–7). Gel columns were cut to slices 1 mm thick, and antibodies were eluted by saline. Pooled fractions designated by numbers were analyzed by RL1:RL2 ratio and affinity properties. Reprinted by permission of Rokhlin *et al.* (1975).

showed that almost all fractions contained molecules of both allotypes, which were heterogeneous in affinity. However, fraction I was homogeneous by both criteria; it contained antibody molecules of only one allotype (RL1), and they eluted after adsorption on the AB adsorbent at a particular concentration. The most important result of these experiments was the fact that, in all F_1 under study, one antibody population presented a somewhat fixed position in the IEF spectrum (pH 5.45–5.5) and was characterized by having only RL1 allotype molecules and a particular affinity.

These experiments suggested that the structural genes coding the specificity of fraction I antibodies were germ-line genes, since one would hardly expect that somatic processes could produce antibody molecules with related properties in F_1 rats of two different parental strains. That is, these experiments were in good accord with the above experiments on inbred animals having similar idiotypic properties.

IEF was also applied to the study of antibody properties in other species such as mice and guinea pigs, and it was shown that heterogeneity of the response varied with the experimental conditons. The results of other studies closely resembled those we had obtained. Haimovich et al. (1974) found that guinea pigs responded to DNP uniformly and anti-DNP spectra were rather similar among the animals studied. McMichael et al. (1975) found that, during early primary responses, about 80% of C57 mice formed homogeneous antibodies against NP-hapten with a characteristic IEF spectrum which was inherited as a dominant trait. Finally, we wish to mention that studying the properties of antibodies in different inbred animals has already yielded important data. At the present time, investigations into the primary structure of chains of antibody fractions isolated from different inbred animals appear to be most promising. Ultimately this work could provide an answer as to whether different animals of one inbred strain can form identical antibody molecules.

VIII. IgM-TO-IgG SWITCH AS STUDIED BY MEANS OF RAT ALLOTYPES

Genes controlling the formation of μ- and γ-chains are known to be closely linked (Mage et al., 1973). At early stages of the immune response, predominantly IgM antibodies are synthesized as a rule (Nezlin, 1964; Mäkelä, 1970). The fact that IgM production switches to IgG is not in doubt; however, it is not yet clear whether this switch proceeds in the same cell or whether IgM and IgG are synthesized by separate cells (Mäkelä et al., 1970; Catty et al., 1969; Kim and Karush, 1974; Pink et al., 1971).

To study the IgM-to-IgG switch, the phenomenon of allelic exclusion was used. IgM and IgG classes differ in the structure of their H chains but have

similar L chains. Thus it became possible to study the IgM-to-IgG switch by comparing the ratio of RL1 to RL2 allelic variants in IgM and IgG antibody fractions. The following were considered. First, if the ratio of allelic variants is approximately similar in IgM and IgG antibody fractions, cells synthesizing these
antibodies should have a common origin. Second, if the ratio of allelic variants
of L chains in the IgM fraction is different from that in the IgG fraction, IgM
and IgG antibodies could be synthesized by separate populations of antibody-
producing cells.

The percentage of RL1 and RL2 allelic variants was estimated in IgM and
IgG fractions from antibodies to p-aminophenyl-β-D-lactoside (Rokhlin, 1976).
The mean ratio in the antibodies ranged, respectively, from 50:50 to 60:40, like
the ratio commonly found in unimmunized heterozygous animals (Section VIA).
Yet, whereas normal Ig of individual animals showed practically no differences
in their ratio of allelic variants in antibodies to lactoside, a rat at one extreme
had 70-90% of RL1 antibody molecules and 10-30% of RL2 molecules and a rat
at the other extreme had the opposite ratio of 70-90% of RL2 and 10-30% of
RL1 chains.

Figure 10 shows deviations from the mean amount of RL1 molecules for
IgM and IgG fractions of antibodies with a high affinity to lactoside. As seen in
Fig. 10, the shift in the ratio of allelic variants was similar for IgM and IgG fractions of antibodies. Thus cells which synthesized IgM antibodies had the same
allotypic markers as did cells synthesizing IgG antibodies. It could therefore be
concluded that the two cell types had a common origin and that the IgM-to-
IgG switch took place in one cell during the development of the particular population of antibody-producing cells. Similar results were obtained for antibodies
to lactoside with low affinity.

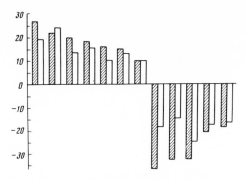

Figure 10. Individual variability in allotypic composition of IgM and IgG fractions of high-
affinity antilactoside antibodies isolated from MWF$_1$ rats. Deviation of content of RL1 IgM
molecules (hatched bars) and RL1 IgG molecules (white bars) from the mean value. Each
pair of columns reflects data obtained from a single rat. From Rokhlin (1976).

IX. CONCLUSION

The results reported in this review on allotypes of rat Ig L chains concern several problems. Chemical and immunochemical studies have unambiguously designated the allotypic light-chain determinants under study as genetic markers of C_κ genes. The multiple amino acid differences between two allelic variants of these chains were indicated and have now been confirmed by amino acid sequencing.

It is also clear that the use of genetic markers combined with the quantitative immunoadsorption method has contributed greatly to the study of the important problems of antibody biosynthesis. It has, for example, been shown that lymphoid cell differentiation according to allelic genes is antigen independent. It has also been found that one of the allelic genes is more active in Ig biosynthesis than the alternative allele and that the formation of a particular fraction of anti-hapten antibodies is most likely to be controlled by germ-line V genes.

In the near future, the rat will undoubtedly become one of the main objects of investigation in the field of genetic regulation of antibody biosynthesis. This species has all the necessary prerequisites for such a study such as a large number of inbred strains, genetic markers of light as well as of heavy α- and γ-chains (Bazin *et al.,* 1974; Beckers and Bazin, 1975), and availability of myeloma Ig-producing tumors.

ACKNOWLEDGMENTS

Original work from the authors' laboratory has been supported in part by the World Health Organization. The paper was translated by Professor A. L. Pumpianski.

X. REFERENCES

Armerding, D., 1971, *Eur. J. Immunol.* 1:39.
Atassi, M.S., 1975, *Immunochemistry* 5:423.
Bazin, H., Beckers, A., Deckers, C., and Moriamé, M., 1973, *J. Natl. Cancer Inst.* 51:1359.
Bazin, H., Beckers, A., Vaerman, J.-P., and Heremans, J. F., 1974, *J. Immunol.* 112:1035.
Beckers, A., and Bazin, H., 1975, *Immunochemistry* 12:671.
Beckers, A., Querinjean, H., and Bazin, H., 1974, *Immunochemistry* 11:605.
Björk, J., Karlsson, F.A., and Berggård, I., 1971, *Proc. Natl. Acad. Sci. USA* 68:1707.
Binz, H., and Lindenmann, J., 1974, *Cell. Immunol.* 10:260.
Catty, D., Humphrey, J.H., and Gell, P.G.H., 1969, *Immunology* 16:409.

Cooper, A.G., and Steinberg, A.C., 1970, *J. Immunol.* **104**:1108.
Dray, S., and Nisonoff, A., 1965, *Molecular and Cellular Basis of Antibody Formation*, p. 175, Academia, Praha.
Eichmann, K., 1972, *Eur. J. Immunol.* **2**:301.
Eichmann, K., Tung, A.S., and Nisonoff, A., 1974, *Nature (London)* **250**:509.
Gutman, G.A., and Weissman, I.L., 1971, *J. Immunol.* **107**:1390.
Gutman, G.A., Loh, E., and Hood, L., 1975, *Proc. Natl. Acad. Sci. USA* **72**:5046.
Haimovich, J., Jaton, J.-C., and Pink, J.R.L., 1974, *Eur. J. Immunol.* **4**:290.
Karlsson, F.A., Peterson, P.A., and Berggård, I., 1969, *Proc. Natl. Acad. Sci. USA* **64**:1257.
Kim, Y.D., and Karush, F., 1974, *Immunochemistry* **11**:147.
Kindt, T.J., Mandy, W.J., and Todd, C.W., 1970, *Biochemistry* **9**:2028.
Kitagawa, M., Yagi, Y., and Pressman, D., 1965, *J. Immunol.* **95**:446.
Mage, R.G., 1974, *Curr. Topics Microbiol. Immunol.* **63**:131.
Mage, R., Lieberman, R., Potter, M., and Terry, W.D., 1973, *The Antigens* (M. Sela, ed), p. 300, Academic Press, New York.
Mäkelä, O., 1970, *Transplant. Rev.* **5**:3.
Mäkelä, O., Ruoslanti, E., and Seppälä, I.J.T., 1970, *Immunochemistry* **7**:917.
McMichael, A.J., Phillips, J.M., Williamson, A.R., Imanishi, T., and Mäkelä, O., 1975, *Immunogenetics* **2**:161.
Milstein, C.P., Steinberg, A.G., McLaughlin, C.L., and Solomon, A., 1974, *Nature (London)* **248**:160.
Nezlin, R.S., 1964, *Biokhimia* **29**:548.
Nezlin, R.S., 1976, *Structure and Biosynthesis of Antibodies*, Plenum Press, New York.
Nezlin, R.S., and Kulpina, L.M., 1967, *Immunochemistry* **4**:269.
Nezlin, R.S., and Rokhlin, O.V., 1969, *FEBS Symposium*, Vol. 15 (F. Franĕk and D. Shugar, eds.), p. 117, Academic Press, New York.
Nezlin, R.S., Rokhlin, O.V., and Vengerova, T.I., 1974a, *Ann. Immunol. (Inst. Pasteur)* **125c**:93.
Nezlin, R.S., Vengerova, T.I., Rokhlin, O.V., and Machulla, H.K.G., 1974b, *Immunochemistry* **11**:517.
Nezlin, R.S., Vengerova, T.I., Rokhlin, O.V., and Machulla, H.K.G., 1975, *Antibody Structure and Molecular Immunology, FEBS Symposium*, Vol. 36 (J. Gergely and G.A. Medgyesi, eds.), p. 93, Akadémiai Kiadó, Budapest.
Pink, R., Wang, A.-C., and Fudenberg, H.H., 1971, *Annu. Rev. Med.* **22**:145.
Poljak, K.J., Amzel, L.M., Chen, B.L., Phjzackerley, R.P., and Saul F., 1974, *Proc. Natl. Acad. Sci USA.* **71**:3440.
Polmar, S.H., and Steinberg, A.G., 1967, *Biochem. Genet.* **1**:117.
Potter, M., and Lieberman, R., 1970, *J. Exp. Med.* **132**:737.
Reisfeld, R.A., and Inman, J.L., 1968, *Immunochemistry* **5**:503.
Rokhlin, O.V., 1976, *Mol. Biol. USSR* **10**:206.
Rokhlin, O.V., and Nezlin, R.S., 1969, *Probl. Med. Chem. USSR* **15**:439.
Rokhlin, O.V., and Nezlin, R.S., 1973, *Eur. J. Immunol.* **3**:732.
Rokhlin, O.V., and Nezlin, R.S., 1974, *Scand. J. Immunol.* **3**:209.
Rokhlin, O.V., Vengerova, T.I., and Nezlin, R.S., 1970, *Mol. Biol. USSR* **4**:906.
Rokhlin, O.V., Vengerova, T.I., and Nezlin, R.S., 1971, *Immunochemistry* **8**:525.
Rokhlin, O.V., Vengerova, T.I., and Nezlin, R.S., 1972, *Mol. Biol. USSR* **6**:263.
Rokhlin, O.V., Nezlin, R.S., and Machulla, H.K.G., 1975, *Immunochemistry* **12**:311.
Schiffer, M., Girling, R.L., Ely, K.R., and Edmundson, A.B., 1973, *Biochemistry* **12**:4620.
Sela, M., 1969, *Science* **166**:1365.
Solomon, A., and McLaughlin C.L., 1969, *J. Biol. Chem.* **12**:3393.
Starace, V., and Querinjean, P., 1975, *J. Immunol.* **115**:59.

Vengerova, T.I., Rokhlin, O.V., and Nezlin, R.S., 1972a, *Immunochemistry* **9**:413.
Vengerova, T.I., Rokhlin, O.V., and Nezlin, P.S., 1972b, *Immunochemistry* **9**:1239.
Waterfield, M.D., Morris, J.E., Hood, L., and Todd, C.W., 1973, *J. Immunol.* **110**:227.
Wigzell, H., 1973, *Scand. J. Immunol.* **2**:199.
Williamson, A.R., Premkumar, E., and Shoyab, M., 1975, *Fed. Proc.* **34**:28.
Wistar, R., 1969, *Immunology* **17**:23.
Zappacosta, S., and Rossi, G., 1972, *Immunochemistry* **9**:689.
Zeeuws, R., and Strosberg, A.D., 1975, *Arch. Intern. Physiol. Biochem.* **83**:41.

Genetic and Structural Studies of a V-Region Marker in Mouse Immunoglobulin Light Chains

Paul D. Gottlieb

Department of Biology and Center for Cancer Research
Massachusetts Institute of Technology
Cambridge, Massachusetts

I. INTRODUCTION

This chapter describes the characteristics and strain distribution of a genetic marker discovered by Edelman and Gottlieb (1970) in the V regions of serum Ig L chains of unimmunized mice. Gottlieb (1974) demonstrated that expression of this V-region marker (called the I_B-peptide marker) is closely linked to the Ly-3 genetic locus governing expression of a thymocyte surface antigen (Boyse *et al.*, 1971). The Ly-3 locus resides in linkage group XI on chromosome 6 of the mouse (Itakura *et al.*, 1972). If the locus governing expression of the I_B-peptide marker is a structural locus for L-chain V regions, then it too resides in linkage group XI, and this would be the first instance in any species in which structural genes for an Ig chain have been placed in a particular linkage group. The possibility exists, however, that the locus which maps in linkage group XI does not contain structural genes for light-chain V regions, but rather is a regulatory locus which governs the expression of structural genes encoded in this linkage group or elsewhere in the genome.

In order to evaluate the I_B-peptide marker with respect to other genetic polymorphisms in Ig chains, it is necessary to determine whether it represents single or multiple amino acid substitution in L-chain V regions. Such studies have been hampered by the presence of the marker in less than 5% of the serum Ig L chains of I_B-positive strains. This is in marked contrast to the rabbit group a allotypes, in which 70–90% of the H chains of serum Ig are allotype positive

(Mage *et al.*, 1973). Because of the paucity of I_B-positive Ig's in serum, it is important to enrich for this material, and the approaches being explored at present are described in this review.

The Ly-3 locus, to which the I_B-peptide marker is genetically linked, is one of a series of loci determining mouse lymphocyte surface antigens (Ly-1, Ly-2, and Ly-3) discovered by Boyse and Old (Boyse *et al.*, 1968a, 1971), and recent studies by these and other workers are adding to this number (Komuro *et al.*, 1975). The Ly-1, Ly-2, and Ly-3 antigens are detected with antisera produced by immunizing allogeneic inbred or F_1 mice with thymic lymphocytes or leukemic cells (Shen *et al.*, 1975) and they can be quantitated by the use of cytotoxic or absorption techniques. Each Ly locus contains two recognizable alleles: *Ly-1ᵃ* and *Ly-1ᵇ*, *Ly-2ᵃ* and *Ly-2ᵇ*, and *Ly-3ᵃ* and *Ly-3ᵇ*. These determine the cell surface antigenic specificities Ly-1.1 and Ly-1.2, Ly-2.1 and Ly-2.2, and Ly-3.1 and Ly-3.2, respectively. The function of these antigens on the cell surface is unknown, but they are present in highest concentration on thymic lymphocytes, and are also present on peripheral lymphocytes

Some information is available concerning the genetic linkage of the various Ly antigens with each other and with other loci in the mouse. Ly-1 resides in linkage group XII of the mouse (Itakura *et al.*, 1971); it segregates from the loci governing Ly-2 and Ly-3 expression, which are very closely linked to each other in linkage group XI. Among 370 backcross progeny, no recombinants between the Ly-2 and Ly-3 loci were observed (Itakura *et al.*, 1972). Moreover, studies with the antibody-blocking technique (Boyse *et al.*, 1968b) suggest that these antigens are adjacent on the cell surface as well. It has been suggested that Ly-2 and Ly-3 may be part of a complex Ly-2, Ly-3 locus and that the Ly-2 and Ly-3 antigenic specificities may even be on the same molecule (Itakura *et al.*, 1972).

Recent studies by Boyse, Cantor, and co-workers (Kisielow *et al.*, 1975; Shiku *et al.*, 1975; Cantor and Boyse, 1975a,b; Cantor and Simpson, 1975; Simpson and Cantor, 1975) have indicated that several functional classes of thymus-derived lymphocytes in the peripheral lymphoid organs may be distinguished by their Ly antigens. About 45% of peripheral T lymphocytes bear only Ly-1 antigenic determinants, and these cells appear to perform as "helpers" in the humoral immune response. Approximately 5% of peripheral T cells bear only the Ly-2 and Ly-3 surface antigenic specificities, and this population of cells appears to contain all the prekiller and killer cell activities of cellular immunity. The remaining 50% of peripheral T cells contain all three Ly-antigenic specificities (Ly-1, Ly-2, and Ly-3) and may represent a population of immature T cells not yet committed to mutually exclusive functional activities (Cantor and Boyse, 1975a). There is also evidence that the Ly-1 peripheral T cells may play a helper role in the cellular immune response as well (Cantor and Boyse, 1975b), and that suppressor T cells may be Ly-2, Ly-3 positive and Ly-1 negative (V. Sato and V. Herzenberg, unpublished results). Determination of the molecular properties of the Ly antigens may open the way to discovering whether they are responsible

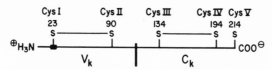

Figure 1. Overall structure of a mouse κ-chain. V_κ and C_κ refer to the variable and constant portions of the chain, respectively, and half-cystinyl residues are numbered from I to V. The black region encompassing Cys I indicates the position of the Cys I hexapeptides which constitute the I_B-peptide marker.

for the helper or killer functions of the cells that bear them. These and other studies to be described should reveal whether the genetic linkage of the I_B-peptide marker in V_L regions and the Ly-2 and Ly-3 loci is fortuitous, or whether there is some structural or regulatory relationship among the products of these linked loci.

II. DETECTION OF THE I_B-PEPTIDE MARKER

A genetic marker is detectable in peptide maps of light chains isolated from normal serum IgG of several inbred strains of mice (Edelman and Gottlieb, 1970). Normal serum IgG from unimmunized mice is prepared by starch zone electrophoresis and two successive gel filtrations on Sephadex G200. Fully reduced and [14C]iodoacetic acid-alkylated light chains* are digested with trypsin, and two-dimensional peptide maps are prepared by high-voltage paper electrophoresis (pH 4.7) and descending chromatography (n-butanol–acetic acid–water–pyridine, 15:3:12:10, v/v). Autoradiograms of the maps indicate the positions of peptides containing 14C-alkylated half-cystinyl residues. The positions of the five half-cystinyl residues in mouse κ light chains are indicated in Fig. 1.

Comparisons of such autoradiograms revealed two classes of maps (Fig. 2). The roman numerals refer to the light-chain half-cystinyl residue from which peptides in each radioactive zone are derived (see Fig. 1) as shown by amino acid

---

*Fully reduced and [14C]iodoacetic acid-alkylated light chains are obtained by either of two protocols, depending on the objectives of the experiment. L and H chains may be first separated after partial reduction by gel filtration on Sephadex G 100 in 1 N propionic acid. L chains may then be fully reduced and alkylated. When the IgG of interest is in short supply, 1 mg or less can be fully reduced and alkylated with [14C]iodoacetic acid of high specific activity and then pooled with carrier mouse IgG which has been fully reduced and alkylated with unlabeled iodoacetic acid. Chains are then separated by gel filtration on Sephadex G100 in 1 N propionic acid–6 M urea.

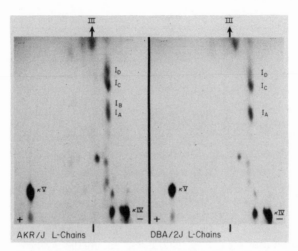

Figure 2. Autoradiograms of peptide maps of L chains from mice of the AKR/J and DBA/2J strains. High-voltage paper electrophoresis at pH 4.7 was in the horizontal direction with the anode (+) at the left of each map; descending chromatography was from bottom to top. The position of sample application is not shown but is indicated by a vertical black line at the bottom of each map. Roman numerals indicate the half-cystinyl residues from which peptides in each radioactive zone are derived (see Fig. 1). From Gottlieb (1971).

analysis and amino acid sequence determination (Edelman and Gottlieb, 1970). As described in detail below, radioactive zones labeled I_A, I_B, I_C, and I_D are all derived from Cys I in the V region of mouse light chains, and it is apparent (Figs. 2 and 3) that the zone labeled I_B in the AKR/J light-chain peptide map is not detectable in the DBA/2J map. The presence or absence of the I_B zone of

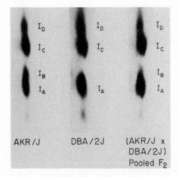

Figure 3. Radioactive zones I_A through I_D peptide maps of AKR/J, DBA/2J, and pooled (AKR/J × DBA/2J)F_2 L chains. The presence or absence of the I_B zone of radioactivity constitutes the presence or absence of the I_B-peptide marker. It is apparent that the hybrid contains an intermediate quantity of I_B relative to the parental strains. From Gottlieb (1971).

radioactivity represents the presence or absence of the V-region genetic marker, and the marker is therefore called the "I_B-peptide marker."

In F_1 mice derived from a genetic cross between the I_B-positive AKR/J strain and the I_B-negative DBA/2J strain, the expression of the I_B-peptide marker is about one-half that of the AKR/J parent (Fig. 3). Peptide maps of light chains from individual animals of an F_2 generation of this cross fell into three groups—the two parental types and the F_1 type. This suggested that expression of the I_B-peptide marker might be segregating as a classical codominant Mendelian marker (Edelman and Gottlieb, 1970).

III. PEPTIDES DERIVED FROM Cys I

Radioactive spots I_C and I_D (Fig. 2) were subjected to further high-voltage paper electrophoresis at pH 1.9, and were then eluted and their amino acid sequence determined by the dansyl-Edman procedure (Fig. 4). I_C was shown to be a mixture of hexapeptides which terminated in lysine, and I_D proved to be a mixture which terminated in arginine. Since the resolution between radioactive zones I_A and I_B was not complete (Fig. 2), the I_A-I_B complex was cut in half, and the halves were subjected to pH 1.9 high-voltage paper electrophoresis. Elution and subsequent amino acid analysis indicated that both halves contained mixtures of tryptic peptides terminating in both arginine and lysine. These could be resolved by high-voltage paper electrophoresis at pH 10.6 (Edelman and Gottlieb, 1970). The I_A-I_B complex of the AKR/J L-chain peptide map was compared with the comparable region of the DBA/2J map by high-voltage paper electrophoresis at pH 10.6 (Fig. 5) (Gottlieb, 1971). As shown by amino acid sequence determination, both AKR/J and DBA/2J have lysine-containing tryptic hexapeptides in the area labeled I_{A1} and arginine-containing hexapeptides in the area labeled I_{A2}. The area labeled I_B is occupied by lysine-containing radioactive hexapeptides in the case of AKR/J, but contains no ^{14}C-labeled peptides in DBA/2J. These peptides in AKR/J overlap I_{A1} and I_{A2} just enough to give an observable difference between I_B-positive and I_B-negative strains in two-dimensional peptide maps.

Dansyl-Edman analysis clearly indicated that the peptides in I_{A1}, I_{A2}, I_B, I_C, and I_D regions of AKR/J light-chain maps were hexapeptides and likely to be derived from the Cys I region of mouse κ-chains. This was apparent when these sequences were compared with the Cys I region of a number of mouse myeloma κ-chains (Fig. 4). These analyses further indicated that, with the exception of I_{A2}, all were *mixtures* of hexapeptides. Since the dansyl-Edman procedure as performed was not quantitative, the relative amounts of the several amino acids at each position in I_{A1}, for example, could not be determined, except for cases where there was an overwhelming amount of one amino acid. Such cases are in-

AKR/J Hexapeptide Group	Dansyl-Edman Analyses					
I_{A1}	Val	Thr Ser	**Val** Met	Ser Thr	Cys	(Lys)
I_{A2}	Ala	Thr	Ile	Ser	Cys	(Arg)
I_B	Val	Thr Ser	**Ile** Met	Ser Thr	Cys	(Lys)
I_C	Val	**Thr** Ser	**Ile** Leu	**Thr** Ser	Cys	(Lys)
I_D	Val	**Thr** Ser	Ile	**Ser** Thr	Cys	(Arg)

Balb/c Myeloma K-chain	No. with hexapeptide sequence						
70	(16)	Ala	Thr	Ile	Ser	Cys	Arg
41	(1)	Val	Ser	Leu	Thr	Cys	Arg
21	(1)	Val	Thr	Leu	Thr	Cys	Lys
773	(5)	Val	Thr	Ile	Ser	Cys	—
M29	(1)	Val	Thr	Met	Thr	Cys	—
T29	(1)	Val	Ser	Met	Ser	Cys	—
157	(1)	Val	Ser	Val	Thr	Cys	—
603	(3)	Val	Thr	Met	Ser	Cys	—
10	(2)	Val	Thr	Ile	Thr	Cys	—
Residues from NH$_2$-terminus		19	20	21	22	23	24

Figure 4. Amino acids found in each position of Cys I hexapeptides isolated from normal AKR/J L chains as revealed by dansyl-Edman amino acid sequence analysis (from Edelman and Gottlieb, 1970). Amino acids presented in boldface type are predominant at a position. Lysine and arginine residues are assigned on the basis of amino acid compositions. Included for comparison are the amino acid sequences of residues 19–23 (or 24, where possible) of mouse myeloma V_K regions which yield Cys I hexapeptides upon tryptic digestion (from Gally, 1973). The identification number of a representative myeloma κ-chain which yields each hexapeptide sequence is given, along with the number of myeloma κ-chains known to contain each sequence. (Note: Not all κ-chains containing a given hexapeptide sequence are identical in sequence in the rest of their V_K regions.)

dicated in boldface type in Fig. 4. As yet, definitive determination of actual amino acid sequences has not been completed. The fact that under the chromatography conditions employed these hexapeptides appear to migrate in resolvable groups probably reflects the sensitivity of the chromatographic system to certain integral features of the peptide compositions and sequences.

Peptide I_{A2} represents the only instance in which dansyl-Edman analysis of Cys I derived hexapeptides revealed a unique amino acid sequence. The amino acid sequence observed is identical to that of mouse 70 myeloma light chain

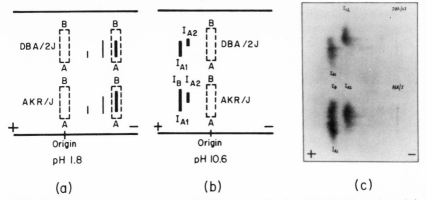

(a)   (b)   (c)

Figure 5. Comparison of AKR/J and DBA/2J L-chain Cys I peptides in the region of the I_A-I_B complex by high-voltage paper electrophoresis. (a) The regions of the I_A-I_B complex of AKR/J (I_B-positive) and DBA/2J (I_B-negative) peptide maps after parallel high-voltage paper electrophoresis at pH 1.8. (b) The major radioactive peptides of (a) after parallel high-voltage paper electrophoresis at pH 10.6. (c) Photograph of autoradiogram of (b). From Gottlieb (1971).

(Dreyer *et al.*, 1967), and its presence in readily detectable quantities in normal serum IgG light chains suggests that it denotes a particular commonly occurring subpopulation of serum IgG light chains. Results to be discussed below involving the fractionation of AKR/J normal serum IgG by ion exchange chromatography suggest that light chains containing I_{A2} are associated most frequently with the more negatively charged IgG molecules.

The detection of the I_B-peptide marker was made possible by a relatively constant structural feature of κ light chain V regions, which is shown in Fig. 6. In most light chains (~80%), the residue following the Cys I appears to be lysine or arginine. Similarly, five residues amino terminal to Cys I arginine or lysine also commonly occurs. The result is that tryptic digestion of a heterogeneous population of light chains yields Cys I largely in the form of hexapeptides. The I_B-peptide marker is a group of such hexapeptides which is apparently expressed in sufficient quantity for detection in the serum IgG light chains of several in-

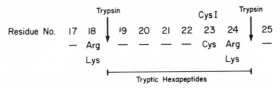

Figure 6. The relatively constant structural feature of the V_κ regions in the neighborhood of Cys I which gives rise upon tryptic digestion to Cys I hexapeptides.

bred strains, but is either lacking or expressed at an undetectable level in most others. Rough calculations suggest that in I_B-positive strains less than 5% of the light chains bear this marker (Edelman and Gottlieb, 1970). Thus this six-residue segment of mouse light-chain V regions, which precedes the first L-chain hypervariable region described by Wu and Kabat (1970), contains a considerable amount of amino acid sequence heterogeneity.

IV. FRACTIONATION OF AKR/J IgG ON DEAE-SEPHADEX

In order to determine whether light chains bearing the I_B-peptide marker might be associated with a population of IgG molecules which might be purified by some unique physical property, normal AKR/J serum IgG was subjected to ion exchange chromatography on DEAE-Sephadex A50 under conditions similar to those used by Takasugi and Hildemann (1969). As shown in Fig. 7, nearly all of the IgG loaded on the column could eventually be eluted with the starting buffer

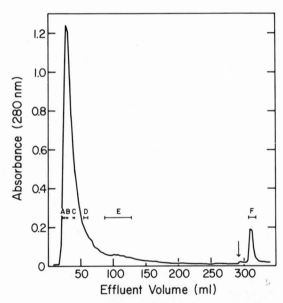

Figure 7. Ion exchange chromatography of AKR/J IgG on DEAE-Sephadex A50. AKR/J IgG (20 mg) in 0.015 M tris, 0.15 M NaCl, pH 8.4, was applied to a column (1.1 by 55 cm) of DEAE-Sephadex A50 (Pharmacia Inc., Piscataway, N.J.) which had been equilibrated with the same buffer. The column was then washed with the same buffer, and effluent fractions were monitored for absorbance at 280 nm. At the position noted by an arrow, all remaining bound protein was eluted with 0.015 M tris, 0.5 M NaCl, pH 7.8. Fractions A–F were taken for peptide mapping.

(0.015 M tris, 0.15 M NaCl, pH 8.4) and what little remained bound was eluted with 0.015 M tris, 0.5 M NaCl, pH 7.8. Preliminary subclass analysis of fractions of the eluted IgG by Ouchterlony double diffusion suggested that partial subclass fractionation was achieved. Thus, although little IgG actually bound to the DEAE-Sephadex under the conditions employed, some degree of fractionation was obtained by chromatography in the starting buffer. Immunoelectrophoresis clearly indicated that this resolution was on the basis of charge, the more negative IgG species being retarded more than the more positively charged species.

Several fractions of the column profile were pooled as indicated in Fig. 7, and peptide maps of the light chains were prepared. Autoradiograms of the Cys I hexapeptide region of these maps are shown on the right side of Fig. 8. This is

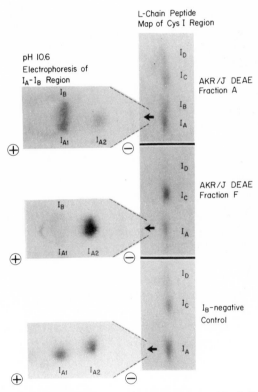

Figure 8. Right: Cys I hexapeptide regions of peptide maps of L chains from fractions A and F of AKR/J IgG obtained after ion exchange chromatography on DEAE-Sephadex A50 (see Fig. 7). The comparable region of a peptide map of L chains from I_B-negative strains (C57BL/6J plus DBA/1J) is shown for comparison. Left: The Cys I_A-I_B regions of the peptide maps shown on the right after parallel high-voltage paper electrophoresis at pH 10.6 (see Fig. 5).

the only region of the maps in which a clear difference between the fractions is visible.

The earliest fraction from DEAE-Sephadex, which by Ouchterlony analysis and by radioimmunoassay (Epstein and Gottlieb, in preparation) seems to be almost entirely IgG_{2a}, appears to contain light chains slightly enriched in the I_B-peptide group as compared with unfractionated AKR/J IgG (Fig. 8). In addition, in all instances in which this fractionation scheme was followed and maps of various fractions were compared, there appeared to be significant resolution between I_A and I_B, suggesting that perhaps the I_{A2} hexapeptide which overlaps I_{A1} and I_B in unfractionated AKR/J light chains was depleted. This suggestion is strengthened by the observation that as we proceed to the more retarded fractions (i.e., less positively charged) (Fig. 8) the amount of I_B and possibly I_{A1} decreases relative to the earlier fractions and relative to unfractionated AKR/J IgG. The fraction of IgG retained by DEAE-Sephadex in starting buffer and recovered by changing the buffer contains very little if any I_B.

In order to further investigate the differences in the I_A-I_B region apparent in the two-dimensional peptide maps, the I_A-I_B regions were subjected to high-voltage paper electrophoresis at pH 10.6. The results, presented on the left side of Fig. 8, indicate that the fraction retained by DEAE-Sephadex is greatly enriched in the arginine hexapeptide I_{A2} and greatly depleted in both I_{A1} and I_B. The earlier fractions from DEAE-Sephadex have normal quantities of I_{A1} and I_B, but are depleted in I_{A2} [e.g., compare Fig. 8 (left), fraction A, with Fig. 5c, AKR/J I_A-I_B].

The results obtained from DEAE-Sephadex fractionation of AKR/J IgG are of interest for two reasons:

1. The slight enrichment for I_B-positive light chains in the early fraction may be useful in providing antigenic material for producing antibodies specific for the I_B-peptide group, or in providing starting material for further fractionation.

2. The concentration of I_{A2}-positive chains in the later fractions from DEAE-Sephadex, which contain very little total protein, provides convenient starting material for investigations of the V-region sequence heterogeneity of these light chains, and perhaps the biological activity and recognition specificity of the immunoglobulins that contain them.

V. L CHAINS OF AKR/J IgG_{2a}

The observation that the early fractions from DEAE-Sephadex, which by Ouchterlony analysis appeared to be almost entirely IgG_{2a}, were enriched in the I_B-peptide group suggested the possibility that perhaps I_B-positive light chains were restricted to the IgG_{2a} subclass. The abnormally high proportion of λ_1 light chains in the IgD class of human myeloma proteins (Fahey *et al.*, 1968) is a precedent for such a restriction, and the enrichment in I_{A2}-positive light chains seen in the later DEAE fractions may be a similar kind of restriction. To investigate this possibility, the IgG from specific goat anti-mouse IgG_{2a} (Gateway Immunosera Co., Cahokia, Illinois) was purified by ammonium sulfate precipitation and gel filtration on Sephadex G200, and was then conjugated to Sepharose 4B using cyanogen bromide. AKR/J IgG from normal serum was passed slowly over the immunoadsorbent until the absorbance at 280 nm had returned to background. Material retained on the column was recovered by pulsing with 0.1 M glycine-HCl, pH 2.5, and the effluent was immediately neutralized with tris buffer. Preliminary Ouchterlony double-diffusion analysis indicated that the retained IgG was rich in IgG_{2a} and showed no trace of IgG_{2b}. The material which was not retained was somewhat depleted in IgG_{2a} but rich in IgG_{2b}, indicating that the affinity column was effective in specifically retaining IgG_{2a}. Light-chain peptide maps were prepared as usual, and the results indicated that the IgG_{2a} retained was not enriched in I_B-positive light chains as compared with unfractionated AKR/J IgG and with the IgG which passed through the affinity column. Thus I_B-positive light chains are present in but do not appear to be restricted to immunoglobulins of the IgG_{2a} isotype. Direct testing of IgG_{2b} and IgG_1 isotypes of AKR/J serum IgG has not yet been completed.

VI. FRACTIONATION OF Fab FRAGMENTS

It therefore appeared that (1) I_B-positive light chains are slightly more prevalent in the more positively charged IgG molecules and (2) they are probably present in at least two and possibly all IgG subclasses. The several subclasses of mouse IgG differ slightly in their electrophoretic and ion exchange properties (Williams and Chase, 1967), and this is likely to be due primarily to differences in the constant portions of γ_1, γ_{2a}, and γ_{2b} heavy chains. It was therefore possible that fractionation of Fab fragments from I_b-positive strains might yield some greater enrichment in I_B-positive light chains than fractionation of intact IgG. Fab fragments from AKR/J and C57BL/6-*Ly-2ª*, *Ly-3ª* IgG were prepared and several fractions were obtained by starch zone electrophoresis at pH 8.6 (see Appendix). In order to prepare peptide maps of light chains from the separate Fab fractions, it was first necessary to separate the light chains from the Fd fragments, which have similar molecular weight. This was achieved by ion exchange chromatography of partially reduced and [^{14}C]iodoacetic acid-alkylated Fab on SP-Sephadex C25 in 8 M urea. Similar fractionation conditions have been employed for separating κ- and λ-chains in man (Skavril *et al.*, 1967) and mouse

(W. Geckeler, personal communication). In addition, purified AKR/J L chains were subjected to ion exchange chromatography under identical conditions. Peptide maps of L chains and Fd fragments were prepared as usual after full reduction and [^{14}C]iodoacetic acid alkylation of fractions from SP-Sephadex, and these studies are described in more detail in Appendix.

Peptide maps of L chains isolated from Fab fragments indicated that there are equivalent amounts of I_B-positive light chains in the several Fab fractions which were obtained by starch zone electrophoresis. Thus the apparent slight enrichment in I_B-positive light chains seen in the more positively charged AKR/J IgG fractions obtained from DEAE-Sephadex does not seem to be a function of Fab alone and is not enhanced by producing Fab fragments.

VII. PURIFIED L CHAINS

The three fractions obtained from the purified light chains by ion exchange chromatography on SP-Sephadex all had equivalent amounts of the I_B-peptide, indicating that I_B-positive light chains do not appear to be restricted in their overall charge. That I_B-positive L chains are not monoclonal was evident from dansyl-Edman analysis of I_B-peptides which indicated the presence of amino acid sequence heterogeneity (Fig. 4). Moreover, their presence throughout the portion of the column profile known to contain κ-chains suggests (although does not prove) that I_B-positive light chains are of the κ type. According to W. Geckeler (personal communication), mouse λ_1 light chains elute as a sharp peak considerably earlier in the gradient than κ-chains. Additional observations suggest the κ nature of I_B-positive light chains:

1. Peptide maps of the λ_1 mouse myeloma light-chain λ_{2020} (obtained from Dr. M. Weigert) indicated that the quantity of λ_1 light chains present in normal AKR/J IgG is too small to account for the I_B-peptide (Cunningham et al., 1971) (Fig. 9).

2. Of the three types of mouse light chains known (κ, λ_1, and λ_2), only κ-chains have ever been shown to yield Cys I in the form of a tryptic hexapeptide. The λ_1-chains studied to date have demonstrated extremely limited amino acid sequence variability in their V regions, and all have yielded Cys I in the form of identical 23-residue tryptic peptides which terminate in–Cys Arg (Weigert et al., 1970; Cohn et al., 1974). In addition, Cys I of the light chain of mouse IgA myeloma MOPC-315, the only example of a λ_2 light chain observed to date (the gift of H. N. Eisen), is also present in a 23-residue tryptic peptide terminating in–Cys Arg (Dugan et al., 1973). The peptide map of the MOPC-315 λ_2-chain is distinctly different from that of λ_1 L chains and normal serum L chains.

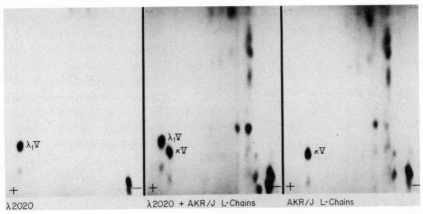

Figure 9. Autoradiograms of peptide maps of mouse myeloma λ_1-chain λ_{2020}, normal AKR/J L chains, and a mixture of λ_{2020} and AKR/J L chains. High-voltage paper electrophoresis at pH 4.7 was in the horizontal direction with the anode (+) at the left of each map; descending chromatography was from the bottom to top. The notations $\lambda_1 V$ and κV refer to the tryptic peptide containing Cys V of λ_1- and κ-chains, respectively. From Cunningham *et al.* (1971).

VIII. L CHAINS OF SPECIFIC ANTIBODIES

It is apparent from the above discussion that fractionation of normal AKR/J serum IgG, Fab fragments, and light chains has not yielded a preparation significantly enriched in I_B-positive light chains. By the criteria used to date, I_B-positive light chains appear to be of the κ type and demonstrate amino acid sequence and overall charge heterogeneity. It is likely that they reflect a genetic polymorphism in otherwise normal κ-chains of the inbred strains that express them, and that immunization of I_B-positive strains of mice with the appropriate antigen may elicit antibodies enriched in I_B-positive light chains. Preliminary studies in this direction have been reported (Cunningham *et al.*, 1971) which in-involved immunization of I_B-positive and I_B-negative strains of mice with the hapten–protein conjugate, DNP-BSA. The antibodies were isolated by specific precipitation with antigen, and peptide maps of purified L chains were prepared. The Cys I peptides contained in these light chains were a subset of those expressed in normal serum, providing a graphic demonstration of clonal selection. The presence of a significant amount of radioactivity in the position of the Cys V constant-region peptide of λ_1-chains further suggested that these chains, which are present at a very low level in normal serum IgG, contributed significantly to the anti-DNP-BSA immune response.

We are at present screening a number of other hapten–protein conjugates for their ability to stimulate the production of antibodies enriched in I_B-positive light chains. The present protocol involves the use of two successive affinity columns, the first containing the protein carrier, and the second containing the hapten–protein conjugate. This allows recovery of anticarrier and antihapten antibodies separately, and comparison of light-chain peptide maps with each other and with those of light chains from immunoglobulins whose production was stimulated by other antigens. Preliminary results indicate (P. D. Gottlieb, E. Raefsky, and S. Epstein, manuscript in preparation) that peptide maps of light chains from the anti-BSA antibodies resulting from stimulation of AKR/J mice with tosyl-BSA, p-azophenylarsonate-BSA, picryl-BSA and p-iodobenozyl-BSA are very similar, containing similar amounts of Cys I peptides and little or no λ_1-chain. However, light chains from the different antihapten antibodies are markedly different, demonstrating different subsets of the standard Cys I peptides and apparently containing a significant quantity of λ_1-chains. In addition, peptide maps of light chains from specifically purified AKR/J anti-streptococcal group A polysaccharide (kindly provided by Dr. Klaus Eichmann) also demonstrate a restricted subset of Cys I peptides, although not containing the I_B-peptide marker.

IX. GENETIC LINKAGE OF THE I_B-PEPTIDE MARKER

In order to identify the genetic locus or linkage group responsible for expression of the I_B-peptide marker, its inbred strain distribution was compared with the strain distributions of other murine genetic markers. As shown in Table I, the four inbred strains that express the I_B-peptide marker in their immunoglobulin L chains (AKR/J, C58/J, RF/J, and PL/J) also express the Ly-3.1 antigenic

Table I. Characteristics of Inbred Mouse Strains

I_B positive Ly-3.1 positive	I_B negative Ly-3.1 negative		
AKR/J	DBA/1J	SWR/J	ST/bJ
C58/J	DBA/2J	C57L/J	BDP/J
RF/J	A/J	CBA/J	129/J
PL/J	A/HeJ	C57BL/6J	MA/J
C57BL/6-Ly-2^a, Ly-3^a	C3H/HeJ	C57BL/KsJ	SEA/GnJ
AKR.B6/1	CE/J	C57Br/cdJ	AKR.M
	SJL/J	NZB	AL/N
	BALB/cJ	RIII/J	

specificity on the surface of their thymocytes. The expression of the Ly-3.1 antigenic specificity on thymocytes and peripheral T lymphocytes is determined by *Ly-3ᵃ*, one of the two alleles at the Ly-3 locus described by Boyse *et al.* (1971).

The similarity in strain distribution of these two genetic markers suggested the possibility that the genetic locus governing expression of the I_B-peptide marker might be closely linked genetically to the Ly-3 locus. Peptide maps were prepared of normal serum IgG light chains obtained from mice of the C57BL/6-*Ly-2ᵃ*, *Ly-3ᵃ* strain. This strain (Ly-2.1 and Ly-3.1 positive) was derived by Boyse and co-workers to be congenic with the C57BL/6 strain (Ly-2.2 and Ly-3.2 positive) at all but the region of the Ly-2 and Ly-3 loci. The *Ly-2ᵃ* and *Ly-3ᵃ* alleles were supplied by the RF inbred strain, and the mice were inbred after 16 backcrosses to C57BL/6 (Klein, 1973). The congenic C57BL/6-*Ly-2ᵃ*, *Ly-3ᵃ* strain was constructed on the basis of Ly-antigen typing without consideration of the I_B-peptide marker. Nevertheless, light chains from these mice proved to be I_B positive, indicating that expression of the I_B-peptide marker is closely linked to the Ly-2 and Ly-3 loci.

Itakura *et al.* (1972) have shown that the Ly-3 locus is very closely linked to the Ly-2 locus in linkage group XI of the mouse. Since the *Ly-3ᵃ* allele appears always to be associated with the *Ly-2ᵃ* allele in laboratory mice, all I_B-positive strains detected to date have the *Ly-2ᵃ*, *Ly-3ᵃ* genotype and display the Ly-2.1, Ly-3.1 phenotype (E. A. Boyse, personal communication). That the I_B-peptide marker is correlated with the *Ly-3ᵃ* allele rather than *Ly-2ᵃ* is demonstrated by strains such as CE/J with the genotype *Ly-2ᵃ*, *Ly-3ᵇ* whose phenotype is Ly-2.1 and Ly-3.2 positive and I_B negative (Gottlieb, 1974).

X. THE NATURE OF THE GENETIC LOCUS GOVERNING EXPRESSION OF THE I_B-PEPTIDE MARKER

The nature of the genetic locus governing expression of the I_B-peptide marker in L-chain V regions is not known. The simplest hypothesis is that it consists of structural gene(s) coding for L-chain V regions. The expression in I_B heterozygotes of approximately half as much I_B-peptide marker as in I_B-positive homozygotes is consistent with a gene dosage effect. However, an alternative possibility is that the *Ly-3ᵃ* allele or a gene linked to it may regulate the expression of L-chain V-region genes. It is therefore possible that all inbred strains contain structural genes which can give rise to I_B-positive L chains but that production of such L chains is under the regulation of a polymorphic locus in linkage group XI. Evidence obtained from investigations of other genetic markers in immunoglobulin V and C regions of mice and other species suggests that allelism at regulatory loci might explain the existence of different Ig phenotypes. This evidence is discussed below.

A number of testable hypotheses can be formulated to account for the observed genetic linkage of an L-chain V-region genetic marker with a particular allele determining a T-cell surface antigen. Such hypotheses are relevant to *all* V-region genetic markers which might owe their polymorphism to structural or regulatory loci. Several such hypotheses are described below.

A. A Structural Locus for L-Chain V Regions

As discussed above, the genetic locus in linkage group XI which governs expression of the I_B-peptide marker may contain structural genes coding for L-chain V regions. Most of the information responsible for our present view of Ig structural genetic loci comes from the study of apparent polymorphisms of Ig chains and intact molecules. These polymorphisms take several forms:

1. Single amino acid substitutions in C regions of Ig L- and H-chains.

2. Multiple amino acid substitutions in V regions and C regions of Ig chains.

3. Antigenic determinants present in V and/or C regions of Ig molecules which are detected by serological methods but which very likely reflect single or multiple amino acid substitutions in the polypeptide chains (i.e., allotypes).

4. Antigenic determinants present on Ig molecules which involve structures in or near the antigen-binding site (i.e., idiotypes).

The inheritance of these polymorphisms is studied by testing the progeny resulting from genetic crosses of parents of differing phenotype. If a polymorphism demonstrates simple Mendelian inheritance (as the I_B-peptide marker appears to), the simplest interpretation is that it is determined in the germ line by a single structural gene. Since the I_B-peptide marker appears to be present in approximately 5% of the L chains of serum IgG from unimmunized mice, one could argue that mouse V_K regions are encoded in the germ line by a small number of genes (~20). This order of magnitude is consistent with the nucleic acid hybridization studies of Leder *et al.* (1975) and of Tonegawa (1976) and would be consistent with the generation of extensive L-chain V-region diversity by somatic mechanisms (Smithies, 1967, 1970; Brenner and Milstein, 1969; Gally and Edelman, 1970; Baltimore, 1974). The I_B-peptide marker involves, at the present limit of our detection, only so-called framework positions preceding the first hypervariable region (Wu and Kabat, 1970). It therefore might reflect a particular germ-line gene (or group of genes) not present (or not expressed, see below) in I_B-negative strains which give(s) rise to a particular subgroup of V_K regions distinguishable by our peptide mapping methods.

Thus the apparent behavior of this V-region genetic marker as a Mendelian codominant gene can by straightforward reasoning lead to the conclusion consistent with nucleic acid hybridization data that the mouse has a small number of germ-line V_κ genes. For the purpose of this review, *structural genes for Ig V regions* consist of all germ-line genes which give rise to all possible V-region amino acid sequences that an animal could ever synthesize. The actual polypeptide sequences observed may come about in two ways. The structural genes in the germ line may be faithfully transcribed and translated in the somatic cells. Alternatively, these structural genes may be operated upon in the somatic cells by mechanisms which alter their nucleotide sequence. Such alteration is stable in the sense that mitosis transmits the altered nucleotide sequence faithfully to daughter cells. The altered nucleotide sequence gives rise, through transcription and translation, to V-region amino acid sequences which are not directly contained in germ-line genes but which are the direct consequence of information present in the nucleotide sequences of the germ-line structural genes.

The reason for being so explicit in defining structural genes is that it is not my purpose here to argue the merits or faults of germ-line and somatic theories for the origin of antibody diversity. Studies of the gene products have given much information, but in all likelihood will never reveal the answer. Nucleic acid hybridization experiments have yielded information on the C regions suggesting few germ-line genes (as suspected from inheritance of simple amino acid substitutions in C regions), and there is evidence to suggest small numbers of germ-line V genes as well, favoring somatic hypotheses. It is possible that the synthesis of large quantities of immunoglobulin genes in bacteria will allow direct assessment and counting of germ-line genes for Ig V regions. My point is to simply say that there must be structural genes for V regions, and whether there are many or few, and whether they are directly transcribed or first modified, it would be of great interest to map them genetically. In order to do so, it is necessary to use good criteria to distinguish between structural and regulatory genes (see below).

Proof of the somatic origin of V region diversity will require elucidation of the mechanisms (e.g., enzymes) by which it occurs. The genetic and structural characterization of polymorphisms in Ig chains has been and will continue to be extremely useful in designing appropriate experiments to identify these mechanisms.

B. Are the I_B-Peptide Marker and Ly-3 Determined by the Same Genetic Locus?

When we first noted the extremely close genetic linkage between the genetic locus governing the expression of the I_B-peptide marker and the Ly-3 locus, we considered the possibility that these loci were *identical* (Gottlieb, 1974). We hypothesized that the Ly-3.1 antigenic specificity on the surface of thymic lymphocytes might be due to the presence of I_B-positive L chains on the thymocyte surface. Thus the Ly-3 locus might contain structural genes coding for L-chain V regions.

There are several reasons for seriously considering this possibility. It is probable that T lymphocytes contain on their surface some kind of antigen receptor, and there is provocative evidence that such receptors might bear some structural homology with conventional immunoglobulins, the products of B cells (Marchalonis, this volume; Binz and Wigzell, 1975; Eichmann and Rajewsky, 1975). Moreover, the extremely close association between the Ly-2 and Ly-3 loci in linkage group XI (Itakura *et al.*, 1972) and evidence for a close topological relationship between the Ly-2 and Ly-3 antigenic specificities on the thymocyte surface (Boyse *et al.*, 1971) led to the suggestion that Ly-2 and Ly-3 may reside on the product of a single gene (Itakura *et al.*, 1972). These characteristics of the Ly-2,3 chromosomal region are remarkably similar to what one might expect for a gene complex coding for immunoglobulin V and C regions (Gally and Edelman, 1970). Thus it seems possible that the I_B-peptide marker in immunoglobulin L-chain V regions may be determined by the *Ly-3^a* allele, and that the Ly-3 and perhaps Ly-2 antigenic specificities might reside on molecules structurally related to immunoglobulins (Gottlieb, 1974).

However, there is at present no direct evidence to suggest that the molecule bearing the Ly-3.1 antigenic specificity is structurally or serologically related to I_B-positive L chains. Experiments designed to detect reactivity of anti-Ly-3.1 antiserum with I_B-positive immunoglobulins were inconclusive. If an antiserum specific for I_B-positive immunoglobulins were available, it could be tested for reactivity with Ly-3.1-positive thymocytes. However, attempts to produce such antisera have been hampered by the extremely low levels of such molecules in serum IgG, and by the failure of standard methods of protein fractionation to significantly enrich in this material. Such enrichment may be achieved by the immunization experiments discussed earlier and by the induction of I_B-positive myelomas (see below).

Characterization of the thymocyte surface molecules which bear the Ly-2 and Ly-3 antigenic determinants may reveal whether or not they are structurally related to immunoglobulins and the I_B-peptide marker. We are therefore utilizing specific anti-Ly antisera and the C57BL/6 congenic strains derived by Boyse and co-workers to determine the molecular structure of these antigenic molecules (Durda and Gottlieb, 1976). The basic design of these experiments as is follows: the thymocytes' surface is iodinated with ^{125}I using lactoperoxidase; the plasma membrane is dissociated using the nonionic detergent NP-40; specific anti-Ly antiserum or control serum is added; and antigen–antibody complexes are precipitated with rabbit anti-mouse IgG. Precipitates are dissolved and subjected to polyacrylamide gel electrophoresis in sodium dodecylsulfate (SDS). For studies of the Ly-3.1 antigenic specificity, thymocytes of the C57BL/6-*Ly-2^a*, *Ly-3^a* strain (Ly-2.1, Ly-3.1, I_B positive) are iodinated. Thymocytes of the congenic partner C57BL/6 (Ly-2.2 and Ly-3.2 positive, I_B negative) and another congenic strain C57BL/6-*Ly-2*^{a} (Ly-2.1 and Ly-3.2 positive, I_B-negative) provide excellent specificity controls. Specific precipitation of protein has been obtained with anti-Ly-3.1 antisera, and there is no evidence for a subunit with the molecular weight of conventional L chains. It is possible, however, that detailed structural analysis of the major polypeptide species with an apparent molecular weight of 35,000 daltons will reveal immunoglobulinlike properties and perhaps an L-chain V region. While this remains a possibility, the evidence to date would suggest that the molecules bearing the Ly-3.1 antigenic determinant and I_B-positive L chains are not identical.

C. A Regulatory Locus Governing Expression of L-Chain V Regions

It is possible that the presence or absence of the I_B-peptide marker in serum IgG L chains of inbred strains of mice is governed by a *regulatory locus* which maps in linkage group XI. Thus it is possible that all inbred strains have in their germ lines structural genes for V_K regions which could, if expressed, give rise to I_B-positive L chains. These structural genes may or may not be genetically linked to the regulatory locus, and therefore may or may not reside in linkage group XI.

Such a regulatory locus need not have as its primary function the regulation of which structural germ-line genes for V_K regions should or should not be expressed. It may be a locus which, by the performance of its normal function (or the function of its protein product), gives rise to serum IgG molecules containing I_B-positive L chains. One can conceive of several kinds of loci which could effect the phenotype (or clonotype) (Gally and Edelman, 1972) of a strain of mice in such a way.

1. The possibility was considered that the IgG containing I_B-positive L chains in the serum of Ly-3.1-positive mice might be autoantibody to the T-cell surface molecule bearing this antigenic specificity. Autoantibodies are known to exist in certain inbred strains (Shirai and Mellors, 1971). If this were so, then polymorphism at the Ly-3 locus itself might govern expression of I_B-positive L chains by stimulating expansion of clones of B cells committed to this antibody. This seems unlikely since extensive absorption of serum containing I_B-positive IgG with washed Ly-3.1-positive thymocytes failed to remove molecules bearing the I_B-peptide marker (Gottlieb, 1974).

2. A genetic locus closely linked to Ly-3 might, by stimulating the production of antibody to its product, cause increased amounts of I_B-positive IgG to be synthesized. An example of such a locus might be an *endogenous virus* which, through complete or partial expression in some tissue(s) of Ly-3.1-positive hosts, stimulates a host humoral immune response. This is an intriguing possibility since the four standard inbred strains which express I_B-positive L chains (AKR/J, RF/J, C58/J, PL/J) all demonstrate a high incidence of spontaneous leukemia (Staats, 1972). In this regard, it might be of great interest to investigate the

incidence of spontaneous leukemia in the C57BL/6-*Ly-2ª*, *Ly-3ª* strain as compared with its congenic partner, C57BL/6, which shows a very low incidence. Our own fragmentary observations of six C57BL/6-*Ly-2ª*, *Ly-3ª* female mice for approximately 2 years suggest no increased incidence. This does not rule out the possibility that the *Ly-3ª* allele or a locus closely linked to it might be contributory to the high incidence of spontaneous leukemia in these strains. Leukemogenesis might be under multigenic control and therefore require the presence of certain alleles at loci unlinked to *Ly-3ª* and the I$_B$-peptide marker. We are observing, for example, C57BL/6-*H-2^k*, *Ly-2ª*, *Ly-3ª* mice produced by breeding the two C57BL/6-congenic strains C57BL/6-*H-2^k* and C57BL/6-*Ly-2ª*, *Ly-3ª*.

3. The Ly-3 locus or a closely linked locus might act as an immune response gene (Ir gene) in allowing the host to respond to some environmental antigen or autoantigen. This response might involve synthesis of IgG bearing I$_B$-positive L chains. The product of such an Ir gene and the mechanism by which it might act are of course unknown. It is known from the work of Benacerraf and of McDevitt (see Shreffler and David, 1975; Klein, 1975) that Ir genes governing the ability to respond well or poorly to a wide range of antigens map within the H-2 complex in linkage group IX of the mouse. It is also known that this same complex chromosomal region determines so-called Ia-antigens which are present on B cells and/or T cells and which may be products of or involved in the mechanism of action of Ir genes (Shreffler and David; 1975; Klein, 1975). Other loci which behave like Ir genes do not map in the H-2 complex (Gasser, 1969). At one time, Taylor and co-workers (personal communication) suspected a possible correlation of the level of chicken red cell agglutinins in the serum of recombinant-inbred AKXL mice with the *Ly-3ª* allele. These workers ultimately demonstrated absolute correlation with the H-chain locus and observed inconsistencies with the *Ly-3ª* correlation. Dorf and Boyse (personal communication) observed no correlation of the GAT immune response with Ly-3. It would be of great interest to investigate the possible correlation of other genetically regulated immune responses with Ly-3.

4. It is possible that all mice have the genetic information for synthesizing I$_B$-positive L chains, but that the regulation of synthesis of such chains occurs at the level of T cell–B cell cooperation. Cooperation with an Ly-3.1-positive T helper cell might be required in order for antigen to stimulate a I$_B$-positive B cell. One method of testing this hypothesis would be to infuse C57BL/6 mice (Ly-3.2 positive, I$_B$ negative) with purified T cells from C57BL/6-*Ly-2ª*, *Ly-3ª* mice (Ly-3.1 positive, I$_B$ positive), and to monitor the serum for the appearance of IgG-containing I$_B$-positive L chains. Alternatively, neonatally thymectomized lethally irradiated C57BL/6 mice could be reconstituted with bone marrow (treated with anti-θ serum to destroy T cells) from C57BL/6 mice and purified T cells from C57BL/6-*Ly-2ª*, *Ly-3ª* mice, and the serum monitored as above. The reciprocal experiment could be used to test whether C57BL/6-*Ly-2ª*,

Ly-3^a B cells can synthesize I_B-positive L chains in the absence of Ly-3.1-positive T cells. These studies are in progress in our laboratory.

There is reason to believe that this is not the reason for the existence of I_B-positive and I_B-negative phenotypes. In collaboration with Dr. E. A. Boyse and Dr. F.-W. Shen, we tested whether hybrid mice homozygous for the Ly-3^a allele (donated by the AKR strain) but athymic due to homozygosity for the *nude* mutation expressed I_B-positive L chains in their normal serum IgG. AKR female mice were crossed with BALB/c males which were homozygous for the nude mutation. Thymic biopsies were performed on F_2 progeny, and thymocytes were assayed for Ly-2.1 and Ly-2.2 antigenic specificities by cytotoxic assay. Typing was for Ly-2 rather than the closely linked Ly-3 due to the relative convenience of this assay. Males and females of genotype Ly-2^a/Ly-2^a were mated, and nude progeny (*nu/nu*) were obtained at the expected frequency. These were bled, normal serum IgG was prepared, and a peptide map of the L chains was prepared as usual. The I_B-peptide marker was expressed in quantity equivalent to that of the AKR/J parental strain, indicating that the presence of a thymus and the normal complement of peripheral T lymphocytes is not a prerequisite for its expression. This conclusion must be qualified, however, because of observations that mice of the *nu/nu* genotype do contain θ-positive lymphocytes and thus may have some limited T-cell function.

In addition, recent evidence of Cantor and Boyse (1975a,b) suggests that in the C57BL/6 mouse (Ly-1.2, Ly-2.2, Ly-3.2 positive), peripheral T cells which perform the helper function are Ly-1.2 positive and Ly-2.2, Ly-3.2 negative (see Section I). The Ly-2.2 and Ly-3.2 antigenic specificities appeared to mark peripheral T cells with killer or prekiller activity. If the products of the Ly loci mark peripheral T cells of the C57BL/6-Ly-2^a, Ly-3^a mouse in an analogous fashion, then the helper T cell would be expected to lack Ly-3.1.

5. Finally, a regulatory locus linked to the Ly-3 locus may have as its primary function the regulation of expression of V_K-region genes. Such loci have been postulated for several Ig allotypes, and these are discussed below.

XI. OTHER Ig GENETIC MARKERS: POLYMORPHISM AT STRUCTURAL OR REGULATORY LOCI?

Genetic polymorphisms in V- and C-regions of Ig chains from several species have been the subject of several useful reviews (Gally, 1973; Mage *et al.*, 1973; Weigert *et al.*, 1975; Kindt, 1975). Much of our knowledge of these structural polymorphisms comes from studies of the antigenic properties of the immunoglobulins when used to immunize animals of the same or different species.

If the recipient animal lacks antigenic determinants present on the donor's immunoglobulins, it will usually respond by producing antibodies specific for these determinants. Such antisera can then be used in suitable assays to detect and quantitate molecules which bear the antigenic determinants in question.

Allotypes are genetic markers on immunoglobulins which can be detected serologically and which are not restricted to antibody molecules having a particular ligand-binding specificity (the latter being *heritable idiotypes*) (Mage *et al.*, 1973). Allotypic determinants result from the existence of multiple forms of immunoglobulin V and C genes which are thought to be alleles at V-gene and C-gene loci. Such allotypes are generally detected using allogeneic antisera (i.e., antisera produced in the same species as the antigen donor but of a different inbred strain). In general, allotypic differences among proteins of a single species can be correlated with differences in the primary structure of polypeptide chains. Detailed amino acid sequence analysis of allotypically different immunoglobulins has resulted in the definition of two categories of allotypes. *Simple allotypes* are alternative forms of immunoglobulin chains which differ by one or a few amino acid substitutions and which segregate in a classical Mendelian fashion (Gutman *et al.*, 1975). Examples of simple allotypes are the Gm markers of the human $C\gamma_1$ region, and the Inv marker of the human C_K region (Mage *et al.*, 1973; Solomon, 1976). Alternative forms of *complex allotypes* differ by multiple amino acid residues, and until relatively recently they were also thought to segregate in a classical Mendelian fashion. Examples of complex allotypes are the group a V_H-region allotypes of the rabbit (a1, a2, a3) and the rabbit group b C_K-region allotypes (b4, b5, b6, b9) (Mage *et al.*, 1973), and the C_K-region allotypes determined by the RI-1 locus (a and b serotypes) of inbred rats (Gutman *et al.*, 1975).

It is easy to account for the evolution of simple allotypes by the conventional genetic mechanisms of point mutation and selection. It is much more difficult to explain the extensive divergence of multiple differences at a single locus. Gally and Edelman (1970) have suggested local inversions to account for the divergence of the rabbit group a allotypes, and Gutman *et al.*, (1975) have discussed other possible mechanisms.

However, as in the case of the I_B-peptide marker in mouse V_L regions, polymorphism at structural genetic loci is not the only way to explain the heritable differences in phenotype that we call allotypes. It is possible that members of a species which express only one or the other allotype actually possess structural genes for all allotypic variants, but contain different codominant alleles at a locus which *regulates* the expression of these structural genes. In such a situation, the genetic locus exhibiting simple Mendelian segregation would be a *regulatory locus*, and mapping of such a locus may say nothing about the location of the structural genes coding for the protein in question.

If allotypy is due to polymorphism in allelic structural genes, an individual can have no more than two allotypic forms of a given immunoglobulin V or C region. However, if allotypy results from polymorphism at a regulatory locus, and, further, if that regulatory control is "leaky," an individual might under certain circumstances express more than two allotypes. That the latter explanation may be correct is suggested by several instances in which animals shown to be homozygous or heterozygous at a particular locus by conventional allotypic testing either express constitutively or can be stimulated to express allotype(s) which they were thought not to contain. Strosberg et $al.$ (1974) detected separate Ig molecules containing Aa^2 and Ab^6 specificities in the serum of a rabbit of "nominal allotype" Aa^1/Aa^2 Ab^4/Ab^5 which was producing antibodies of restricted heterogeneity to $Micrococcus$ $lysodeikticus.$ Mudgett et $al.$ (1975) introduced the term "nominal allotype" to designate those experimental typings of animals by qualitative tests and breeding data and "latent allotype" to refer to allotypes present in such animals but detectable only by sensitive assays. Using sensitive radioimmunoassays, these workers detected small quantities of latent group a allotypes (less than 1% of the nominal allotype) in the serum of about 50% of rabbits thought to be homozygous for allotype. In other experiments, Bosma and Bosma (1974) have reported transient appearance of the BALB/c IgG_{2a} allotype in the serum of ICR CB-17 inbred mice thought to be congenic with BALB/c but containing the Ig-1 allogroup of the C57BL/Ka inbred strain. Pothier et $al.$ (1974) detected, during the passage of a human lymphoid tumor line in newborn Syrian hamsters, intermittent expression of a Gm allotype not present in the donor phenotype. Also, Rivat et $al.$ (1973) detected in the supernatants of human mixed leukocyte cultures allotypes not present in the donor serum.

Observations of the apparent nonallelic behavior of allotypes are consistent with the possibility that, within a species, a haploid set of chromosomes may contain structural genes for several or all of the immunoglobulin allotypes characteristic of that species. The expression of nominal allotypes might be governed by allelic regulatory genes, and experimental or other perturbations might cause sporadic appearance of what might be interpreted as latent allotypes. It must be remembered that whenever antisera are used to characterize complex antigens (in this case, allotypes) the possibility of $cross-reactions$ must be considered. It is therefore possible that the allotypes are indeed specified by alleles at a genetic locus, but that, at least in the case of the V regions, the generation of sequence diversity by somatic means or expression of a small number of diverging germline V genes might produce varying quantities of Ig molecules which cross-react with the antiallotype reagent. For this reason, the amino acid sequences of purified proteins identified as possessing latent allotypes must be compared with material from an animal of that nominal allotype.

In the case of latent C-region allotypes, the above explanation cannot apply, since there is no a $priori$ reason to suspect that C-region sequences do not result from the faithful transcription and translation of germ-line genes. However, the serological findings must nonetheless be verified by the purification of proteins bearing the latent allotype and by subsequent primary structural analysis.

A number of cases are known in which the same individuals of a species express two or three forms of a particular C region presumably coded by separate C genes. Three structural genes for the human C_λ region have been postulated on the basis of the Kern and Mcg sequence markers and the Oz serological markers (Solomon, 1976). In this case, all three sequences are expressed in an apparently equal fashion in each individual and expression is therefore apparently not under alternative regulatory control. Landucci-Tosi *et al.* (1973) have reported serological evidence which suggests that individual hares express the Ab^4, Ab^5, and Ab^6 C_K-region antigenic specificities which show allotypic behavior in the rabbit. One possible interpretation is that hares and rabbits both have at least three different C_κ genes, but that expression of these is equal and unregulated in the hare (similar to the three human C_λ genes) and under strict alternative regulatory control in the rabbit (Strosberg, 1974).

It is well known that rabbits are able to synthesize V_H-region sequences which do not bear antigenic determinants characteristic of their nominal allotypes. Dray and Nisonoff (1963) and Stemke (1965) determined that 10-30% of IgG molecules from individual rabbits did not react with antisera specific for group a allotypes. Moreover, this group a negative population of IgG was greatly enriched in the serum of rabbits subjected to homozygous allotype suppression by zygote transfer (David and Todd, 1969; Vice *et al.*, 1970). Rabbits bearing each of the three nominal group a allotypes constitutively synthesize a-negative H chains (Tack *et al.*, 1973). Moreover, there exists serological evidence that among the a-negative molecules there are two or more allotypic V_H groups (group x and group y) distinct from those bearing group a allotypes and genetically linked to the V_Ha locus (Dray *et al.*, 1974). The structural correlates of group x and group y allotypes on group a negative heavy chains are not known. There is considerable evidence, however, which suggests that the Fc_γ region of a-negative chains is indistinguishable from that of a-positive chains (Kindt, 1975). This speaks strongly against the notion that a-negative molecules may constitute different subclasses of rabbit IgG. On the other hand, a-negative H chains are known to contain structural differences from a-positive chains in their amino terminal region (Prahl *et al.*, 1973).

Large amounts of a homogeneous a-negative IgG molecules specific for streptococcal carbohydrate were produced by a rabbit in response to immunization with this antigen (Kindt *et al.*, 1970). The amino terminal sequence of the group a negative H chain is pGlu-Glu-Gln (Waterfield *et al.*, 1972), whereas a-positive H chains begin with pGlu-Ser-Val or pGlu-Ser-Leu (Jaton and Braun, 1972; Fleischman, 1971; Mole *et al.*, 1971; Porter, 1974; Kindt, 1975). The a-negative sequence had been observed earlier in H-chain pools by Wilkinson (1969a,b). This and the amino acid composition data of Prahl *et al.* (1973) suggest that significant differences exist among V_H regions bearing group a allotypes and those with group x and y allotypes.

XII. CAN I_B-NEGATIVE STRAINS PRODUCE I_B-POSITIVE L CHAINS?

It is therefore clear that the V_H-region sequences which are expressed by rabbits are not limited to those bearing the group a allotypes. If the latent allotypes detected serologically are confirmed to be such by structural studies, then they may indicate quantitative differences in gene expression which are governed by regulatory loci. Such regulatory control of group b allotypes may have a selective advantage in the rabbit but not in the hare (Gutman *et al.*, 1975). The expression of the I_B-peptide marker in mouse L-chain V regions may be under similar regulatory control. Just as the definitive demonstration of the latent allotype might be taken as evidence against allelism at a structural genetic locus, so the expression of I_B-positive L chains by nominally I_B-negative strains would suggest that regulatory control might be operative in this system as well. We are therefore exploring experimental systems in which breakdown of such control might be detected:

1. We are screening BALB/c myeloma L chains for the presence of the I_B-peptide marker. Even if I_B-positive B cells exist but are unable to be stimulated under normal circumstances due to regulatory control, they may nonetheless undergo neoplastic transformation.

2. We are immunizing BALB/cJ and other I_B-negative strains of mice with various antigens in an effort to stimulate clonal expansion of I_B-positive clones and to obtain expression of the I_B-peptide marker.

3. Green and Schultz (1975) have reported that homozygous motheaten (*me/me*) mice are immunologically impaired, and they have presented serological evidence that the serum immunoglobulins of these mutant mice contain λ_2 light chains (Schultz and Green, 1976). The only known example of such an L chain, distinguishable by both its V anc C regions, is the L chain of the murine DNP-binding IgA molecule MOPC-315 described by Dugan *et al.* (1973). It is possible that abnormal regulation of immunoglobulin gene expression in these mutant mice allows expression of Ig genes normally silent or only minimally expressed (like the latent rabbit group a allotypes discussed by Mudgett *et al.*, 1975). Thus even though the C57BL/6J background strain is I_B negative, we are attempting to obtain sufficient quantities of C57BL/6J-*me/me* serum to test for expression of the I_B-peptide marker.

XIII. INDUCTION OF I_B-POSITIVE MYELOMA

If I_B-negative strains lack structural genes capable of giving rise to I_B-positive L chains, I_B-positive strains would be the only ones from which an IgG population enriched in I_B-positive L chains could be obtained. Screening of myeloma proteins from the I_B-negative BALB/c strain would be to no avail.

We have therefore begun to place upon the BALB/c genetic background the locus governing expression of the I_B-peptide marker. The strains AKR/J and C58/J are serving as donors in the derivation of two such BALB/c-I_B-positive strains. Instead of testing each backcross generation for the I_B-peptide marker, we are typing for the closely linked Ly-3^a allele by cytotoxic assay of thymocytes obtained by thymic biopsy since this assay is considerably more convenient than peptide mapping. When suitable inbred strains have been established, we shall induce plasmacytomas and screen by peptide mapping for homogeneous immunoglobulins containing I_B-positive L chains. These should provide ample material for detailed primary structural analysis of L chains bearing this genetic marker, and for use in immunizations to produce antisera specific for I_B-positive immunoglobulins. Such antisera should considerably facilitate genetic experiments to map the locus governing expression of the I_B-peptide marker with respect to the Ly-3 and other loci in linkage group XI. In addition, such reagents would allow examination of lymphoid cells from I_B-positive animals to determine the frequency, distribution, and class of cells which express this genetic marker.

XIV. CHANGING VIEWS OF GENETIC MARKERS: ISOTYPES, ALLOTYPES, IDIOTYPES

It is interesting to note the changes in our view of immunoglobulin genetic markers which have been developing over the past several years. The different subclasses of Ig's distinguished by their C_H regions have been considered to be *isotypes*, determined by different (although closely linked) genetic loci. Each such locus appears to have alternative alleles, and these were considered to determine *allotypes* of C regions. Rabbits had been shown to have what appeared to be allotypes in their V_H regions (group a) and their C_κ regions (group b) (Mage *et al.*, 1973). Since alternative forms of these so-called allotypes differed from each other by multiple amino acid substitutions, they were viewed as more complex than simple allotypes, but were nonetheless considered as the products of alternative alleles at a single, albeit complex, locus. The finding that small amounts of latent allotypes were detectable in rabbits nominally lacking in these allotypes raised the possibility that all rabbits might contain structural genes for all alternative forms, but that alleles at regulatory loci might determine which of these loci would be expressed. Thus the alternative forms may be encoded by different genetic loci, and would really be *more like isotypes than allotypes*.

The observations that certain strains synthesize immunoglobulins with characteristic *idiotypes* suggested that the different strains might differ considerably in their germ-line genes determining, either directly or after somatic alteration, immunoglobulin V genes. Evidence has recently been obtained which suggests that T cells may have on their surface molecules which bear these characteristic idiotypes and which are likely to function in antigen recognition (Binz and Wigzell, 1975; Eichmann and Rajewsky, 1975).

In several cases, genetic linkage has been established between the locus for the H-chain C region (IgC_H) and the expression of Ig's bearing certain idiotypes (Blomberg et al., 1972; Lieberman et al., 1974; Pawlak et al., 1973; Eichmann, 1973). The segregation of apparent recombinants from crosses between inbred strains known to express different patterns of idiotypes and at least one case of apparent recombination within the V_H gene complex during construction of a congenic strain are allowing construction of a genetic map of the mouse V_H-gene complex (Weigert et al., 1975). It is worth noting that while the apparent recombination events being detected in these linkage studies may well be occurring within a complex of V_H structural genes, this complex may also contain regulatory genes which determine which V_H genes are to be expressed. It is therefore possible that inbred strains which differ in various idiotypes might contain identical sets of V_H genes but differ at regulatory loci linked to IgC_H. Heritable idiotypes may be similar to the rabbit group a allotypes in that both may be isotypes whose expression is under strict regulatory control. This is consistent with the suggestion of Weigert et al. (1975) that since the T15 idiotype is distinct from the site-specific idiotype of anti-PC antibodies (Claflin and Davie, 1975), its presence in preimmune serum may reflect the genetically determined expression of a V_H subgroup analogous to the rabbit V_H-region allotype (or isotype). Similarly, the I_B-peptide marker in mouse V_L regions may be a V-region isotype which is under strict regulatory control.

It is apparent from the above discussion that it is important to distinguish the contributions of structural and regulatory genes to the observed phenotypes. Our hope is that structural and functional studies of I_B-positive immunoglobulins and the Ly-2 and Ly-3 antigens, combined with studies of the genetic loci governing these markers in linkage group XI of the mouse, will help to distinguish between the roles of structural and regulatory loci in immune phenomena.

XV. APPENDIX: FRACTIONATION OF Fab FRAGMENTS INTO Fd FRAGMENTS AND L CHAINS

Separation of L chains from Fd fragments was achieved by ion exchange chromatography of partially reduced and alkylated Fab on a column (1 by 20 cm) of SP-Sephadex C25 in 8 M urea using a salt gradient from 10^{-4} M KCl, pH 3.0, to 0.25 M KCl, pH 3.0. Similar procedures were employed by Škavřil *et al.* (1967) for the separation of human κ and λ light chains and by W. Geckeler (personal communication) for mouse κ- and λ-chains. Alkylation was performed with [¹⁴C] iodoacetic acid, and effluent fractions were monitored by scintilla-

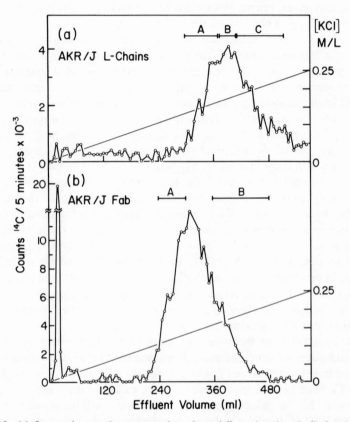

Figure 10. (a) Ion exchange chromatography of partially reduced and alkylated AKR/J L chains on SP-Sephadex C25. Approximately 3 mg of partially reduced and [¹⁴C] iodo-acetic acid-alkylated AKR/J L chains dissolved in 8 M urea, 10^{-4} M KCl, pH 3.0, was applied to a column (1.1 by 15 cm) of SP-Sephadex C25 (Pharmacia Inc., Piscataway, N.J.) which had been equilibrated with the same solvent. After washing with the same solvent (100 ml), the bound protein was eluted with a linear gradient of 8 M urea, 10^{-4} M KCl, pH 3.0 (300 ml), to 8 M urea, 0.25 M KCl, pH 3.0 (300 ml). Fractions of 55 drops were collected, and aliquots of 50 μl each were counted for ¹⁴C in a liquid scintillation counter. (b) Ion exchange chromatography of partially reduced and alkylated AKR/J Fab on SP-Sephadex. Approximately 2.5 mg of a fraction of AKR/J Fab obtained from starch zone electrophoresis was partially reduced and alkylated with [¹⁴C] iodoacetic acid, and was subjected to ion exchange chromatography under conditions identical to those described for AKR/J L chains (a).

tion counting. Amounts of Fab loaded per column ranged from 2.5 to 10 mg. Yields as determined by ^{14}C recovery were quantitative. Representative column profiles of purified light chains and of Fab are presented in Fig. 10. It is apparent that purified light chains are eluted late in the gradient, while the elution profile of partially reduced and alkylated Fab begins in the earlier portion of the gradient and extends through the light-chain region.

Fractions from SP-Sephadex were pooled as indicated in Fig. 10, and after complete reduction and alkylation with [^{14}C] iodoacetic acid and digestion with trypsin, peptide maps were prepared in the usual way. Representative autoradiograms of peptide maps are presented in Fig. 11. It is apparent that the fractions which are eluted late from the column are rich in light chains, while peptide maps of fractions eluted early are quite different from those of mouse light chains. The probable Fd identity of these early fractions is suggested by comparison of their peptide maps with that of AKR/J γ_{2a}-chains obtained from IgG$_{2a}$ purified by affinity chromatography on anti-IgG$_{2a}$/Sepharose (Fig. 11c). Evidence to be published elsewhere (P. D. Gottlieb and S. Epstein, manuscript

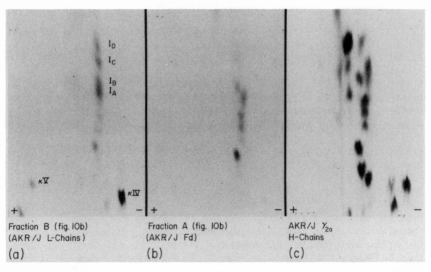

Figure 11. Peptide maps of L chains and Fd fragments obtained from partially reduced and alkylated Fab by ion exchange chromatography on SP-Sephadex C25 (Fig. 10). Fractions A and B (Fig. 10) were fully reduced and alkylated with [^{14}C] iodoacetic acid and digested with trypsin, and peptide maps were prepared. The anode (+) is at the left of each map and descending chromatography was from bottom to top. (a) Map of fraction B (Fig. 10); Cys V of the L chains is less intense than Cys IV due to the use of [^{14}C] iodoacetic acid of lower specific activity for alkylation of the partially reduced Fab before ion exchange chromatography. (b) Map of fraction A; the Fd identity of this fraction is suggested by comparison with the peptide map of AKR/J γ_{2a} H chains shown in (c).

in preparation) demonstrates conclusively that the early fractions contain pure Fd fragments. Intermediate fractions contain mixtures of light chains and Fd framents, and these can possibly be resolved further by the use of a more shallow gradient of KCl. It appears, however, that some Fd fragments may still elute late in the gradient and it may not be possible to separate them from κ-chains by this procedure.

ACKNOWLEDGMENTS

This work was supported in part by a U.S. Public Health Service Research grant (CA 15808) from the National Cancer Institute to Paul D. Gottlieb and by a U.S. Public Health Service Research grant (CA 14051) from the National Cancer Institute to the Massachusetts Institute of Technology Center for Cancer Research.

XVI. REFERENCES

Baltimore, D., 1974, *Nature (London)* **248**:409.
Barstad, P., Rudikoff, S., Potter, M., Cohn, M., Konigsberg, W., and Hood, L., 1974, *Science* **183**:962.
Blinz, H., and Wigzell, H., 1975, *J. Exp. Med.* **142**:197.
Blomberg, B., Geckeler, W., and Weigert, M., 1972, *Science* **177**:178.
Bosma, M., and Bosma, G., 1974, *J. Exp. Med.* **139**:512.
Boyse, E.A., Miyazawa, M., Aoki, T., and Old, L.J., 1968a, *Proc. Roy. Soc. London Ser. B* **170**:175.
Boyse, E.A., Old, L.J., and Stockert, E., 1968b, *Proc. Natl. Acad. Sci. USA* **60**:886.
Boyse, E.A., Itakura, K., Stockert, E., Iritani, C.A., and Miura, M., 1971, *Transplantation* **11**:351.
Brenner, S., and Milstein, C., 1969, *Nature (London)* **211**:242.
Cantor, H., and Boyse, E.A., 1975a, *J. Exp. Med.* **141**:1376.
Cantor, H., and Boyse, E.A., 1975b, *J. Exp. Med.* **141**:1390.
Cantor, H., and Simpson, E., 1975, *Eur. J. Immunol.* **5**:330.
Claflin, J.L., and Davie, J.M., 1975, *J. Immunol.* **114**:70.
Cohn, M., Blomberg, B., Geckeler, W., Raschke, W., Riblet, R., and Weigert, M., 1974, in: *The Immune System, Genes, Receptors, Signals* (E.E. Sercarz, A.R. Williamson, and C.F. Fox, eds.), p. 89, Academic Press, New York.
Cunningham, B.A., Gottlieb, P.D., Pflumm, M.N., and Edelman, G.M., 1971, in: *Progress in Immunology* (B. Amos, ed.), pp. 3–24, Academic Press, New York.
David, G.S., and Todd, C.W., 1969, *Proc. Natl. Acad. Sci. USA* **62**:860.
Dray, S., and Nisonoff, A., 1963, *Proc. Soc. Exp. Biol. Med.* **113**:20.
Dray, S., Kim, B.S., and Gilman-Sachs, A., 1974, *Ann. Immunol.* **125**:41.
Dreyer, W., Gray, W.R., and Hood, L., 1967, *Cold Spring Harbor Symp. Quant. Biol.* **32**:353.
Dugan, E.S., Bradshaw, R.A., Simms, E.S., and Eisen, H.N., 1973, *Biochemistry* **12**:5400.

Durda, P.J., and Gottlieb, P.D., 1976, *J. Exp. Med.* **144**:476.

Edelman, G.M., and Gottlieb, P.D., 1970, *Proc. Natl. Acad. Sci. USA* **67**:1192.

Eichmann, K., 1973, *J. Exp. Med.* **137**:603.

Eichmann, K., and Rajewsky, K., 1975, *Eur. J. Immunol.* **5**:661.

Fahey, J.L., Carbone, P.O., Rowe, D.S., and Bachmann, R., 1968, *Am. J. Med.* **45**:373.

Fleischman, J.B., 1971, *Biochemistry* **10**:2753.

Gally, J.A., 1973, in: *The Antigens*, Vol. I (M. Sela, ed.), p. 161, Academic Press, New York.

Gally, J.A., and Edelman, G.M., 1970, *Nature (London)* **227**:341.

Gally, J.A., and Edelman, G.M., 1972, *Annu. Rev. Genet.* **6**:1.

Gasser, D.L., 1969, *J. Immunol.* **103**:66.

Gottlieb, P.D., 1971, Ph.D. thesis, Rockefeller University.

Gottlieb, P.D., 1974, *J. Exp. Med.* **140**:1432.

Green, M.C., and Schultz, L., 1975, *J. Hered.* **66**:250.

Gutman, G.A., Loh, E., and Hood, L., 1975, *Proc. Natl. Acad. Sci. USA* **72**:5046.

Itakura, K., Hutton, J.J., Boyse, E.A., and Old, L.J., 1971, *Nature (London) New Biol.* **230**:126.

Itakura, K., Hutton, J.J., Boyse, E.A., and Old, L.J., 1972, *Transplantation* **13**:239.

Jaton, J.C., and Braun, D.E., 1972, *Biochem. J.* **130**:539.

Kindt, T.J., 1975, in: *Advances in Immunology*, Vol. 21 (F.J. Dixon, and H.G. Kunkel, eds.), p. 35, Academic Press, New York.

Kindt, T.J., Todd, C.W., Eichmann, K., and Krause, R.M., 1970, *J. Exp. Med.* **131**:343.

Kisielow, P., Hirst, J.A., Beverley, P.C.L., Hoffman, M.K., Boyse, E.A., and Oettgen, H.F., 1975, *Nature (London)* **253**:219.

Klein, J., 1973, *Transplantation (Baltimore)* **15**:137.

Klein, J., 1975, *Biology of the Mouse Histocompatibility-2 Complex*, Springer-Verlag, New York.

Komuro, K., Itakura, K., Boyse, E.A., and John, M., 1975, *Immunogenetics* **1**:452.

Landucci-Tosi, S., Tosi, R., and Perramon, A., 1973, *J. Immunol.* **110**:286.

Leder, P., Honjo, T., Swan, D., Packman, S., Nau, M., and Norman, B., 1975, in: *Molecular Approaches to Immunology*, Vol. 9 (E.E. Smith and D.W. Robbins, eds.), pp. 173–188, Miami Winter Symposia, Academic Press, New York.

Lieberman, R., Potter, M., Mushinski, E.B., Humphrey, W., and Rudikoff, S., 1974, *J. Exp. Med.* **139**:983.

Mage, R., Lieberman, R., Potter, M., and Terry, W.D., 1973, in: *The Antigens*, Vol. I (M. Sela, ed.), p. 299, Academic Press, New York.

Mole, L.E., Jackson, S.A., Porter, R.R., and Wilkinson, J.M., 1971, *Biochem. J.* **124**:301.

Mudgett, M., Fraser, B.A., and Kindt, T.J., 1975, *J. Exp. Med.* **141**:1448.

Pawlak, L.L., Mushinski, E.B., Nisonoff, A., and Potter, M., 1973, *J. Exp. Med.* **137**:22.

Porter, R.R., 1974, *Ann. Immunol (Inst. Pasteur)* **125C**:85.

Pothier, L., Borel, H., and Adams, R.A., 1974, *J. Immunol.* **113**:1984.

Potter, M., and Lieberman, R., 1970, *J. Exp. Med.* **132**:737.

Prahl, J.W., Tack, B.F., and Todd, C.W., 1973, *Biochemistry* **12**:5181.

Rivat, L., Gilbert, D., and Ropartz, C., 1973, *Immunology* **24**:1041.

Schultz, L.D., and Green, M.C., 1976, *J. Immunol.* **116**:936.

Shen, F.-W., Boyse, E.A., and Cantor, H., 1975, *Immunogenetics* **2**:591.

Shiku, H., Kisielow, P., Bean, M.A., Takahashi, T., Boyse, E.A., Oettgen, H.F., and Old, L.J., 1975, *J. Exp. Med.* **141**:227.

Shirai, T., and Mellors, R.C., 1971, *Proc. Natl. Acad. Sci. USA* **68**:1412.

Shreffler, D.C., and David, C.S., 1975, *Adv. Immunol.* **20**:125.

Simpson, E. and Cantor, H., 1975, *Eur. J. Immunol.* **5**:337.

Škavřil, F., Brummelová, V. and Franěk, F., 1967, *Biochim. Biophys. Acta* **140**:371.

Smithies, O., 1967, *Science* **157**:267.

Smithies, O., 1970, *Science* **169**:882.

Solomon, A., 1976, *N. Engl. J. Med.* **294**:17.

Spring, S.B., and Nisonoff, A., 1974, *J. Immunol.* **113**:470.

Staats, J., 1972, *Cancer Res.* **32**:1609.

Stemke, G.W., 1965, *Immunochemistry* **25**:359.

Strosberg, A.D., Hamers-Casterman, C., Van der Loo, W., and Hamers, R., 1974, *J. Immunol.* **113**:1313.

Tack, B.F., Feintuch, K., Todd, C.W., and Prahl, J.W., 1973, *Biochemistry* **12**:5172.

Takasugi, M., and Hildemann, W.H., 1969, *J. Natl. Cancer Inst.* **43**:843.

Tonegawa, S., 1976, *Proc. Natl. Acad. Sci. USA* **73**:203.

Vice, J.L., Gilman-Sachs, A., Hunt, W.L., and Dray, S., 1970, *J. Immunol.* **104**:550.

Waterfield, M.D., Prahl, J.W., Hood, L.E., Kindt, T.J., and Krause, R.M., 1972, *Nature (London) New Biol.* **240**:215.

Weigert, M., Cesari, I.M., Yonkovich, S.J., and Cohn, M., 1970, *Nature (London)* **228**:1045.

Weigert, M., Potter, M., and Sachs, D., 1975, *Immunogenetics* **1**:511.

Wilkinson, J.M., 1969a, *Biochem. J.* **112**:173.

Wilkinson, J.M., 1969b, *Nature (London)* **223**:616.

Williams, C.A., and Chase, M.W., eds., 1967, in: *Methods in Immunology and Immunochemistry*, Vol. I, Academic Press, New York.

Wu, T.T., and Kabat, E.A., 1970, *J. Exp. Med.* **132**:211.

Multivalent Binding and Functional Affinity

Fred Karush

Department of Microbiology
School of Medicine
University of Pennsylvania
Philadelphia, Pennsylvania

I. INTRODUCTION

The evolutionary development of the architecture of the antibody molecule has provided in its contemporary form a distinctive structure superbly suited for multivalent interaction. In addition to multivalence, the general occurrence of multiple and identical antigenic determinants on the surfaces of infectious agents and neoplastic cells has led to the emergence of two further structural features. These, indeed, are required for the effective utilization of the multivalence of antibody. They comprise the property of intramolecular structural symmetry, i.e., identical subunits, resulting in the identity of the antigen-binding sites of the antibody, and the segmental flexibility of the Fab portions of the molecule. The conjunctive effect of these properties is the capacity of the antibody molecule to adjust the separation and relative orientation of its binding sites to the generally fixed distances between the identical complementary groups of the complex ligand. The biological utility of the resulting multivalent interaction is undoubtedly linked to the enhanced affinity which is associated with multivalent binding.

The concept of the enhancement of intrinsic affinity by virtue of multiple attachment has become widely recognized among immunologists only within the past decade, although its possible significance was pointed out as early as 1937 (Burnet *et al.*, 1937) and the bivalence of 7 S antibody clearly demonstrated in 1949 (Eisen and Karush, 1949). The quantitative description of the enhancement is usefully specified as a factor which represents the multiple by which the intrinsic affinity, expressed as an association constant, is increased by virtue of multivalent interaction. Operationally, the enhancement factor is evaluated by the ratio of affinities for the interaction of a particular antibody population with a monovalent ligand and a multivalent one. The ligands should, of course, possess as nearly identical reactive groups as is chemically feasible. The occasional reference in the immunological literature to the notion that multivalent interaction involves nonspecific factors, in implied contrast to monovalent binding, is misleading, since, obviously, both interactions are dependent on such factors as temperature, pH, and ionic strength.

The term "avidity" is widely used in connection with multivalent interaction instead of the conventional and thermodynamically defined quantity "affinity." The compulsion for this substitution is apparently the desire to emphasize the significance of multivalent interaction for the stabilization of antigen-antibody complexes involved in biological systems. However, "avidity" has rarely been defined precisely and in thermodynamic terms, although the reversibility of the formation of multivalently linked complexes provides an adequate basis for a precise thermodynamic characterization. Rather, over the years, the meanings assigned to "avidity" have been varied, often obscure, and frequently unrelated to experimental operations. It appears to me that the conceptual clarity of immunological analysis would benefit greatly from the abandonment of this term.

As an alternative concept I shall employ the term "functional affinity" (Karush, 1970) to characterize those systems involving multivalent linkages. The use of this term implies, of course, a distinction as well as a similarity between "intrinsic affinity" and "functional affinity." Both terms refer to formally identical reversible processes as follows:

$$F_1 + L_1 \rightleftharpoons 1:1 \text{ complex (monovalent)}$$

$$Ab_n + L_m \rightleftharpoons 1:1 \text{ complex (multivalent)}$$

where F_1 is a monovalent antibody fragment, L_1 a monovalent ligand, Ab_n a multivalent antibody, and L_m a multivalent ligand with m identical groups. In each instance, two kinetic units combine reversibly to form one unit and each process can, in principle, be characterized by an association constant. Since the association constant is a measure of the thermodynamic affinity, both processes can therefore be assigned quantitative values of the affinity.

The utility of the distinction between "intrinsic affinity" and "functional affinity" arises from the different emphasis involved in each term. The former is most useful when the structural relationship between the antibody combining site and the complementary region of the ligand is under scrutiny or when kinetic mechanisms of the specific interaction are under investigation. On the other hand, the latter is particularly significant when the quantitative measurement of the enhancement of affinity is being examined or when this enhancement is relevant to a biological process, such as viral neutralization and cell stimulation.

The quantitative evaluation of the enhancement factor has been possible for only a few systems. The main difficulties in the determination are the selection of a system in which multivalent binding does not proceed beyond the formation of the 1:1 complex and the measurement of association constants in excess of 10^9 M^{-1}. A further restriction has emerged since 1972 from the recognition that the distance of closest approach between the binding sites of a 7 S antibody is about 9 nm (Werner et al., 1972). This geometrical limitation requires, therefore, that on multivalent ligands one or more pairs of reactive groups exist with a separation between members of the pair that falls within 9 nm to approximately 20 nm. The failure of several bivalent lactose-containing ligands to exhibit enhanced binding with 7 S anti-lactose antibody (Gopalakrishnan and Karush, 1974a) has demonstrated the significance of this requirement.

II. STUDIES WITH BIVALENT ANTIBODY

Several studies have been concerned with the functional affinity of the interaction of bivalent antibody with multivalent ligand. The earliest of these which provided an estimate of the enhancement factor was described by Greenbury et al. (1965) in a study of the interaction of bivalent (7 S and 5 S) rabbit antibody and monovalent (5 S and 3.5 S) antibody specific for blood group A with human A_1 cells. Although association constants of these interactions were not obtained, the relative values of K_0 were estimated from the difference in the quantity of red cells required to bind 50% of the labeled antibody. On this basis, it was estimated that the enhancement factor for this system ranged between 150 and 450.

Another experimental approach for the analysis of multivalent interaction is based on viral neutralization. This method provides the advantage that the multivalent ligand, i.e., the virus, can be used at extremely low concentrations (10^{-17} M) and the extent of neutralization of the virus quantitatively assessed. It carries the additional simplification that the concentration of uncombined antibody remains perceptibly unchanged in the course of the reaction. The earliest studies of viral neutralization with antiviral antibody revealed a substantial loss of neutralizing capacity when bivalent antibody was converted to monovalent fragments (Klinman et al., 1967). However, it was not possible to determine association constants for the formation of the neutralized complexes. Subsequently, the utility of viral neutralization for the quantitative evaluation of the multivalent interaction of antihapten antibody with hapten conjugated to bacteriophage emerged from the demonstration that hapten-conjugated bacteriophage was subject to neutralization by antihapten antibody (Haimovich and Sela, 1966; Mäkelä, 1966). This method has been the most fruitful one to date in providing a quantitative measure of the enhancement factor.

The first application of this method for the measurement of functional affinity and for the evaluation of the enhancement factor in bivalent interaction ("monogamous bivalency") was made with rabbit anti-DNP IgG antibody and DNP-conjugated ϕX174 (Hornick and Karush, 1969). In this system, it was possible to determine the association constant both by equilibrium measurements and by the evaluation of the rate constants for neutralization and reactivation. The measurement of the reactivation kinetics was feasible because the antibody which dissociated from the bacteriophage was rendered inactive by the presence of a relatively high concentration of DNP-lysine. The equilibrium value of 3.5×10^{11} M^{-1} ($37°C$) was in excellent agreement with the calculated value of 1.1×10^{11} M^{-1} ($37°C$) from the rate constants (3.7×10^7 $M^{-1} \cdot s^{-1}/ 3.4 \times 10^{-4}$ s^{-1}). The association constant for the binding of DNP-lysine was measured by equilibrium dialysis at $37°C$ to yield a K_0 of 6×10^6 M^{-1}. The enhancement factor for this system was thus found to lie between 2×10^4 and 6×10^4. The decisive element responsible for this striking value is, as would be expected for bivalent binding, the decreased rate of dissociation compared to monovalent binding. The value of 3.7×10^7 $M^{-1} \cdot s^{-1}$ for the rate of association is comparable to that found with monovalent ligands but the dissociation rate constant is several orders of magnitude lower (Froese and Sehon, 1965).

In a later study with anti-DNP antibody, the interaction with rabbit 7 S antibody was compared with that of bivalent 5 S antibody and monovalent 7 S and 3.5 S antibodies at $25°C$ (Hornick and Karush, 1972). The purified preparation of rabbit anti-DNP IgG in this case gave an enhancement factor of about 10^3 with a K_0 for the intrinsic affinity of approximately 1×10^7 M^{-1}. The 5 S fragment prepared by peptic digestion of the 7 S antibody gave the same values for functional and intrinsic affinity as the parent preparation. On the other hand, the monovalent 3.5 S fragment and the monovalent hybrid 7 S sample exhibited a greatly reduced K_0 for the neutralization reaction as anticipated. However, in both instances, there was a tenfold disparity between the K_0 measured by equilibrium dialysis and that determined by bacteriophage neutralization. For the 7 S monovalent antibody, the values were 3.3×10^7 M^{-1} and 3.3×10^8 M^{-1}, respectively. Since the antibody concentration was manyfold higher than the bacteriophage concentration (10^{-9} M vs. 10^{-17} M), it is quite likely that the apparent discrepancy was due to a secondary equilibrium involving the preferential binding of high-affinity molecules. The generally heterogeneous nature of the anti-DNP response would provide the basis for such selective interaction. A similar reequilibration reaction appears to have been involved in the study by Blank et al. (1972) of the neutralization of DNP-T_4 bacteriophage with anti-DNP antibody. Although this system did not permit quantitative measurement of functional affinity and therefore of the enhancement factor, the wide variation in the apparent neutralization rate constants was in accord with a decisive role for multivalent interaction.

The uncertainty of interpretation arising from the heterogeneous nature of the anti-DNP populations was avoided in a later study with anti-lactoside antibody (Gopalakrishnan and Karush, 1974b). In addition, the latter system served to confirm the energetic importance of multivalent interaction for antibodies in general. In this study, multiple lactoside groups were conjugated to ϕX174 to render the bacteriophage susceptible to neutralization with antilactoside antibody. Purified antibody was obtained from a rabbit immunized with a vaccine prepared by conjugating the R36A strain of pneumococcus with p-aminophenyl-β-lactoside. The antibody was fractionated by preparative isoelectric focusing to yield one and, possibly, a second functionally homogeneous population. Binding measurements with a monovalent ligand, N-acetyl-p-aminophenyl-β-lactoside, were made at 25°C by equilibrium dialysis. The neutralization reaction was studied at 25°C with an antibody concentration varying between 2.5×10^{-10} M and 5×10^{-10} M. The values for the intrinsic and functional association constants are shown in Table I together with the second-order rate constants for the neutralization reaction. The value of the intrinsic association constant (2×10^5 M^{-1}) is at least thirtyfold smaller than the K_0's for the anti-DNP antibody preparations used in the earlier neutralization studies. Since the K_0's for the functional affinity exceed 2×10^9 M^{-1}, it can be concluded that the enhancement factor for this system is of the order of 10^4. In the light of the similar, but not identical, results from the anti-DNP studies, a reasonable generalization for the enhancement due to bivalent interaction is a factor of the order of magnitude of 10^4.

Table I. Equilibrium and Rate Constants for Neutralization Reaction and Ligand Binding at 25°C with Anti-PAPL Antibody[a]

Preparation	Antibody concentration in neutralization mixture (M)	Rate constant for neutralization, k_t ($M^{-1} \cdot s^{-1}$)	Association constant for neutralization (M^{-1})	Association constant for ligand binding[b] (M^{-1})
IgG antibody	4.3×10^{-10}	7.1×10^5	8.7×10^9	2.4×10^5
Fraction I	5.0×10^{-10}	9.4×10^5	6.7×10^9	2.4×10^5
Fraction I	2.5×10^{-10}	4.3×10^5	2.3×10^9	2.4×10^5
Fraction II	4.0×10^{-10}	1.26×10^6	1.22×10^{10}	1.6×10^5

[a] Adapted from Gopalakrishnan and Karush (1974b) with permission.
[b] The ligand was N-acetyl-p-aminophenyl-β-lactoside (N-acetyl-PAPL).

III. STUDIES WITH IgM ANTIBODY

It is a common observation that IgM antibody is more effective on a molar basis than IgG antibody in such assays as neutralization (Finkelstein and Uhr, 1966) and hemagglutination (Onoue *et al.*, 1965), a difference which is attributed to the higher valence of the IgM antibody. The quantitative measurement of the functional affinity of IgM antibody and the determination of the enhancement factor have been apparently reported only in the study of anti-DNP IgM antibody by Hornick and Karush (1972). In an earlier investigation, Onoue *et al.* (1965) compared rabbit IgM and IgG anti-*p*-azobenzene arsonate antibody. It was observed that, although the intrinsic affinities of these classes of antibody were approximately the same, the IgM antibody was more effective on a molar basis in hemolytic and hemagglutinating reactions than the IgG antibody by a factor of 60–180. This difference was attributed to the greater opportunity for multivalent attachment and enhanced affinity.

In the study of IgM anti-DNP antibody (Hornick and Karush, 1972), both the intrinsic and functional association constants were measured. The latter were obtained by equilibrium measurements of the extent of neutralization of DNP-ϕX174 at known concentrations of purified antibody. Four antibody preparations from three species were evaluated and the relevant results are summarized in Table II. The intrinsic association constants for the binding of DNP-lysine were relatively low as compared to IgG antibody and in accordance with the selective limitation of IgM affinity. On the other hand, the functional association constants reached a level of 2×10^{11} M^{-1}, a value equal to the highest exhibited by IgG antibody. The enhancement factor in the case of IgM appears to range between 10^6 and 10^7. This exceeds the enhancement factor of the bivalent IgG antibody by a factor of at least a hundredfold. It would thus

Table II. A Comparison of Multivalent and Monovalent Affinities at 25°C of Anti-DNP IgM Preparations[a]

Preparation	Antibody concentration in neutralization mixture (M)	Association constant for neutralization (M^{-1})	Association constant for ligand binding (M^{-1})
Rabbit IgM	5×10^{-12}	2.4×10^{11}	$<10^6$
Chicken (M) IgM	1×10^{-9}	2.4×10^9	$<10^4$
Chicken (H) IgM	2×10^{-11}	8.1×10^{10}	4×10^4
Shark IgM	9×10^{-12}	1.7×10^{11}	$\sim 1 \times 10^4$

[a]Adapted from Hornick and Karush (1972) with permission.

appear that in the neutralization of DNP-ϕX174 the IgM antibody molecule utilizes at least three of its combining sites for attachment to DNP groups on the surface of the bacteriophage. In this connection it should be noted that an additional factor contributes to enhanced affinity for IgM binding beyond the use of more than two binding sites. This factor is a statistical one arising from the number of ways in which the ten sites of the IgM molecule can be used to form n linkages. However, there are undoubtedly severe topological restraints involved in the actual expression of these alternatives. It is evident that in interactions permitting a larger number of sites to be occupied the process would appear to be virtually irreversible. Except for the chicken IgM preparation used at a concentration of 1×10^{-9} M, the second-order rate constants for the neutralization reaction were similar to those for IgG antibody, namely, about 10^7 $M^{-1} \cdot s^{-1}$. This value emphasizes again that the increased enhancement factor is due primarily to a reduced rate of dissociation.

An interesting example of a nonantibody multivalent interaction showing enhancement of affinity has been described by Hammarström (1973). The invertebrate agglutinin *Helix pomatia* A hemagglutinin agglutinates human A erythrocytes. It is a hexavalent molecule with a K_0 for the appropriate monovalent ligand of 5×10^3 M^{-1} at 25°C. The binding of the hexavalent molecule to A erythrocytes was studied with the ^{125}I-labeled agglutinin and characterized by a functional association constant in the order of 10^{10} M^{-1}. The approximate enhancement factor of 10^6 is strikingly similar to the corresponding value for IgM antibody. Furthermore, the binding of bivalent subunits showed a reduced K_0 value of about 5×10^{-7} M^{-1}. In this instance also the enhancement factor of 10^4 is in accord with the IgG results.

IV. THEORETICAL ANALYSIS

The theoretical calculation of quantitative values for the enhancement factor is a complex and unsolved problem even for bivalent antibody. Several attempts have been made to develop theoretical equations from which estimates can be made of the enhancement (Greenbury *et al.*, 1965; Crothers and Metzger, 1972; Schumaker *et al.*, 1973). The simplest system to consider is the formation of a bivalently linked complex between bivalent antibody and a bivalent ligand. This process may be formulated as follows:

complex I   complex II

The formation of complex I is a second-order process involving the loss of one kinetic unit. The association constant for this reaction is measured, at least approximately, by the intrinsic affinity for complex formation between the corresponding monovalent antibody and monovalent ligand. In addition, there is a small favorable statistical factor (4) adding to the stability of complex I. The analysis of the stabilization achieved in complex II by the formation of a second S–L linkage requires attention to several additional considerations. Since the conversion from complex I to complex II is a first-order process, the free energy difference between these forms does not include a decrease in the entropy of mixing (Karush, 1962). On the other hand, since association constants for the binding of monovalent ligand almost invariably use molar concentrations, this entropy loss is a significant factor in the quantitative value of K_0 and in the corresponding value of the standard free energy. This value of the standard free energy, without appropriate correction, is not therefore the proper value to use as a first approximation to the free energy change resulting from the formation of the second linkage of complex II.

Beyond the proper value for this required starting point in all of the theoretical analyses, the formation of complex II involves other contributions to the free energy change. From a topological point of view, it is clear that the accessibility of a second specific group and the number available enter directly into consideration. These factors and related structural aspects can be formulated in terms of (1) the loss of internal degrees of freedom of both the bivalent antibody and bivalent ligand, (2) the strain or distortion of intramolecular linkages introduced into each of the two molecules, and (3) the statistical factors associated with the multiplicity of accessible ligand groups in the case of multivalent antigens, e.g., cell surfaces. It may be noted also that with IgM antibody additional statistical enhancement is provided by the decavalence of this molecule.

In the earliest and most simplified attempt at a mathematical formulation of the enhancement effect, Greenbury *et al.* (1965) assumed that the forward rate constant for the formation of complex I was equal to the rate constant for the formation of complex II and that the corresponding rate constants for dissociation were equal. With these questionable assumptions, the enhancement factor was given by the product of the intrinsic association constant and a factor representing the concentration of membrane groups available to the free site of the monovalently linked antibody. With reasonable estimates of the parameters determining the value of this concentration factor, a crude approximation to the observed enhancement values was obtained.

The theoretical analysis of Crothers and Metzger (1972) includes both statistical-mechanical and structural considerations. It represents a more sophisticated version of the earlier model employed by Greenbury *et al.* (1965) and avoids the questionable assumptions of the latter. The form of the approximate equations for the calculation of the enhancement factor is, however, the same in both cases. The primary difference in the equations is the assumed most probable separation of the combining sites of the bivalent antibody. Greenbury *et al.* used a distance of 25 nm based on the model of a rod-shaped molecule with one site at each end. Crothers and Metzger calculated a most probable distance of 8.7 nm, taking into account the dimensions of the Fab fragment but assuming complete flexibility between the Fab arms. In both cases, the enhancement factor is given by a product which includes the intrinsic association constant and the distance between antibody sites.

There remains an unresolved difficulty associated with the use of the intrinsic association constant in this calculation. The problem arises from the fact that the intrinsic constant includes a contribution from the loss of translational and rotational entropy due to the conversion of two kinetic units into one. Although there may also be some loss of entropy arising from constraints generated in the bivalently linked complex, this is likely to be much smaller (Jencks, 1975). The result is that the intrinsic association constant is not the appropriate quantity for the calculation of the enhancement factor. Further application and, perhaps, a more critical test of the utility of the formulation of Crothers and Metzger will be possible when studies are done with well-defined bivalent ligands and homogeneous bivalent antibody.

The analysis of the interaction of bivalent antibody and bivalent ligand by Schumaker *et al.* (1973) was made strictly in thermodynamic terms. The basic equation relating the association constants for the variety of possible complexes to the thermodynamic and statistical parameters is

$$K(m, n) = S(m, n)e^{-[b\delta F + \zeta(m,n)]/RT}$$

where $K(m,n)$ is the equilibrium constant for the formation of a complex, $HmAn$, containing m bivalent ligands denoted H and n bivalent antibody molecules denoted A, and is related to the free concentrations as follows:

$$[HmAn] = K(m, n) [H]^m [A]^n$$

where $[H]$ and $[A]$ represent the free concentrations of ligand and antibody, respectively. $S(m,n)$ is the statistical factor equal to the number of distinct ways of assembling the complex divided by the number of distinct ways of taking it apart (V. N. Schumaker, personal communication). All of the free energy contributions arising from steric restrictions, loss of internal degrees of freedom, loss of translational entropy, and other changes which make the total free energy of interaction different from $b\delta F$ are included in the term $\zeta(m, n)$. The number of occupied antibody sites is b, and δF, in effect, is the intrinsic affinity. The value of δF is obtained by setting $\zeta(2,1)$ equal to zero, i.e., assigning zero strain to the complex $H2A1$ and using the following relation, including the statistical factor of 4 for this complex:

$$2\delta F = -RT \ln [K(2,1) / 4]$$

With the aid of a computer program and judicious choices of the thermodynamic parameters δF and $\zeta(m,n)$ guided by available experimental data, the distribution of antibody and ligand among various complexes can be calculated as a function of concentration of reactants and the selected thermodynamic quantities. One of the distinctive features of this analysis is that it provides explicitly for the existence of circular (i.e., closed) complexes as well as linear ones. It is of particular interest that in the absence of strain the $1:1$ closed complex, i.e., bivalently linked, is a thousandfold more stable than the next most stable form which is the closed dimer, the $2:2$ complex, with all sites occupied. The approach used by Schumaker et al. (1973) will probably find fruitful application when suitable experimental systems are developed.

An alternative version of the formulation of Schumaker et al. may be suggested in which the contribution of the entropy of mixing is explicitly included rather than contained in the strain term $\zeta(m, n)$. Since this contribution is simply statistical and dependent on the composition of the complex, its separation from $\zeta(m,n)$ would relate the latter directly to the structural properties of the reactants.

The correction for the entropy of mixing (ΔS_{mix}) depends on the standard states chosen for the reactants and products, i.e., the concentration units. For the formation of the complex $HmAn$ the value of ΔS_{mix} may be expressed by

$$\Delta S_{mix} = -R \ln (f/f^m f^n)$$

where f is the factor required to convert the concentration unit used to define the standard state to mole fraction. For the usual case of dilute solutions in which the concentration of the solutes is expressed in moles per liter, the factor f is $1/55.6$ and ΔS_{mix} is given by

$$\Delta S_{mix} = -(m + n - 1) R \ln 55.6$$

The modified equation for obtaining δF is given by

$$2\delta F = -RT \ln [K(2, 1)/4] - 2RT \ln 55.6$$

The value of δF given by the above equation is the unitary free energy (Kauzmann, 1959). It is calculated from the value of the equilibrium constant $K(2, 1)$ with concentrations expressed in moles per liter. The corresponding modification required in the general equation is as follows:

$$K(m, n) = S(m, n) \frac{e^{-[b\delta F + \zeta(m,n)]/RT}}{(55.6)^{m+n-1}}$$

In the computation of $K(m,n)$, the unitary free energy (δF) must be used and the value of $K(m, n)$ would be given in units of $(moles/liter)^{1-m-n}$.

V. CLOSING STATEMENT

The large values of the enhancement factor observed in systems studied to date point to the importance of multivalent interaction in processes involving cell surface membranes. For example, the interaction of antigen with the immunoglobulin receptors of bone marrow derived lymphocytes and the consequent signals for proliferation and differentiation may depend critically on the functional affinity of the interaction. The affinity in turn may depend on the density and mobility of cell surface receptors, which properties may differ between virgin and memory cells (Klinman, 1972). The molecular analysis of the cellular processes associated with the immune response depends significantly, therefore, on the development of techniques for the measurement of the functional affinity of cell surface interactions.

ACKNOWLEDGMENT

The author is the recipient of a Public Health Service research career award (5-K6-AI-14, 012) from the National Institute of Allergy and Infectious Diseases.

VI. REFERENCES

Blank, S.E., Leslie, G.A., and Clem, L.W., 1972, *J. Immunol.* **108**:665.
Burnet, F.M., Keogh, E.V., and Lusk, D., 1937, *Aust. J. Exp. Biol. Med. Sci.* **15**:226.
Crothers, D.M., and Metzger, H., 1972, *Immunochemistry* **9**:341.
Eisen, H.N., and Karush, F., 1949, *J. Am. Chem. Soc.* **71**:363.
Finkelstein, M.S., and Uhr, J.W., 1966, *J. Immunol.* **97**:565.
Froese, A., and Sehon, A.H., 1965, *Immunochemistry* **2**:135.
Gopalakrishnan, P.V., and Karush, F., 1974a, *Immunochemistry* **11**:279.
Gopalakrishnan, P.V., and Karush, F., 1974b, *J. Immunol.* **113**:769.
Greenbury, C.L., Moore, D.H., and Nunn, L.A.C., 1965, *Immunology* **8**:420.
Haimovich, J., and Sela, M., 1966, *J. Immunol.* **103**:45.
Hammarström, S., 1973, *Scand. J. Immunol.* **2**:53.
Hornick, C.L., and Karush, F., 1969, *Isr. J. Med. Sci.* **5**:163.
Hornick, C.L., and Karush, F., 1972, *Immunochemistry* **9**:325.
Jencks, W.P., 1975, *Adv. Enzymol.* **43**:219.
Karush, F., 1962, *Adv. Immunol.* **2**:1.
Karush, F., 1970, *N.Y. Acad. Sci.* **169**:56.
Kauzmann, W., 1959, *Adv. Protein Chem.* **14**:1.
Klinman, N., 1972, *J. Exp. Med.* **136**:241.
Klinman, N.R., Long, C.A., and Karush, F., 1967, *J. Immunol.* **99**:1128.

Mäkelä, O., 1966, *Immunology* **10**:81.

Onoue, I., Tanizahi, N., Yagi, Y., and Pressman, D., 1965, *Proc. Soc. Exp. Biol. Med.* **120**:340.

Schumaker, V.N., Green, G., and Wilder, P.L., 1973, *Immunochemistry* **10**:521.

Werner, T.C., Bunting, R., Jr., and Cathou, R.E., 1972, *Proc. Natl. Acad. Sci. USA* **69**:795.

Index